Y0-BTB-781

MALNUTRITION

Its causation and control

MALNUTRITION
Its causation and control
(with special reference to protein calorie malnutrition)

Volume 1

John R. K. Robson
School of Public Health
University of Michigan

in collaboration with

Frances A. Larkin
Anita M. Sandretto
Bahram Tadayyon

GORDON AND BREACH

NEW YORK   LONDON   PARIS

Copyright © *1972 by*

Gordon and Breach, Science Publishers, Inc.
440 Park Avenue South
New York, N.Y. 10016

Editorial office for the United Kingdom

Gordon and Breach, Science Publishers Ltd.
42 Willian IV Street
London W.C.2

Editorial office for France

Gordon & Breach
7–9 rue Emile Dubois
Paris 14ᵉ

John R.K. Robson, M.D. (Newcastle), D.T.M. & H. (Edinburgh), D.P.H. (London), is Professor of Human Nutrition, and Director of the Nutrition Program, at the School of Public Health, The University of Michigan, U.S.A;

Frances A. Larkin, Ph.D. (Cornell), M.S. (Minnesota), is Associate Professor of Nutrition, at the School of Public Health, The University of Michigan, U.S.A.;

Anita M. Sandretto, M.P.H. (Michigan), is Instructor in Nutrition at the School of Public Health, The University of Michigan, U.S.A.; and

Bahram Tadayyon, Ph.D. (Cornell), M.S. (American University of Beirut), is Associate Professor of Biochemistry, Faculty of Sciences, at Mashad University, Mashad, Iran.

Library of Congress catalog card number 71–162626. ISBN 0 677 03980 8. All rights reserved. No part of this book may be reproduced or utilized in any form or by any means, electronic or mechanical, including photocopying, recording, or by any information storage and retrieval system, without permission in writing from the publishers. Printed in east Germany.

To Benjamin Stanley Platt (1903–1969)
Professor of Human Nutrition

Contents

Preface

We have been involved in various aspects of nutrition work in every continent of the world. This experience, which covers a range of eighteen years, has included the planning of nutrition programs at national and local levels and the delivery of nutrition services in the richest and the poorest countries of the world. Our experience has covered laboratory and field research, and teaching nutrition in a variety of settings from graduate and undergraduate programs in nutrition in the United States and elsewhere, to the training of local auxiliaries in the field.

It is our impression that a vast amount of information has been accumulated but there is less evidence of application through the establishment of effective nutrition programs. We believe that an understanding of the environment is a prerequisite for the application of knowledge to nutrition problems regardless of whether the site is in Africa, Asia, or in an "inner city ghetto" in the United States. We perceive that one of the greatest needs is a better understanding of the interrelationships of the various factors which influence nutritional status. Knowledge of nutritional science will not be used effectively unless it is related to physiology, pathology, human behavior, and the many factors constituting the ecology of food and nutrition. Our combined experiences have led us to believe that there is a need for a textbook that will examine some basic principles in nutrition as related to the environment. The causation and control of malnutrition differs little in principle between the developing and sophisticated areas of the world. The latter situation is more complex and therefore it is more difficult to isolate and identify all the factors related to causation and control. In an attempt to recognize the breadth of the problem, we have therefore addressed ourselves to discussing several questions. What are the manifestations of malnutrition, what is the setting? What is normal nutrition and what nutrients does the body require to maintain health? How do we know if adequate nutrition has been achieved? How do we promote better nutrition and relieve existing malnutrition? These questions are discussed separately in each chapter. A systematic approach to the study of each disease has been avoided, as we believe such an approach tends to inhibit an understanding of the interrelationships. We make no apologies for the fact that the reader has to consult separate sections of the book in order to obtain a complete understanding of one specific problem such as the causation and control or protein calorie malnutrition.

It seems apparent to us that a broad concept of nutrition is required but we hope that we have made it clear that breadth does not necessarily mean that depth of understanding has to be sacrificed. Our attitudes, views, and understanding of nutrition have been acquired through an exposure to a number of scholarly and human personalities in nutrition and we would like to acknowledge their role in stimulating the writing of this book. In addition to the late Professor B. S. Platt to whom this book has been dedicated, we would like to express our particular appreciation to Dr. George Wadsworth, Professor Emeritus, University of Singapore, and A. G. van Veen, Professor Emeritus, Cornell University who have provided us with guidance, counsel, and an understanding of human nutrition. We would also like to acknowledge the help of colleagues scattered throughout the world including Professor H. A. P. C. Oomen, Dr. David Morley, Dr. J. M. Tanner, Mrs. Joyce Doughty of the London School of Hygiene and Tropical Medicine, Dr. J. M. Bengoa of the World Health Organization and Dr. Marcel Autret and Dr. Bruce Nicholl of the Food and Agriculture Organization who have provided photographs or figures. Finally we would like to thank Simon Robson for his help with art work, and our respective wives, husbands, and relatives for their support. We also wish to express our appreciation to our indefatigable secretary Mrs. Gertrude Flint, our associate Mrs. Elodia Jones, Cleland Child and Tom Raboine who always helped when help was most needed.

J. R. K. R.

Introduction

Nutrition is an exceedingly complex subject based on pure, applied and social sciences including chemistry, biology, physiology, medicine, agriculture, education, sociology, economics, anthropology and politics. Knowledge provided by these sciences has to be applied by nutrition workers who may be physicians, nurses, nutritionists, dietitians, home economists, agricultural and social workers, and educators.

There has been a tendency for each person to pursue his or her interests within their own particular brand of science. Consequently, the meaning of nutrition has been interpreted independently, and differently by individual personalities, sciences and disciplines. For example, to the biochemist, nutrition may mean the study of metabolic pathways, to the gastro-enterologist it may mean the study of deficiency states resulting from inadequate digestion, or the absorption, of food materials. To the public health nutritionist it may mean the provision of services to alleviate a community nutrition problem, to the social worker it may mean filling an empty belly, and to the anthropologist it may mean the study of food habits which are part of the cultural behavior of a society.

One of the initial tasks of this book will be to define some of the terms used in public health nutrition.

Health has been defined by the World Health Organization as "a state of complete physical, mental and social well-being and not merely the absence of disease or infirmity."[1] The definitions of nutrition are legion; that given in a recent text book typifies the approach of nutrition scientists — "Nutrition is the science that interprets the relationships of food to the functioning of the living organism, it includes the uptake of food, liberation of energy, elimination of wastes and all the syntheses essential for maintenance, growth, and reproduction".[2]

While the ultimate aim is to ensure that every cell receives a constant supply of the nutrients required for its proper function, there is actually much more to nutrition. Nutrition in its broadest sense must be concerned with food itself and those factors which influence its quality, quantity and availability to the body.[3] Due attention must be given to the production and distribution of food throughout the country, the community and the family.

The social, cultural, environmental and economic factors involved in this process and which affect the intake of food are of prime importance, but they tend to be overlooked. The quantity and quality of the food pattern is influenced not only by physiological demands but by many other factors which are controlled by custom, habit and necessity. Once food is taken into the body, finely integrated physiological processes determine the nutritive value of the diet. Nutrition is therefore concerned with the provision, ingestion, mastication, insalivation and digestion of food. It is concerned with the absorption of nutrients into the body where they are transported to the tissues to be stored or utilized according to body demands. Finally, nutrition must be concerned with the removal of the products of the above process by excretion by the lungs, kidneys, skin and intestines. If the whole cycle from food production to proper utilization of nutrients and excretion of waste products is completed then good nutrition is the result. The process is not, however, an automatic affair and much depends on human beliefs, attitudes and behaviour expressed through the individual, the community, the society, or social, industrial or political organizations.

Hunger is a symptom or a sensation which is expressed as a craving for food.

Food is composed of *nutrients* which fulfill certain functions such as providing energy for the body, for growth and the maintenance and repair of body tissues, and for regulating body function.

Undernutrition is a state of the body and is the result of an inadequate intake of food or utilization of nutrients. It is frequently associated with the symptom of hunger.

Malnutrition is the result of an imbalance of nutrient intake; the consumption of too little or even too much of one nutrient can lead to malnutrition. Malnutrition may appear as a clinical syndrome with typical symptoms and signs, depending on the nutrients responsible for the disease.

Overnutrition is a state of the body and is the result of an overindulgence of food or perhaps of one or more nutrients; it is therefore possible to consider overnutrition as a manifestation of malnutrition.

Food has been the subject of learned discussion for thousands of years, but the study of nutrients depended on the acquisition of chemical methodologies and these had not become sufficiently sophisticated until the end of the 19th century. At that time however, the preparation of relatively purified food stuffs lead to the discovery of accessory food factors later known as vitamins. The peak of the "Chemical era" of nutrition was reached between 1930 and 1940 during which time discovery after discovery was made; these not only contributed to knowledge but they had great commercial implications also. Consequently, enthusiasm over-rode restraint and attention was diverted from the human aspects of nutrition to the more scientific, sterile laboratory, and the rich commercial world of the vitamin industry.

Commenting on the transfer of the study of nutrition to the sphere of the chemist, Galdston noted[4]"... we have gained enormously in particular knowledge and lost as enormously in humanity. We became so preoccupied with the subject that we have forgotten the man to whom the subject relates." Recently however, the human side of nutrition has begun to receive the attention it deserves. It is being recognized increasingly that despite the huge volume of knowledge relating to nutrition, the true nature and extent of malnutrition throughout the world is largely unknown.[5] Whereas it had formerly been assumed that nutritional problems were those of the underprivileged or those living in developing countries, now they are seen to be affecting communities in the richest country in the world. While this fact alone is disturbing, it is of even greater concern that we do not have certain knowledge of effective ways to prevent malnutrition.

The time is long overdue for this unsatisfactory state of affairs to be remedied, but in order to do so community nutrition problems will have to be approached in a far more practical, methodical and logical fashion than has been the custom in the past.

It is the teacher, the nurse, the physician, the nutritionist, the dietitian, the home economist and the social worker who will be coming into contact first with malnutrition in the community. They should, therefore, be familiar with the basic causes of malnutrition and recognize their existence in the community as early signs of real or potential nutrition problems.

If the presence of the basic causes or indeed, malnutrition itself, can be detected, then the prospects of defining its true nature and extent will be greatly enhanced. This should enable more realistic nutrition programs and services to be planned and implemented. Hopefully, such services will help to prevent further malnutrition and control those which already exist.

Undernutrition and malnutrition constitute the greatest threat to public health in the world today.[6] It is commonly believed that these conditions are the result of inadequacies of food supplies and impoverishment caused by "population explosions". While this may be responsible in some countries, (for example, Central Java in Indonesia), population pressures cannot

1*

always be blamed. Libya has a low population density but malnutrition is still a childhood problem, poverty is not entirely responsible because Libya's relatively high per capita income has increased ten fold over the last 14 years.[7]

The more malnutrition is studied as a community problem rather than a clinical problem, the more apparent it becomes that it is not due to one or two isolated events but to a number of factors which are often interrelated. Identifiable factors could include the size, health status and productivity of the population, and perhaps even the politics of the community. The interrelationships of these factors are part of the ecology of food and nutrition in any given situation and until they are studied and understood it is unlikely that a realistic, practical and acceptable remedial program will materialize. Seeking the cause, rather than treating the effect, might seem a sensible and logical approach to solving community nutrition problems. However, these procedures have not always been followed and the world is full of problem areas where the effects alone have been noted and treated symptomatically, while the causal factors have been left to perpetuate sickness and death.

One of the reasons the ecology of food and nutrition has been neglected lies in the recent history of nutrition research. During the "Chemical era" much of the pioneering investigative work was centered in academic institutions and laboratories, mostly situated in highly developed countries. Attention was focused on the effects of the deficiency states rather than the cause; the investigations were *centripetal* in nature and frequently remote from the community. Since the second world war, however, the investigations of malnutrition have become more *centrifugal* with investigators moving out into the community where causal relationships are much easier to see and understand.

It has already been pointed out that malnutrition is world wide and affects both affluent and poor societies. The ecology of malnutrition in developing and impoverished countries is relatively simple. To facilitate an understanding of this important subject the reader will now be introduced to a real life situation which gives an insight first, into the causation of malnutrition in a rural community in a remote area of East Africa, and second, into the development of a remedial program based on the causes of the problem.

The area concerned is in South West Tanganyika (now Tanzania) in Songea District of the Southern Province (Plate 1). Government officials assigned to this very remote area had formed a District Team consisting of the District Administrator, the District Medical, Agriculture and Edu-

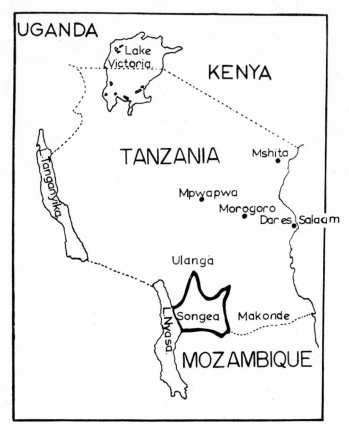

Plate 1   Tanzania showing Songea District

cation Officers, and others on detachment from the Departments of Public
Works, Co-operative Development and Community Development. The
team met at regular intervals to discuss problems encountered during the
Administrative and Development programs for the District. During one
of these meetings the District Medical Officer reported the presence of
severe and wide-spread malnutrition in the village of Maposeni near Songea
(Plate 2). This lead to an enquiry into the nature, extent and cause of the
malnutrition and the development of a remedial program. The latter
centered around the promotion of health through better infant care and
education, the development of natural and local resources through an agricultural program. This included the establishment of a model farm, citrus
culture, fish and poultry production and by improving animal husbandry.
    The project will now be described in detail.

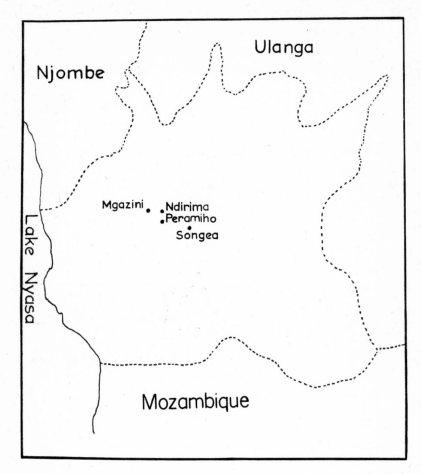

Plate 2   Songea District

Background

Approximately 66,000 Africans in the central part of Songea District bear
the tribal name of *Ngoni* (See Fig. 1). They are the descendants of a group
of *Nguni* who declined to form an alliance with the *Zulu* of Natal. Assuming
the tribal name of *Ndwandwe*, they forayed north over the Zambesi in the
middle of the 19th century and eventually reached South West Tanganyika
where they split up into three groups, the *Zulu,* the *Mbonani* and the
Maseko.

  Individually, and in alliances they continued to raid the local tribes and
to engage in inter-group intrigue and murder. The conflicts against others

and themselves terminated in the formation of two main groups, the *Njelu Ngoni* and the *Mshope*. The former, who assumed undisputed control over most of South West Tanganyika had adopted a very efficient military type of organization for their wartime activities, but it proved to be unsuited to peace.

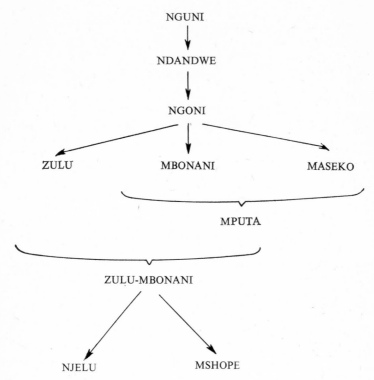

Figure 1   The tribal origins of the Songea Ngoni

In the normal life of conflict the chief was in supreme command. After he had taken his share of conquered land, the remainder was divided among his subchiefs who took what land they required and divided the remainder among their headmen. In return the headmen kept the chief and the subchiefs supplied with warriors or labor as required. During years of peace the Chief became more of a figurehead and the day to day leadership was shared between the sub-chiefs.

The German colonists who arrived in East Africa towards the end of the 19th century were concerned at the looseness of control of some of the subchiefs on the fringes of the tribal areas and appointed an *Akida* who assumed the role of headman. Some of the existing headmen were replaced by the appointed *Akida* and others were not, so leadership in a particular village might be influenced by tribal, governmental or selfish interests. During these maneuverings some subchiefs had obtained proprietary rights over large areas of land, the acquisition of which required an agreement in cash or barter between the buyer and the subchiefs. This unstable situation was perpetuated by the British colonists who appointed *Jumbes*, who were another cadre of appointed headmen similar in function to the subchiefs and the *Akida*. The *Ngoni* traditional authority suffered a final setback following their participation in the *Maji Maji* rebellion against the Germans in 1906.

The punitive measures which followed swept away their traditional mode of life for all time. Gulliver[8] describes the impact of this event:

> "At a blow the Ngoni were humiliatingly deprived of their military
> power and pride and were thrust into a modern world in which local
> warfare was banned and in which they were totally unfitted by custom
> and training to live. Bereft of their military activities and prestige, they
> could find little to put in their place as a cultural ideal or as a basis of
> a political system."

In topography, Songea District is fertile and well watered with reliable rainfall and free running perennial streams. Reports of malnutrition caused by food inadequacy in such circumstances were viewed with some skepticism by the government, but in view of undoubted evidence of childhood malnutrition, it was decided that a team of officials from Songea would investigate the nature, extent, and cause, of the problem.

The survey was made on a total of 98 families who were living in 88 homesteads in an area of some four square miles (Plate 3). This particular site was chosen because all the cases of protein calorie malnutrition which had been observed had come from within that area. It also included the tribal headquarters of the *Njelu Ngoni* at Maposeni. The agricultural methods were typical of those used elsewhere in *Ungoni* (the land of the *Ngoni*), and it also included three schools which could be used in subsequent education programs.

Each family was visited and questioned on their tribal origins, occupation, employment, manual skills, earnings and educational attainment, and each child was medically examined—particular attention being given to overt signs of malnutrition. The clinical survey confirmed a high prevalence of malnutrition of a type associated with a deficiency of protein and calories.

An attempt was then made to relate the clinical signs to the food intake of the *Ngoni*. It was found that the main staple foods were cereal, usually

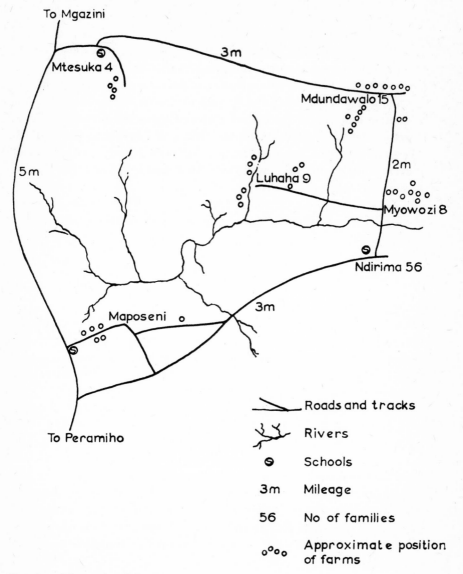

To Mgazini

3m

Mtesuka 4

Mdundawalo 15

5m

2m

Luhaha 9

Myowozi 8

Ndirima 56

3m

Maposeni

To Peramiho

Roads and tracks

Rivers

Schools

3m   Mileage

56   No of families

Approximate position of farms

Plate 3   Maposeni and the survey area

maize or cassava, eaten with side dishes of beans or green leaves. Both maize and cassava are nutritionally inadequate; their nutritional deficiencies are not completely compensated by the other components of the diet—beans and green leaves. Animal foods would have improved the quality of their diet but foods of animal origin were consumed only on very rare occasions.

Monotony was a feature of the diet, it was relieved only by occasional interludes of consuming grubs and wild honey and the gleanings from groundnut gardens. The nutrient intake for the population was calculated and it was found to conform reasonably well with the averages for the whole of Tanganyika, but such averages do not take into account inequalities in distribution of food, within the community and within the family.

Because infants and children have special needs, attention was directed towards their nutrient intake and the infant feeding practices of the *Ngoni*. The study showed that breast feeding was the only form of infant feeding practised and it was prolonged for several years. Weaning was difficult because the only foods available were cereal gruels and doughs which were bulky and had a low concentration of essential nutrients. Foods of animal origin were either unobtainable or, in the case of eggs, taboo or forbidden as they were believed to cause sterility. It seemed that the *Ngoni* child could only survive if he received breast milk as a supplement.

The clinical picture of protein calorie malnutrition in infants and children could certainly be explained by the diet. The questions which had to be answered were: Was the malnutrition due to a deficiency of intake of foods of animal origin? Was this deficiency due to an absolute shortage of animal foods or was it because the *Ngoni* mothers had insufficient knowledge of proper infant feeding practices? The next phase of the enquiry sought answers to these questions.

Fish were available in the rivers but were considered as unsuitable food for such a prestigious tribe as the *Ngoni*. The usual village in East Africa has chickens and goats in abundance but at Maposeni a survey of the live-stock showed that there was an extreme shortage of animals of any sort. Further research revealed the reasons for the shortage of cattle. First, there had been outbreaks of the fatal cattle disease rinderpest, following the first and second world war. These latter events had also opened up communications and facilitated the entry of the *tsetse* fly into the area— the sleeping sickness which followed further reduced the numbers of do-mestic cattle. The survivors of these two scourges were finally decimated during a well-intentioned campaign carried out against rinderpest in 1949, when the vaccine that was being used proved to be *live* and not *attenuated*. The poultry population had also been wiped out on several occasions by outbreaks of disease. It was not surprising that the *Ngoni* were short of animals and were skeptical of the value of animal husbandry.

The possibility that hunting was providing a source of food was con-sidered but the *Ngoni* are not, by tradition, hunters. The only available weapons were bush knives or stones — they did not know how to trap animals and they had no firearms. Game animals that were reported as plentiful at one time had largely disappeared. It was therefore concluded, that the community was lacking animal food sources; even if the mothers knew how to utilize animal food in their weaning practices it was unlikely that there would be adequate amounts available.

The productivity of the farms was investigated further. A land utilization survey showed that on average there was only threequarters of an acre of land per person under cultivation; this is a figure far below the three acres usually considered necessary for subsistence farming in East Africa. Not only was insufficient land being cultivated but that which was being used, was of poor quality. Soil analyses were described as being typical of "worked out" land. This provided an explanation why the crop yields were about one half of that achieved in other parts of Tanganyika.

Productivity was also being retarded by the patterns of cultivation which allowed crops to grow in competition with one another. The final yields and variety of crops grown were such that during the month of January only cow peas, cassava and bananas were available.

If cash is available then some of the deficiencies in productivity may be compensated. The generation of cash within the community was minimal however, and restricted to the Chief and some of his tribal government assistants. There were more people consuming cassava than growing it; indicating that some bartering was taking place. Overall however, there was little evidence that the deficits in productivity could be compensated by the purchase of food.

At this stage it was concluded that a shortage of food, especially that of animal origin was the main problem. The shortage was seen to be related to low productivity, associated with poor farming methods, and a series of unfortunate accidents which had greatly reduced the availability of animal foods.

The community which was living at a subsistence level could not generate either at that time, or in the forseeable future, enough cash to supplement its own food supply. It was believed, therefore, that remedial measures should concentrate on increasing food production and adjusting the agricultural program so that it might ensure food during the "hungry months".

In order to meet the problems of protein calorie malnutrition in the infants and children it was imperative that the production drive should make food available. The food should supply plenty of good quality protein as well as calories.

As a prelude to the food production campaign several factors affecting productivity were examined. These are summarized as follows:

Population pressure and land shortage

According to the most recent census there was no evidence of overpopulation; the population density being only six persons per square mile. A study of land availability made two years previously, concluded that land was plentiful everywhere and more than enough to meet the modest demands of the *Ngoni* who still had proprietary rights over large tracts of fertile, arable land.

The land and the work force

The farmland around Maposeni was worked out and "rock hard", and no form of mechanical cultivation was available. Land preparation was the traditional responsibility of the women and when the farm land or *shamba* became unproductive and difficult to work, new land was opened up. This involved bush clearing and tree felling which is extremely hard work and the usual responsibility of the men. If land was available, could not new land be opened up? A study of the population showed that there was an apparent shortage of males between the ages of 20 and 35 years of age. This was the result of migration of fit young men in search of work. The situation is similar to that seen elsewhere in rural Africa where the only means of supporting the population is exporting labor. The absence of the males undoubtedly placed additional work loads on the men and women who remained behind.

Labor Resources in the future

A long term program aimed at increased productivity must depend on the availability of manpower. A study of the sex ratio of the population showed that there was an overwhelming preponderance of females in preschool years. This was partly due to the practice of farming out boys into the care of grandparents, a practice which greatly increases the risk of malnutrition, but there was no obvious biological reason for the disparity between the sexes.

It is possible to speculate that girls are viewed with greater favor than boys for they are useful as domestic help, whereas the boys tend to concentrate on play. Females also carry the prospect of a dowry, so males may have come to be regarded as an economic burden. This could serve as a justification for practicing male infanticide, a custom reported in neighboring tribes.

In normal circumstances life expectations continue to be poorer for males than females so the future prospect for developing an adequate work force with a proper balance of the sexes is poor.

The health of the work force

Productivity must depend on health. There was adequate evidence of severe malnutrition in the children, and nutrient intakes in adults were marginal so that their nutritional status was likely to be affected.

The malnourished child of today makes up the work force of the future. It is well documented that malnutrition is associated with impairment of mental and physical function that can continue into adult life. Infections aggravate malnutrition, and malnutrition in turn makes infections more serious. There was plenty of evidence of communicable disease risks in the vicinity of Maposeni.

Malaria was endemic and there were no organized malaria control measures. Over 90 per cent of the school children were infested with hookworm. It was estimated that between 10 and 90 per cent of the children were infested with liver fluke. There were the usual epidemics of influenza, typhus, and occasional outbreaks of sleeping sickness in the area. All of these added to the health hazards of the population and inhibited its physical efficiency.

Education

Education could exert an influence in two ways. First, better education could be related to increased productivity, and second, it could be related to improved food intake patterns and better methods of infant feeding. Compared with many other parts of Tanganyika, the community was well endowed with educational facilities. There were three schools in the area with vacant seats for pupils. The introduction of education was recent however, and the population was for the most part illiterate.

Ethnic influences

Literacy is not essential for achievement of reasonably good agricultural practices in this part of the world, for the neighboring *Matengo* tribe had been forced by the marauding *Ngoni* to adapt their farming system to steep slopes. Over the years they have developed an ingenious method of cultivating in pits which is very efficient. The *Matengo* were, however, well motivated. It has been already pointed out that the *Ngoni* had lost group initiative and self-reliance in the face of the repeated demands of the alien conqueror. It is also possible that the nomadic pastoral *Ngoni* may not have had sufficient knowledge of agriculture handed on by tradition. At the commencement of the study of the *Ngoni* nutrition problems, it had been assumed that the community was a homogeneous ethnic group, representing the descendants of the Natal *Nguni*. This assumption was far from correct for it was eventually established that the 98 families were derived from 19 different tribes, and out of a total of 378 persons only 40 claimed true *Nguni* origins. The remainder represented tribes which had capitulated to the *Ngoni* in the past and had become slaves, and in later times they had become accepted as part of the sect. As it was the custom for the *Ngoni* to kill to a man any tribe which offered opposition, it can be postulated that only the weakest groups were absorbed into the *Ngoni*, and it is possible that the *Ngoni* had become a conglomerate of weak tribes adopting the lowest common denominator of the varying cultures which these ex-slaves represented. This loss of power and recent weakness of the *Ngoni* was noted by explorers early in the century, who commented on the affinity of tribes in South West Tanganyika to mimic, but not emulate, the strong war-like attributes of the original *Ngoni*. It is now possible to correlate the various factors and events which had led to the severe malnutrition occuring in this unusual community. To summarize:

The Maposeni *Ngoni* was a subsistence farmer, poorly educated with no real roots, traditions, or heritage enabling him to live and farm efficiently in his environment. The agriculture was of the "slash and burn" – "bush following type" with the accompanying penalties should the crops fail. There were hungry months during the year at which time the community was in real need of outside help, leadership and encouragement from its leaders. The leaders were weak and lacking in direction; there was even some doubt as to where the leadership lay. The Songea farmer had neither the knowledge nor capital to develop new agricultural methods nor could he move on to new land. This he had to purchase from the subchiefs, who had assumed so much control of tribal possessions since the peace imposed by the colonialists.

The cultural background of the *Ngoni*, his recent harsh experiences, and frustrations were such, that it was unlikely that he would have sufficient drive and innovation to better himself. Even should this drive exist, the local opportunities for employment and trade and commerce were very limited. The presence of tribal disunity and poor leadership meant that concerted efforts for improvement of the tribe were improbable. The *Ngoni* were handicapped by ill health, the condition being aggravated by a lack of adequate animal and vegetable foods. The availability of these foods diminished with soil and personal impoverishment. With this background, the vicious circle of malnutrition, ill health, decreased productivity, poverty and more malnutrition was established. Increasing child mortality and morbidity added to the hopelessness of the situation, the sole relief appeared to be labor migration, yet even this offered immediate help only to the worker. The prospects of community benefit from exporting labor were not good and the development of a "rural slum" seemed inevitable. Despite the presence of educational facilities the beneficial effects of education were too remote to affect the community at that time. The complexity of the Maposeni problem pointed out the inadequacy of the usual policies of promoting food sufficiency as the first step towards alleviating malnutrition in the community. The provision of fertilizers, mechanical cultivators, and food handouts was unlikely to solve the problems of the *Ngoni*, for as Cicely William says,[9] "... the well intentioned action program of food supplementation may perpetuate the malnutrition unless constructive action in correcting the total causes of malnutrition accompanies relief measures".

In the opinion of the District Team the problem of malnutrition could be alleviated best by changing the system of land tenure, by promoting better leadership, by the demonstration of better agricultural methods using local resources, by increasing the availability of animal foods for consumption or cash, by introducing an economic incentive through promotion of a cash crop, by educating the adults and children in simple nutrition principles and by providing better maternal and infant care facilities. Although these activities fell into the domain of many of the officials at Songea, including the District and Local Administration and representatives of the Departments of Agriculture, Education and Health, there was considerable interdisciplinary discussion and planning before each part of the program was implemented. For example, the crop rotation at the model farm was based on nutritional considerations as well as agricultural. Fish production in ponds was encouraged with due consideration being paid to the risk of increasing malaria and *schistosoma* transmission. The education of the children involved the development of school gardens as a means of education in nutrition.

The Maposeni Applied Nutrition Project was not planned originally as a formal study. It had its origins in a public health crisis. There were undoubtedly deficiencies in the investigative aspects, but in these days when nutrition problems abound there must be some compromise between the sterility of scientific experiment and the need to meet community health needs. The fact that the project was not a self-limited medical or clinical enquiry probably provided the reason why the ecology of the malnutrition came into the open and why such an excellent understanding of the situation was achieved by the participants from the various disciplines, and why a practical remedial program emerged.

The Maposeni project provides an excellent example of the complexity of community nutritional problems but it is an account of problems affecting only one community in one area. The variety, magnitude and complexity of nutritional problems on a global scale is infinitely greater. However, the approach to the definition, alleviation, and prevention, of community nutritional problems may not be too different anywhere in the world. It is the objective of this book to give an insight into such an approach. The basic principles and concepts of public health will be used with the ultimate goal of promoting health rather than just curing problems as, and when, they arise.

The material has been placed in a particular order; there is first a description of the manifestations of improper nutrition and a review of its immediate and remote cause. This is followed by an account of the chemical, biological and physiological reasons for the clinical characteristics of nutritional disease. The clinical signs of malnutrition are an indication that the body has failed to meet its nutrient requirements. The rationale for defining the requirements will be discussed after which there will be a review of the methods used to evaluate whether the body has in fact succeeded in meeting them. Finally, there will be a discussion of the organization and implementation of nutrition programs and services which are intended to ensure that nutritional requirements are being met. This latter phase of implementation must of necessity take into account the hard, but uncontravertible fact, that planning programs and services alone does not ensure that changes in food habits will take place. Perhaps one of the most difficult tasks in public health nutrition is bringing about change; the change agent will be the subject of discussion in the last chapter.

References

1. Constitution of the World Health Organization. Basic Documents, p. 1, **2/st** Edition. World Health Organization, Geneva, 1970.
2. Pike, R. L., Brown, M. L. *Nutrition: An Integrated Approach.* p. 1, New York: Wiley, 1967.
3. Norman, E. C., Robson, J. R. K. Nutrition and Mental Health. In *Mental Health Considerations in Public Health.* Ed. Goldston, S. E. Publication No. 1898, U. S. Public Health Service, Washington, D. C., 1969.
4. Galdston, I. "Nutrition from the Psychiatric Viewpoint." *J. Amer. Diet. Ass.* **28**: 405, 1952.
5. Goldsmith, G. A. "More Food for More People." *Amer. J. Public Health.* **59**: 694, 1969.
6. Jelliffe, D. B. *The Assessment of the Nutrition Status of the Community.* W. H. O. Monograph No. **53**, p. 7, World Health Organization, Geneva, 1966.

7. The World Almanac and Book of Facts, Centennial Edition, p. 509. Newspaper Enterprise, New York, New York, 1968.
8. Gulliver, P. H. Labour Migration in a Rural Economy. *East African Studies*, no. 6, p. 2. East African Institute of Social Research. Kampala, 1955.
9. Williams, C. D. "Factors in the Ecology of Malnutrition." *Proceedings, Western Hemisphere Nutrition Congress*, 1965, p. 20. American Medical Association. Chicago 1966.

CHAPTER 1

Global Nutritional Problems

There is little doubt that the population of the world is increasing at an alarming rate. However, the magnitude of this increase is impossible to measure because the exact size, and rate of increase, of the present population is unknown. The estimate of 3.3 billion persons for the population of the world in 1965 is based on inadequate data for a number of countries.[1] For example, there are no recent census figures for many African, Asian and Latin American countries; the uncertainty over the size of the population of mainland China may introduce an error as high as 100 million persons. The populations of the developed countries were probably undercounted so the total population in 1965 was probably some 200 million more than estimated. Estimates of the global growth rate is possibly inaccurate also. Based on the 1951 and 1961 census figures, the population of Pakistan is increasing at a rate of 2.1 per cent per annum. According to calculations based on sample surveys conducted since 1962 the actual rate of increase in this country is probably 3.2 per cent. The United Nations, in 1969 estimated the world population to be increasing at the rate of 1.9 per cent per annum; this is probably an underestimate too.[2]

It is customary to compare the nutrient demands of present and future populations with existing and projected food supplies. The failure of food production to meet the projected needs has provoked gloomy forecasts of global famine in the future. Increases in food production required to meet future needs are believed to be unattainable, because of the capital and technical investments that will be required, and which will not be available to those countries most in need of increased food supplies.

A second school of thought has been more optimistic of the future. The population projections for the future have largely assumed that fertility and mortality rates will be continuing on their present level. The decrease in births resulting from family planning campaigns have been largely offset by the improvements in environmental health and communicable disease control, which have reduced the number of deaths in the reproductive period. It has been suggested recently, that improvements in standards of living do not necessarily lead to population increases.[3] Improved health certainly reduces mortality experience, it also fosters increased productivity and further increases in living standards. The phenomenon of reduced mortality and increased economic wealth is believed to remove uncertainty, and a voluntary reduction in family size, or perhaps reduced fertility, will follow. However, the desired demographic changes do not appear to be automatic, nor is there an indication that these feedback mechanisms will be influencing populations before the final crises caused by too many people and too little food, is with us. The depressing forecasts for the future should not however distract our attention from the problems of today. While whole populations are undoubtedly suffering from the effects of food in-adequacy, others are suffering from the effects of overindulgence. Many populations have a quantitative adequacy of food but they lack food which is adequate in quality. The problems are therefore associated with three situations, the first, where there is too much food, the second where there is too little food, and the third where nutrient quality of the food is inade-quate. These are respectively associated with the clinical states of *over-nutrition, undernutrition* and *malnutrition,* they have been defined in the introduction and which will now be discussed in detail.

Overnutrition

A general overindulgence of foods in a normal healthy individual may result in an *overweight* body having a *normal body composition.* A person is classified as overweight when he or she exceeds by more than two standard deviations the weight of others of the same age; it is assumed that the weight change is unaccompanied by comparable deviations in height. Certain athletes, e.g. wrestlers, weight lifters, may be overweight but they may have normal body compositions. When there is a significant change in the ratio of lean body mass to body weight due solely to an increase in fat then the subject is said to be *obese.* There is a third manifestation of overnutrition which is the result of the excessive ingestion of a particular nutrient.

Obesity

The commonest manifestation of overnutrition is obesity. This is basically a very simple phenomenon occurring when there is a positive balance to the energy equation.

$$Energy\ in = Energy\ out.$$

The reasons for this imbalance which leads to the storage of the excess energy as fat is far from simple, however. Genetic influences are quite strong. For example, matings between obese and average size parents have resulted in half of the offspring being obese. Where both parents were overweight, twothirds of the offspring were obese. Investigations of twins has shown a very high weight correlation between identical twins but less in fraternal twins. It has also been observed that although weights of natural children correlate well with their parents, the weights of adopted children do not.

The effects of geography, climate, and culture, also affect food intake and there is not doubt that obesity is subject to strong social influences.[4] Ethnic origins also have a bearing on the prevalence of obesity; higher prevalence rates have been observed among Czechs and Hungarians than other Europeans living in the United States. Socio-economic status and ethnic background are apparently inter-related. In the U. S. A. obesity is associated with lowering of socio-economic status, whereas in German males it is associated with a high socio-economic status.

Differences have also been observed between the sexes, for in some countriess obesity is prevalent in women but not in the men. The direction and intensity of influence of social factors are far from being fully understood, and many more studies of obesity are required. It is clear however, that overweight infants tend to be born of heavy parents. The overweight infant tends to become an overweight child and the overweight child tends to become an overweight adolescent and adult.

Excessive food intake is the primary cause of obesity hence it might be expected that an examination of the causes of excessive appetite or eating would throw some light on the causation of obesity. The natural control of appetite is extremely complex. It is known to be under the control of the hypothalamus but as this is also under the influence of visual, olfactory and tactile stimuli, as well as gastro-intestinal reflexes and reflexes of chewing, ingestion and swallowing, the total regulation of appetite must project therefore far beyond the hypothalamus.

The weight of animals is stabilized over a wide variety of food intake and energy expenditure levels and it is obvious that many humans too, are able to stabilize their weight over a period of years including times of varying energy demands. The mechanism of control must be very precise to achieve this. It has been suggested that the levels of glucose concentration in the blood might control the appetite, but efforts to show a relationship between blood glucose levels and appetite have not been successful. It is possible that the mechanism, if based on humoral influences, may be controlled by the blood concentrations of a number of metabolites. Fluid shifts within the body compartments and the rise in heat production may also play a part in the control of food intake.

Emotional factors play an important role in the development of obesity, for it has been shown that emotional disturbance is more common in the obese than in the non-obese.

Many studies have noted differences in the metabolic activity of individuals, perhaps the basic fault may lie in having an abnormal number of fat cells,[5] or an abnormality in fat and glucose metabolism and energy utilization. The role of the endocrines and their inter-relationships in obesity is not clear. Raised insulin levels have been observed in the obese, and in response to a carbohydrate load the insulin levels in the blood have risen higher and remained higher for longer periods than has been observed in normal persons. (The role of insulin in carbohydrate metabolism is discussed in Chapter 3.) There is some evidence that the adrenal cortex is also abnormally active.

The adoption of certain eating patterns may affect the metabolism of carbohydrates and fats and may lead to obesity. In animals, the timing of food intake can bring about changes in the metabolic mechanisms responsible for the disposal of ingested energy sources. As a result excess fat can be formed on a given caloric intake. The ingestion of one or two large meals has been associated with obesity in humans and it is possible that this habit may also bring about metabolic changes that causes excessive deposition of fat in the adipose tissues.

The other half of the energy equation is concerned with energy expenditure and it is obvious that on a given intake of food a reduction in activity will result in a positive energy balance and the accumulation of fat. The decrease in energy expenditure may be part of the phenomenon of obesity itself for obese children have been observed to be less active and their movements more economical in the use of energy. The acquisition of extra weight will further reduce activity so a vicious circle may be started.

Exposure to cold will stimulate the thin person to exercise but the obese with better insulation of fat is not so stimulated. The balance of the energy equation in a person of normal weight is particularly vulnerable at times of enforced inactivity, or when activity is reduced. For example, the athlete with a high energy expenditure during his active life may retire and still maintain his normal food intake. His energy equation will certainly become imbalanced and unless his intake is curtailed proportionately, obesity is inevitable. Similarly, the active man in mid-adult life may be promoted to a more sedentary occupation, he too should readjust his calorie intake if he is to avoid gaining weight.

The exact prevalence of obesity throughout the world or even in one country cannot be determined accurately as there are no standardized criteria for obesity. In the definition of obesity, it was stressed that a change in body composition should have taken place: In many studies however, weight has been the sole criterion for obesity and consideration has not been given to the composition of the body. Desirable body weights based on height and body frame have been supplied by the Metropolitan Life Insurance Company. Tables have been compiled from data obtained from policy holders with low mortality experience. As the frame sizes have not been defined, interpretations of weight from this table must be viewed with some caution. On these criteria a person is said to be obese if his body weight is greater than 20 per cent of the desired weight.

The Ponderal Index has also been used: this is calculated from the formula:

$$\text{Ponderal Index} = \frac{3\ \text{Height in inches}}{\sqrt{\text{Weight in pounds}}}.$$

A Ponderal Index of less than 12.4 has been suggested as being indicative of obesity in High School girls in the United States.[6] Skinfold thickness has also been used as an index of obesity. In adolescent girls skinfold thickness over the triceps region in excess of 25 mm is said to be indicative of obesity. However, this may be an over simplification of the use of skinfolds for there are many pitfalls associated with the interpretation of such measurements. This subject is discussed later. Because the measurement of height, weight and skinfold thickness are time consuming, frequently inaccurate, and subject to incorrect interpretation, it has been suggested that a visual assessment of juvenile obesity may be adequate for public health purposes.[7] The shortcomings of the methodology of evaluating obesity prevents an accurate assessment of the prevalence of obesity but the magnitude of the problem in the U. S. A. may nevertheless be judged from the estimate that three million adolescents are seriously ill because of overweight.[8] The immediate effects of obesity are reflected in problems of locomotion and liability to serious injury during falls and accidents around the home. It also produces progressive changes in pulmonary function.[9] In time, changes in the joints are likely to occur because of the excessive weight bearing strains. Cardiovascular and renal disease has been noted to be almost twice as prevalent in the obese as in the non-obese, although this is only an association and not necessarily a cause and effect relationship.

Nutrient overnutrition

Many nutrients are potentially toxic if taken in excessive amounts, but fortunately nutrient overnutrition is not common.

Vitamin and mineral overnutrition

Vitamin D   which is discussed in Chapter 3, controls and facilitates the passage of calcium through the intestinal wall and prevents rickets. In well intentioned efforts to prevent rickets in countries where this disease is likely to occur, it has become the practice to add vitamin D to food stuffs. Over a period of years the number of foods *fortified* or *enriched* in this way has greatly increased, and now ready-to-eat cereals, margarine, milk, chocolate flavorings, and diet foods contain considerable quantities of vitamin D. Sea foods such as shrimp, tuna, sardines, salmon, and herring are natural sources of vitamin D. Studies in the United States have revealed a very wide range of intake of vitamin D; in children the highest level recorded was four times greater than recommended.[10] Although at this level toxic effects are unlikely, little is known of the effects of large quantities of vitamin D consumed over a prolonged period of time. The cumulative vitamin D intake from a wide variety of fortified foods may be causing harmful effects that have yet to be recognized.

The excessive consumption of vitamin D causes withdrawal of calcium from bone and may cause growth retardation. The withdrawal of the calcium leads to high calcium levels in the blood and a tendency for the mineral to be deposited in the soft tissues of the body. A derangement of vitamin D metabolism in infants results in a clinical syndrome characterized by anomalies of dental development and narrowing of the pulmonary and systemic arteries. It may be significant that a similar condition to this can be reproduced in the offspring of rabbits fed high levels of vitamin D during pregnancy.[11]

Vitamin A   When taken into the body in large quantities vitamin A causes fatigue, muscle and joint pains, skin changes, weight loss, and enlargement of the liver. Cases of vitamin A intoxication are rare, mainly because the high intakes required to produce toxic symptoms and signs requires a bizarre diet. For example, massive amounts of vitamin A have been consumed by explorers after eating polar bear liver.[12] A massive single dose such as this, caused nausea, headache and vertigo although the symptoms were transient, and full recovery followed. Large quantities of vitamin A are now available in the form of pharmaceutical preparations and it is not surprising that chronic hypervitaminosis A is reported from time to time. It is possible that milder forms of intoxication are also occuring but perhaps they are not being recognized.[13] The ingestion of large quantities of carotenes, the precursors of vitamin A appear to be compatible with health.[14] Toxic effects resulting from high intakes of both vitamins A and D through an excessive consumption of tunny fish livers has been reported in German fishermen.[15] The symptoms and signs of intoxication included headache, vomiting and marked muscular weakness, facial edema and "grass green" urine. It is unlikely however that the excessive consumption of tunny will constitute a serious threat to health.

Sodium Sodium is an element that is essential for normal body function. It is required in very small amounts and normal diets usually contain more than enough. It is important to note that high levels of sodium intake have been associated with the development of hypertension. Studies in the South Pacific showed that populations with a low salt intake experienced a lower incidence of high blood pressure than a similar ethnic group consuming a high salt intake.[16] Further evidence of the harmful effects of salt is provided by animal experimentation which has shown that hypertension can be induced in rats fed a high salt diet.

Food manufacturers have introduced *convenience* foods based on cereals, strained meat and vegetables that are used in weaning the child on to solid food. Because of the demand by mothers for a "tasty" food, salt has been added by the manufacturers although there is good evidence that the food is equally acceptable to the child unsalted.[17] Studies have shown that the salt intakes in babies fed in this manner may be 5 or 6 times higher than the estimated requirements;[18] although no serious effects are being reported perhaps the effects may be delayed for years. It is not unnatural that reports of the ingestion of large quantities of salt by infants is causing nutritionists some concern.

Fluorine The subject of overnutrition cannot be dismissed without mentioning the role of fluorine in relation to health. Much attention has been given to this element because of its ability to protect teeth from dental caries. However, fluorine is an extremely toxic substance which may harm health when taken into the body in excessive amounts.

Fluorine is normally stored in the bones and the teeth, so not unexpectedly these tissues show the effects of excessive fluorine intake. In the early stages of the disease stage *fluorosis*, or *fluoride poisoning*, the teeth show opaque white flecks in the enamel; in later stages the teeth become stained with a brown pigment (see plate 4). In the advanced stages the teeth are pitted and have a corroded appearance. There is an increase in bone density and overgrowth of bone; joints become immobilized and severe disability is caused when ligaments and tendons become the seat of deposition of calcium. With spinal involvement there may be neurological disturbances caused by the bony overgrowths of the vertebrae interfering with the nerve trunks as they leave the spinal column.

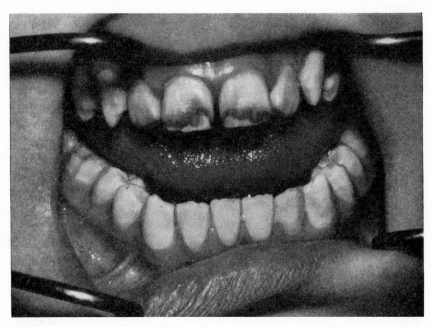

Plate 4   Dental fluorosis showing mottling of upper incisors (Photograph courtesy of Professor A. L. Russell)

Fluorine is present as a naturally occuring *fluoride* in the land and sea. In some volcanic areas the soil may contain large amounts of *fluoride*, which is leached out by the rain and passed into the streams and rivers. Food grown in such areas may contain more fluoride than food grown in normal soils. It has become the custom to express the quantity of fluorine present in food materials and water as a concentration. For example, fluoridated water supplies may be described as containing 1 part per million (abbreviated 1.ppm) of fluoride, tea leaves as 40–400.ppm. However *concentration of fluoride* means little since the *total intake of fluoride* determines whether health is being jeopardized.

Some population groups may have only one source of water; this may contain high concentrations of fluoride but they may suffer no harm because they consume very little water. Conversely, populations with a relatively low concentration of fluorides may exhibit fluorosis. This may be because they consume large quantities of water, or food containing fluoride, or perhaps food contaminated by fluoride emissions from industry.

The actual fluoride content of food, *as consumed*, is difficult to estimate because crops are affected by rain contaminated by atmospheric pollution, and by irrigated water supplies containing fluorides in undesirable amounts. The present system of evaluating fluoride intake by concentration encourages complacency. There is a great need to measure the total intake of fluoride from all sources. The toxicity of trace elements is discussed in Chapter 3.

Undernutrition

Undernutrition can arise in several ways. It may be the result of having too little to eat, or it may be a consequence of severe disease of the digestive tract which prevents the absorption of nutrients. Apart from famines, having too little to eat may occur during acute episodes of personal impoverishment, during labor migrations, or as the result of family breakdown. The absorption of nutrients may be prevented by malignant growths of the gastrointestinal tract or by the malabsorption syndrome, described later in this chapter.

Undernutrition may also be the consequence of a systemic toxemia caused either by the accumulation of waste products in the body, such as occurs in liver and kidney disease, or it may be the result of chronic infections. The toxemia may interfere with metabolism, or reduce the appetite.

In a growing infant or child, a given level of food intake may be able to maintain health. However, the young are continually exposed to infections and injuries which place an extra stress on the body. The intake becomes inadequate and the child enters a state of undernutrition.

The effects of food deprivation

The famine in Egypt and Palestine recorded in the Book of Genesis dates back to 1708 BC. Since that time, until the commencement of the second world war, some 295 famines were documented outside India. These are in addition to some 80 reports of famines in that country between the years 503 BC. and 1907 AD.[19] During the second world war, starvation affected civilian populations in Europe, Asia, and Africa, as well as prisoners-of-war in the Far East and Europe. Despite the cessation of global hostilities, famine and starvation still occur from time to time. They may follow natural disasters such as earthquakes, floods, and droughts, and those made by man such as civil war and rebellion. In Africa, war and civil strife affected Biafra, Somalia, Ethiopia, Sudan, Egypt, Libya and Mozambique in 1970. The cost in human life due to the undernutrition which frequently accompanies these events, must be considerable.

The character of undernutrition and starvation is well known. Individual selfimposed fasts, experimental starvation and the experiences of persons surviving prisoner-of-war camps, detention camps, and sieges, have provided much information and knowledge concerning the effects of acute and prolonged food deprivation. Hunger increases in intensity until the individual becomes completely preoccupied with the thought of food. So strong are these emotions that cravings for food may persist for years after the starvation has been relieved. Mental and physical lethargy become progressive. There may be changes in behavior, characterized by outbursts of violence. In the terminal stages of starvation, there is a final apathy and disinclination to live.

The pathological features of undernutrition may take several weeks to appear. Loss of weight is one of the first features of starvation. At first this is due to the negative energy balance that drains the fat stores. Soon body tissue is sacrificed. This is not equally shared throughout the body however, but in inverse proportion to its importance. The brain and heart lose only 3 per cent of their bulk, the muscle 31 per cent, the liver 54 per cent, and the spleen 67 per cent.[20] The intestinal tract may be affected, consequently its power to absorb nutrients may be seriously diminished. This adds to the problems of treatment and the prospects of recovery.

The general wasting, rapid at first, eventually slows down as the actual decrease in the total body cell mass results in a reduction of nutrient requirements. There is also less energy expenditure involved in movement because of the loss of weight; there is a reduction in all voluntary muscular activity. In severe underfeeding the water content of the body does not decrease in proportion to the loss of tissue, therefore there is a relative state of hydration. The accumulation of fluid at first is insufficient to cause any visible changes but eventually the ankles become swollen and finally there may be generalized edema. The prevalence of this edema, termed hunger or famine edema may be taken as an indication of the severity of the food deficiency. In an individual however, the severity of the edema may not be a reliable index of nutritional status because overhydration may be aggravated by concurrent infections, parasitic infestations, renal, or cardiac disease.

With progressive and continuous starvation, death is an inevitable result. However, 25 per cent of healthy non-obese weight may be lost without immediate danger to life. With greater losses, a fatal termination is likely, although some victims of starvation have survived as much as 50 per cent weight loss.[21]

While starvation is the extreme of undernutrition and tends to be well documented, lesser degrees of undernutrition may be unnoticed. Undernutrition must however, be extremely common for the reasons already given. One of the first effects of undernutrition is cessation of growth. Interruption of growth may be short-lived; when an adequate intake of nutrients becomes available growth is resumed and a "catch up" process takes place. It is uncertain whether the whole deficit is ever made up completely. Undernutrition is critical in certain periods of life and will be discussed in detail in other chapters. At this stage it is sufficient to note that severe undernutrition in females, may lead to temporary sterility. This is probably a protective mechanism for there is ample evidence that abortion or fetal abnormalities are liable to occur if the deprivation takes place after conception. With a lesser degree of deprivation, the baby may be born premature, and be undersize and underdeveloped.

All these conditions add to the hazards of parturition and the neonatal period, and reduce the chances of survival of both the mother and the child. The significance of the nutrition status of the mother during pregnancy is discussed further in Chapter 5.

Apart from retardation of physical growth, undernutrition can lead to defective learning and retardation of mental development.[22] The cumulative effects of these two disabilities on large numbers of individuals in the community must contribute to the perpetuation of inefficiency, lack of productivity and further impoverishment.

Undernutrition in the growing child may not be the direct result of food insufficiency. A syndrome known as *Failure to Thrive* is being recognized increasingly in the developed parts of the world. The causation of the disease is complex (see page 418), but it frequently affects the child who has been deprived of adequate maternal love and attention. In response to this, he may then lose his appetite or refuse food and enter a period of real undernutrition which is reflected in retardation or cessation of growth.

Because of the additional needs for growth, infancy and childhood are particularly dangerous times, but in adolescence, also a time of active growth, there is in addition emotional stress. This may be expressed in anxiety over the normal physiological gain in weight which occurs at this time.

It is widely believed that obese subjects are psychologically disturbed. Occasionally this belief may cause people of normal weight to develop an excessive fear of weight gain. In extreme cases the pathological condition of *anorexia nervosa* may result, a disease characterized by loss of appetite, wasting and emotional disorders.

Malnutrition

The diet may satisfy the appetite but if the food fails to supply sufficient nutrients the diet is nevertheless inadequate and a state of malnutrition will exist.

While the enormity of the global problem of malnutrition can not be denied, it is impossible to estimate its extent with any degree of accuracy. There are several reasons for this. First the clinically recognizable disease and the debilitation caused by body dysfunction, are late phenomena in the

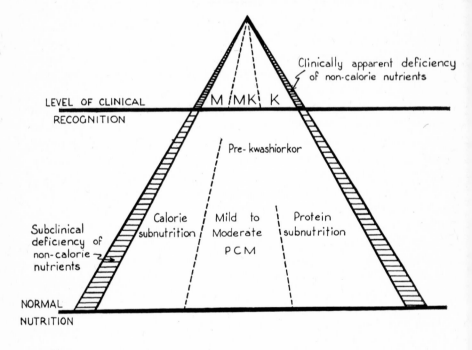

CLINICAL AND SUBCLINICAL MALNUTRITION

Figure 2   The Iceberg Analogy (Reproduced with the permission of Professor J. F. Brock; from *Annals of Internal Medicine*, **65**: 890, 1966)

course of malnutrition. The proper function of the body is affected in an imperceptible way for some time before the patient becomes aware of disturbed function.In some cases there may be no complaint by the patient, or the family. Growth retardation, for example, is symptomless and its presence is not usually recognized by parents or relatives.

The situation has been compared to an iceberg (see Figure 2). The part of the iceberg visible above the water represents clinical malnutrition that is recognizable to the mother or the physician; these are the *clinically apparent* cases. Below the surface of the water there is the much larger mass of the iceberg; this is unseen and represents the large mass of *subclinical* malnutrition in the community. These are the cases which may not have overt signs of malnutrition but perhaps they can be detected by other means. This possibility is discussed in Chapter 5. The recognition of malnutrition in a community is dependant on the presence of some skilled person who can diagnose both the overt and the subclinical cases. Unfortunately the areas where the problems are most likely are also those usually deprived of medical and health services. Even if reports of malnutrition are available it is difficult to make accurate estimates of prevalence because the population *at risk* may not be known. Many developing countries have adopted reporting procedures used in a far more sophisticated situation and these procedures may be quite inappropriate for detecting malnutrition. For example, malnutrition is relatively rare in infants under six months of age and may not in fact really become apparent until late in the first year of life. The Infant Mortality Rate is frequently used to evaluate health and nutritional status. This rate expresses the number of infants dying under one year of age as a proportion of the number of live births in the same period of time. In developing countries infant deaths are more likely to be recorded than live births, so it is probable that the Infant Mortality Rate will be inflated and misleading.

The lack of information on the prevalence of malnutrition is not restricted to developing countries. The failure to recognize the occurence of malnutrition in the United States until recently, has been due to a combination of factors. These include a lack of recognition of the ecological factors associated with malnutrition, a lack of professionals able to recognize early malnutrition, a lack of medical and health services in areas where malnutrition is likely to occur and a reporting system that is geared to reporting the diseases of affluence rather than need. It is apparent that a proper evaluation of the world situation will not possible for many years, it is imperative however, that efforts to deal with malnutrition are not delayed because of this.

The term malnutrition has been associated in the past with the classical clinical conditions which result from deficiencies of vitamins and minerals. There are many comprehensive descriptions of these syndromes in medical and nutritional science texts. For the purposes of this book discussion will be confined to those deficiency diseases that cause serious global public health problems.

Vitamin A deficiency

Hypovitaminosis A produces a wide variety of changes in animals but in man only those affecting the retina of the eye and the conjunctiva and cornea are unquestionably due to a lack of vitamin A. In the early stages of the disease, the efficiency of function of the light-sensitive rod cells in the retina of the eye is impaired; eventually vision in poor light conditions becomes impossible. This is a phenomenon of *night blindness*. In later stages of the disease, the conjunctiva assumes a dry "lack-lustre", thickened, and wrinkled appearance; a condition known as *xerosis conjunctivae*. In darker skinned races diffuse pigmentation may occur.

A silver plaque with a foamy surface is sometimes found on the conjunctiva. Superficial, and readily removed, it is frequently used as a diagnostic criterion for vitamin A deficiency. However, the lesion which is known as a *Bitots spot* may also be found in the absence of vitamin A deficiency. In the severe and rapid deficiency experienced by many infants, the *xerosis* does not have time to develop. In these cases the cornea becomes dry, the protective precorneal film is lost, and a structural damage to the surface epithelium follows. Ulceration, in response to trauma, is a frequent sequel. When infection supervenes, pus may accumulate in the anterior chamber of the eyeball. Eventually the whole integrity of the cornea may be lost. When the anterior chamber of the eye is penetrated, there is a rapid liquefaction, and eventual total destruction, of the contents of the eye. If recovery takes place before this stage is reached, some scarring of the cornea is inevitable; if the iris is also involved, sight may be severely impaired.

The corneal involvement of the eye is termed *xeropthalmia*; it is most serious during, and after, the weaning period. In areas where *xeropthalmia* is prevalent, it exhibits marked seasonal patterns that may follow closely the patterns of protein calorie malnutrition (see Figure 3).

The problem mainly affects the underpriviledged of South and East Asia, and to a lesser extent urban concentrations in the Near East, in Latin America and Africa. A warning note may have been sounded on the possibility of marginal vitamin A adequacy in New York City where low levels of vitamin A storage in the liver have been noted.[23] The skin manifestations associated with vitamin A deficiency are discussed in Chapters 3 and 5.

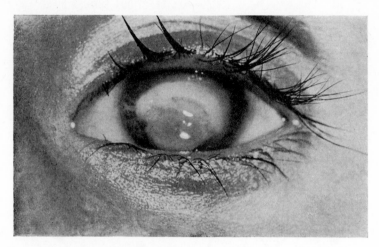

Plate 5   Keratomalacia. The lens of this 12 month old Javanese child is being extruded from the eyeball (Photograph by Professor H. A. P. C. Oomen)

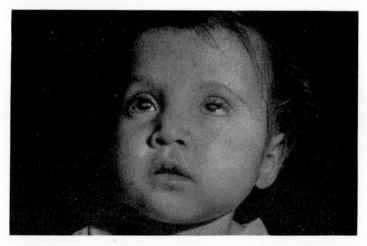

Plate 6   Corneal scars on both eyes following xeropthalmia (Photograph by Professor H. A. P. C. Oomen)

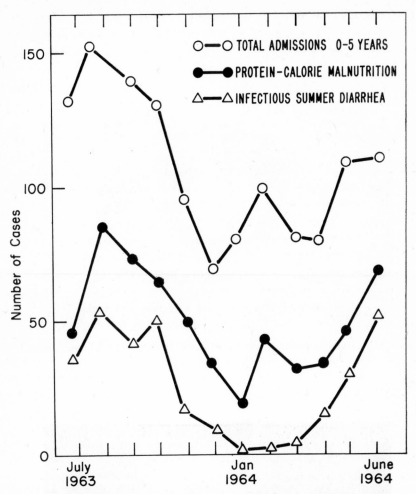

Figure 3   Comparison of total preschool age admissions, those with protein calorie malnutrition, and those with infectious summer diarrhea at Luzmila Hospital, Amman, Jordan, during a typical year. (Redrawn from a figure by Professor D. S. McLaren in the Transactions of the Royal Society of Tropical Medicine and Hygiene, **60**: 449, 1966)

Vitamin B deficiencies

The vitamins in this group and the diseases occuring as a result of deficiency were the focus of attention of nutritional scientists and clinicians for many years. *Beri-beri* is usually described as two distinct clinical entities depending on whether the nervous system or the cardiovascular system is affected. The former type is usually termed *Dry beri-beri*. The polyneuritis in this disease is characterized by muscular weakness, painful muscles, paralyses of the limbs, and sometimes mental confusion. The cardiovascular manifestations are usually referred to as *Wet beri-beri*; this syndrome is typified by edema and cardiac failure. Infants born of thiamine-deficient mothers are also liable to contract the disease because the mothers milk will fail to supply sufficient thiamine to meet the needs of the infant, and *Infantile beri-beri* is a likely sequel. In affected infants, cardiac failure and dyspnea is accompanied by a characteristic cry; when this stage of the disease is reached, death is the usual outcome.

In the past, beri-beri was found where rice was polished before consumption. Thiamine is located in the outer layers of the cereal grain, which is removed during the polishing process; the final *polished* rice product is consequently seriously deficient in the vitamin. Polished rice became a status symbol among rice eating populations and as it became more widely consumed so beri-beri became a serious public health problem. This has been partly solved by the development of a new technology which helps to preserve the thiamine content of the polished cereal. The process known as parboiling involves the treatment of rice with heat and water. Thiamine is soluble in water and is carried by the process from the outer layers of the grain to be distributed more evenly in the inner parts. These are not affected by the subsequent polishing process. The popularity of parboiling is not as high as might be expected, however, for the grain is still not as white, and therefore not as acceptable, as the processed rice.

The desire for a white, highly refined product, has now spread and cereal grains of high extraction rates, but containing minimal amounts of thiamine, are being widely consumed. It is not surprising that reports of diseases resembling dry *beri-beri* are now being reported and causing concern to public health nutritionists. Sensory disturbances and difficulty in walking have been noticed in patients consuming highly refined maize meal.[24] Similar signs and symptoms, with deafness and optic atrophy have been found also in areas where refined maize meal, cassava, and rice are consumed.[25] The deficiency is thought to be multiple with thiamine being predominent.

In the past, cases of thiamine deficiency, have followed classical descriptions. However, as the staple foods have been modified so have the clinical features of the deficiency diseases changed. Again, the *Iceberg Analogy* should be mentioned, and thought given to the subclinical, or non-classical cases, that are unrecognized but nevertheless contributing to much ill health around the world. New clinical syndromes may be unrecognized yet affecting considerable numbers of the population. It has been noticed,

3*

for example, that many East Africans have lost their neuromuscular reflexes, although they exhibit no other signs of neurological disease.[26]

The problem should not be considered as being confined to developing countries. Similar changes in eating habits are taking place elsewhere, and they could herald danger. The potential hazard of consuming highly refined flours has been recognized in the United States and to reduce the risk of occurence of vitamin deficiencies, legislation has been drafted which recommends that all white flour used in the manufacture of bread be fortified with vitamins. Other flours which are used in the manufacture of pastries, pastas and cakes are not so affected. The usefulness of this legislation has been reduced considerably by the changes in eating habits between 1955 and 1965. There is now a trend towards the consumption of an increased amount of pastries and cakes and a decrease in the consumption of bread (see Figure 4).

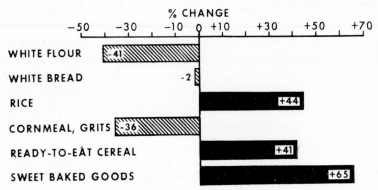

Figure 4   Change in the consumption of grain products in the United States between 1955 and 1965. Percentage change in all households in the US. Data from household food consumption surveys, Spring 1955 and 1965 (Reprinted from the Journal of Agriculture and Food Chemistry, **16**: 155, March–April 1968. Copyright (1968) by the American Chemical Society. Reprinted by permission of the copyright owners)

Pellagra

This deficiency disease is endemic in those parts of the world where populations are poor and where the staple diet is maize; it is caused by a deficiency of nicotinic acid and tryptophan (see page 266). Pellagra is characterised by loss of weight, skin lesions, gastro-intestinal and mental disturbances.

In the fully developed case, the skin lesions are so typical that the diagnosis is beyond doubt; in milder cases, especially where multiple nutrient deficiencies are affecting body function, the diagnosis may not be so obvious. The pellagric skin is abnormally sensitive to sunlight and becomes hyper-

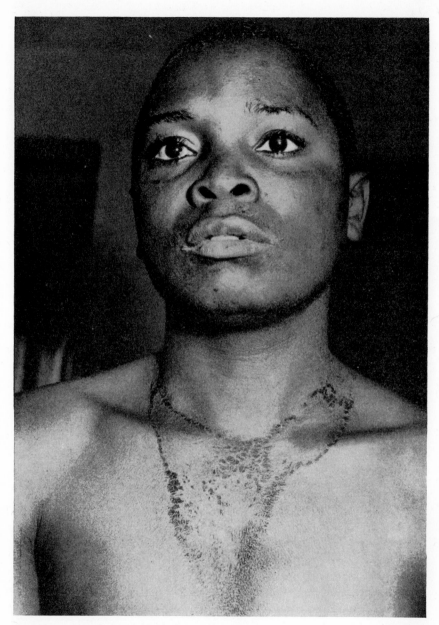

Plate 7 Pellagra in an East African. The Casal's necklace around the neck and upper chest is the result of the light-sensitive skin being exposed to the sun through an open neck shirt (FAO photograph)

pigmented. The increased pigmentation on the exposed parts around the neck is known as *Casals Necklace* after the Spanish physician who first described the disease in 1730 (see plates 7 and 8). The wrists and ankles are also frequently affected but any part exposed to the sun is liable to become abnormally pigmented.

The gastro-intestinal tract is also affected, the tongue becomes red and raw, the mouth may be sore and complaints of abdominal pain are common. The production of gastric and pancreatic digestive juices may be reduced which adds to the digestive and absorptive dysfunction.[27] A watery and profuse diarrhea is symptomatic of the inflamed bowel and may be severe

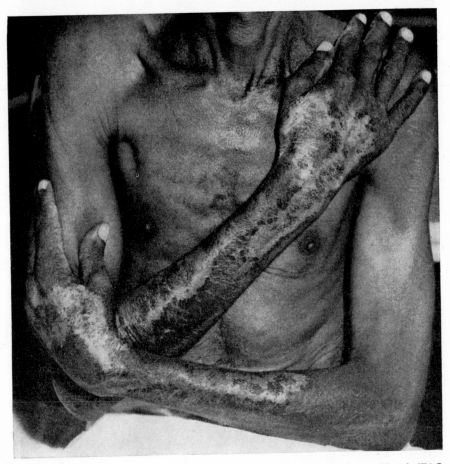

Plate 8   Pellagra. Typical "dermatitis" on exposed forearms, wrists and hands (FAO photograph)

enough for blood and mucus to be passed. This latter sign may lead to an assumption that the primary disease is dysentery.

In mild cases the patients may experience mild disorientation, minor irritability and anxiety; later in the disease the mental disturbances may lead to delirium and dementia. In chronic cases there may be degenerative changes in the nervous system causing disturbances of sensation, muscle paralyses and an abnormal gait.

The epidemiology of pellagra was described in the classical studies of Goldberger and have been reviewed by Terris.[28] The disease occurs all over the world where maize is eaten. The poor are especially prone to pellagra and epidemics are reported from time to time in southern Europe and in Africa; it is especially prevalent in Egypt. Pellagra also occurs sporadically and may be a complication of alcoholism.

The exact relationship of nicotinic acid to pellagra is still not perfectly understood. It has been suggested that the nicotinic acid in maize may not be available to the body. This would explain why it occurs in maize eaters and not in others who consume cereals containing less nicotinic acid than maize. The etiology of pellagra is probably more complicated because not all the symptoms and signs of pellagra respond readily to treatment with nicotinic acid. The mental disturbances for example, may persist after the skin and gastro-intestinal manifestations have disappeared. It has recently been suggested that the syndrome may be caused by an excess of the amino acid leucine which is present in large amounts in the millet staple known in India as *Jowar*.[29]

Pellagra will probably continue to be endemic and a public health problem in many parts of the world; elsewhere sporadic cases may be expected to occur from time to time. Personal experiences have indicated that florid cases may be misdiagnosed when the condition is seen only on rare occasions. In one particular case the arm lesions resembled healing burns; this together with mental state of the patient (an elderly male) had led to a diagnosis of burns sustained during an epileptic episode. It was not surprising that the condition had not responded to local dressings applied to the hands and arms.

Early cases of pellagra are also likely to be missed and perhaps many cases of subclinical pellagra exist but remain undiagnosed in marginally fed communities.

An epidemic of what was most likely subclinical pellagra has been observed personally among a labor force on a sisal plantation in East Africa. Seasonal outbursts of violence and dysentery had occured for several years but an interrelationship had not been suspected. Further investigation revealed however, that the gastro-intestinal symptoms were not infective in origin. A relationship was established between the onset of the symptoms and the end of the dry season when the diet of the labor force, based on maize, was at its poorest.

It was eventually concluded that the irritability, as expressed by the outbursts of unrest and violence on the estate, and the gastro-intestinal symptoms were part of a syndrome of malnutrition and undernutrition with nicotinic acid deficiency playing a major part in its etiology. Such experiences should alert nutritionists to the possibility that malnutrition may be underlying other episodes of community dissent.

Multiple deficiences of vitamins

It is virtually impossible for an inadequate diet to be lacking in one nutrient alone. In most instances the quality of the diet is poor because of a lack of a particular food, or food group, which may be the only source of several essential nutrients. For example, green leaves provide the precursor of vitamin A, vitamin C and riboflavin; cereals are sources of vitamins from the B group.

Skin, eye and oral lesions may be manifestations of mixed deficiences which do not always comply with the classic descriptions offered in textbooks. Riboflavin or vitamin B_2 deficiency may be expected where there is protein malnutrition or where there are signs of other vitamin deficiencies.

Deficiency of riboflavin leads to a seborrheaic condition of the nasolabial region, cracks at the corner of the mouth (*angular stomatitis*) and sore, cracked lips (*cheilosis*). These may be associated with the skin lesions of nicotinic acid deficiency or with the mouth lesions of vitamin C deficiency. Similarly, the eye lesions which occur in vitamin A deficiency may be complicated by the photophobia, lachrymation and vascularization of the cornea that is a feature of riboflavin deficiency.

Vitamin B_{12} and folic acid deficiency

Folic acid is concerned with the formation of hemoglobin. As vitamin B_{12} controls folic acid enzymes, a deficiency of either or both of these vitamins in the tissues can lead to the development of an anemia. This is characterized by a low hemoglobin level and the presence of large and immature red cells in the blood and is designated megaloblastic anemia. There are changes in the gastro-intestinal tract resulting in a sore tongue and diarrhea. Tingling sensations in the hands and feet may be a distressing feature of the disease.

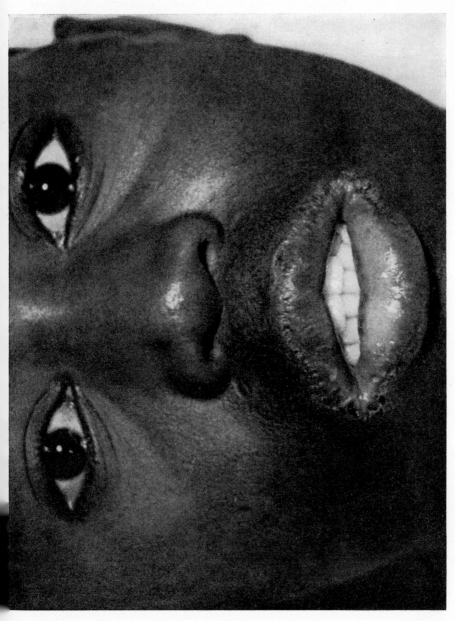

Plate 9   Cheilosis and angular stomatitis (FAO photograph)

Megaloblastic anemia caused by deficiency of vitamin B_{12} may be complicated by severe neurological disturbances following degeneration of the spinal cord. The disabilities from this condition may be serious. Mental disturbances in vitamin B_{12} deficiency are more common than generally believed.[30]

Megaloblastic anemia is rarely the result of a deficiency of folic acid in the diet. Dietary vitamin B_{12} deficiency is similarly rare except in vegetarians. It does occur, however, when there are extra demands for these nutrients, consequently it is common in pregnant females. Lactation also drains the maternal stores because an assured supply of folate in breast milk takes precedence over maternal needs.

Megaloblastic anemia is mainly the consequence of malabsorption. Vitamin B_{12} requires the presence of *Intrinsic Factor* secreted by the gastric mucosa, the factor combines with the vitamin B_{12} molecule and transports it into the intestinal mucosal cells. The Intrinsic Factor may be congenitally absent, or lacking because of surgical removal of the stomach; the resulting megaloblastic anemia is known as *pernicious anemia*. The malabsorption syndrome may be responsible for a failure of absorption of folic acid. In protein calorie malnutrition an inability to absorb folate may be responsible for the megaloblastic anemia that is a common complication of kwashiorkor. The variety of causes indicates the potential of the disease to create public health problems in most areas of the world.

Vitamin C deficiency

Deficiency of vitamin C (ascorbic acid) leads to the development of the clinical condition known as *scurvy*. When ascorbic acid is deficient, the body is unable to develop adequate supporting tissues. This disability produces characteristic pathological changes.

In the bones and teeth, the lack of supporting tissue prevents their growth and further development. The teeth also become loose because the tissue that normally holds them firmly in the jaw is lacking. There is a similar deficiency of supporting tissue in the walls of the smaller blood vessels and capillaries. They are consequently liable to rupture, and blood escapes into the surrounding tissues. In the skin, these lesions show as small hemorrhages and bruises.

Anemia and conjunctival lesions and hemorrhages may also be seen in patients suffering from scurvy.[31] These manifestations may not be attributable to a deficiency of vitamin C alone, but may be one more example of the multiple deficiencies that are liable to occur in humans who are consuming diets generally poor in quality.

Fruits, vegetables, tubers and leaves are the principle sources of vitamin C. They are widespread throughout the world but supplies may be available only in one season. If the community is dependent on seasonal sources their vitamin C status will depend on their knowledge of the technology of storing, or preserving, the raw food. If their knowledge is limited, vitamin C deficiency is liable to be a seasonal event. The ability of the body to accumulate a considerable amount of the vitamin during times of plenty means that a long interval of time may elapse before signs of depletion appear. The storage status of individuals within population groups can not be predicted; it is for this reason (and others) that the human requirements for vitamin C are the subject of controversy.

Vitamin C is unstable and soluble in water, therefore it is liable to be destroyed during processing and cooking. This has importance in communities which are depending, to an increasing degree on processed convenience foods and preserved fruits and vegetables. Freezing of vegetables helps to preserve ascorbic acid and is an excellent method of storing food for retail sale. If however there is a breakdown in the marketing or distributing system, subsequent thawing may cause depletion of the vitamin content.

The food industry can now provide attractive carbonated or non-carbonated fruit drinks which have become highly acceptable to large sections of populations living in developing, as well as the more sophisticated countries. These beverages are replacing drinks made from natural fruit and vegetable juices; it is therefore essential to ensure that they contain adequate amounts of vitamin C, equivalent to that found in natural fruit. Some countries have attempted to protect the consumer by introducing legislation specifying minimal levels for vitamin C in natural or artificial fruit beverages.

In many European countries potatoes provide the main source of vitamin C. In the lower socio-economic groups any factor which causes a reduction in potato consumption should therefore be viewed with concern.

In the recent National Nutrition Survey carried out on low income and poverty groups in the USA 56 per cent of the sample population in Texas and Louisiana had an intake of vitamin C judged to be low. Twelve per cent of the Louisiana group and 14 per cent of the Texas group has unacceptably low serum vitamin C levels.[32] The national food supply in the USA has provided decreasing amounts of ascorbic acid in the last decade; surprisingly farm diets contained less than city diets.[33] Low levels of intake and low serum levels are not necessarily associated with overt deficiency disease but this data goes give a warning that vitamin C deficiency may become a public health problem in certain parts of the USA.

Recent studies suggest that tobacco smokers either have less vitamin C available for utilization or that they use vitamin C differently from non-smokers. This may indicate that smokers may be more at risk to vitamin C deficiency.[34]

Scurvy usually occurs in infants who have been fed on cows milk alone, prevention lies in the provision of a supplementary source of ascorbic acid. Consequently scurvy in infancy is a problem of the indigent and populations who do not have access to welfare food services, or are not informed of the existence of such services.

Vitamin D deficiency

The inter-relationships of nutrients are important but they are frequently overlooked. It is important to realize however, that deficiency, or excess of one nutrient, may affect the function of another. The relationships of vitamin D and the elements calcium and phosphorus are so closely inter-related that they must be considered together. All of these nutrients are involved in the deficiency diseases of rickets and osteomalacia. The former affects infants and children and the latter, adults, usually the pregnant and lactating mother.

Man can obtain vitamin D either by ultra-violet irradiation of sterols in the skin or from ready-made sources in food. If a deficiency of the vitamin occurs through a breakdown in either of these two sources of supply, then both the absorption of calcium and phosphate from the gut is impaired. The deficiency of the vitamin also causes disturbance in the formation of cartilage that would normally become bone. In an attempt to maintain proper calcium levels calcium is drawn out of the matrix of existing bone which then becomes softened.

Rickets The clinical features of the disease may include the following: cessation of bone growth, widening of the wrists due to the extension of the cartilaginous epiphyses of the forearm bones. Because of the same pathological changes, swellings appear at the junction of the rib cartilages and the breast bone. In an advanced stage, the swellings have been likened to the beads of a rosary, hence the expression *Rickety Rosary*. The withdrawal of calcium from areas of the skull bones results in these becoming softened; this can be detected on palpation. Later the skull may become bossed. The development of teeth is affected so the eruption of the primary dentition is delayed.

The continuation of the deficiency is accompanied by secondary complications; the softened bones are unable to support the weight of the body and they become bowed. Similarly, the chest cage may be deformed and the resultant *Pigeon* chest may hinder proper pulmonary ventilation so upper respiratory infections may be an important and terminal feature of the disease. In the female the inability of the pelvic bones to bear the stresses of the body weight can cause pelvic deformities; these may hinder or prevent normal parturition at a later date. The failure to absorb calcium may lead to the formation of soaps in the intestinal tract; these may irritate the bowel therefore diarrhea and other gastro-intestinal upsets are common. During the course of the disease the calcium levels in the blood fall and may reach such a low level that *tetany* appears. This clinical syndrome is characterised by twitchings of the hands and feet and vocal cords. The spasms of the latter leads to difficulty in respiration and causes a distressing cry; in severe cases there may be generalized convulsions.

Osteomalacia   This is a disease of adult life; because of the extra demands for calcium and vitamin D during pregnancy and lactation, women are particularly prone to the disease. The deficiency leads to a failure of the body to lay down calcium in the bone matrix. Pain in the bones of the feet and in the lumbar region is a common feature and may cause the subject to adopt a peculiar gait. The bones are very liable to fracture and if a diagnosis has not been made at this point it will soon be obvious when the radiological examination reveals the typical picture of the *Milkmans Syndrome* of generalized rarifaction and artifacts which resemble bone fractures.

Vitamin D is fat soluble, therefore disturbance in fat absorption will also interfere with vitamin D absorption. As malabsorption of fat is not rare, rickets (celiac rickets) and osteomalacia can occur as secondary phenomena and complicate the clinical picture of the malabsorption syndrome.

Osteoporosis   This clinical syndrome is usually found in the elderly and is currently receiving considerable attention. Until recently it was thought to be due to a dysfunction of calcium metabolism. There is a loss of mineral material from the bones. Although it is a disease that is especially prevalent in post-menopausal women, with advancing age, both sexes may be affected. There is a generalized rarifaction of the bones, accompanied by pain which may be extremely severe.

Recently it has been shown that vitamin D may be playing a part in the etiology of this disease. The *serum anti-rachitic* activity which is a measure of vitamin D levels has been found to be low in some groups of women in the USA; the levels were subject to seasonal variations which coincided with their exposure to ultra-violet activity.[35] In addition to low vitamin D intakes and inadequate irradiation other factors must be taken into consideration; for example, malabsorption and dietary faddism also tend to occur in the senile.

Rickets and osteomalacia occur in populations consuming poor diets and in regions where the opportunities for irradiation of the skin by sunlight are poor. It is primarily considered a disease of temperate climates and was so prevalent in England at one time that it was known as the *English disease*. Diets lacking milk or dairy products are associated with rickets. Cereal diets are especially dangerous since they may interfere with the absorption of

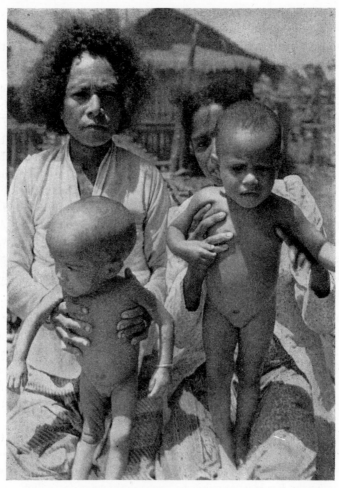

Plate 10   Rickets in New Guinea. On the north coast of New Guinea infants are kept inside the houses and are rarely exposed to the tropical sun. The child on the right is the same age as the child with rickets (Photograph by Professor H. A. P. C. Oomen)

calcium. The other contributory factor, lack of sunlight, is frequently associated with poverty- stricken slum areas where the sun may be blocked out by high buildings and atmospheric pollution. In the tropics, where the diet may be a poor source of vitamin D, the availability of continual sunshine may not prevent the occurence of rickets or osteomalacia. In many places customs and cultural beliefs prevent, or prohibit, exposure of the skin to the sun. The practice of *purdah* among some Moslem groups in the Middle East and Asia limits the women to the confines of dark dwellings or requires them to cover their entire body when walking in public places. Infants and children in some societies are swathed in clothes and may be

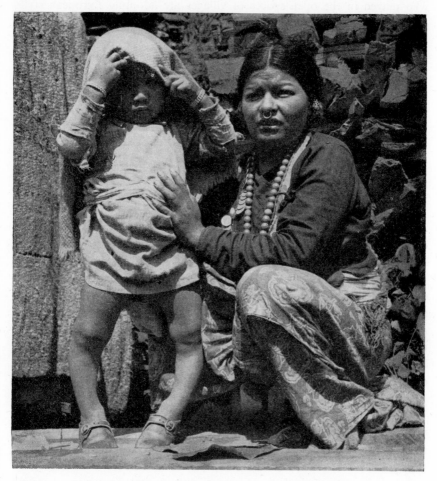

Plate 11   Rickets in a Nepalese child. During the rainy season, which lasts five to six months, children are kept inside very dark huts (WHO photograph)

deprived of sunlight. In many parts of Iran, working mothers spend many hours each day in carpet factories with poor lighting. As they may have to take their family with them, the children are also deprived of sunlight and are especially prone to rickets.

Public health measures have brought about smoke abatement and have made milk and other sources of vitamin D available. These actions have succeeded in eradicating rickets from the industrial areas of Europe and North America, but elsewhere in the world new problems arise. Atmospheric pollution is increasing in the developing countries as they become more industrialized. African children who formerly wore scanty clothing and who played in the open spaces of villages are adopting European styles of clothing. They are moving to urban areas where new industries are opening up. They are living in tall houses and apartment blocks which cut off sunlight from the streets. They are spending more time at school and less time out in the open.

It is therefore, not surprising that rickets is being reported in areas where it was formerly unknown.[36] Where air-conditioning provides relief from tropical temperatures, adults will undoubtedly spend more time indoors. The loss of radiation from sunlight may play an important role in the development of osteomalacia in communities formerly unaffected by the disease.

Iron

A deficiency of iron leads to the clinical condition of anemia which may be extremely severe. In iron deficiency anemia the red cells are normal in size but they are incompletely filled with the oxygen carrying pigment hemoglobin; in advanced stages of the disease the cells are smaller in size than normal cells. Mild anemia produces lassitude but the more severe cases show signs of inadequate cardiac function. Breathlessness, palpitations, swelling of the feet and ankles may become increasingly distressing; the disease may progress until cardiac failure occurs. The deficiency of iron may lead to other disturbances of function caused by a lack of enzymes that depend on iron.

Iron deficiency anemia is extremely prevalent and is a serious public health problem in the under-developed and tropical regions. It is not possible to make a scientific evaluation of the prevalence of anemia for several reasons. First, the size of the population at risk is unknown, second, the criteria for anemia vary in different parts of the world, and third, there are several ways in which the degree of anemia may be measured. These are discussed in Chapter 5, page 444.

Severe symptoms may be expected when hemoglobin levels fall below 7 mg per 100 ml of blood, but the body may be suffering harm long before this low level is reached. Minimum levels for hemoglobin have been established by the World Health Organization. Persons with levels below these are considered anemic[37] (see Table 1).

Table 1 Levels of hemoglobin as a criterion for anemia

Group	Hemoglobin level g per 100 ml of venous blood
Children: 6 months–6 years	11
6–14 years	12
Adults: males	13
females, non-pregnant	12
females, pregnant	11

Source: Nutritional Anemias. Wld. Hlth. Org., Tech. Rep. Ser. No. 405, 1968.

The mean corpuscular hemoglobin concentration of blood at all ages should be 34. The hematocrit value is being used as an additional or alternative method of evaluating levels of anemia. This is obtained by measuring the proportion of the red cells packed by centrifugal force in the total volume of the blood. The hematocrit values corresponding to the hemoglobin concentrations given above may be obtained by multiplying the hemoglobin figures by three.

The criteria for anemia which have been used in the past have differed from those suggested by WHO. Nevertheless, the prevalence rate for anemia in some countries is still extremely high. In Mauritius, for example, 50 per cent of certain groups in the population may be affected by anemia of which 90 per cent is due to iron deficiency. In the United States it has been estimated that 25–30 per cent of infants from 3 to 36 months have a hemoglobin concentration of less than 10 mg per 100 ml of blood; and the US Public Health Service has estimated that 5 per cent of white males and females, 10 per cent of negro males, and 12 per cent of negro females are anemic. Elsewhere in the world there are ample reports of anemia in pregnant women, and in the United Kingdom 35 per cent of a group of 202 apparently fit, healthy people, aged 65 years and over had a hemoglobin level less than 13.0 mg per 100 ml of blood.[38]

Iron deficiency anemia therefore affects all ages and physiological states. Some of the reasons for this will now be discussed. The infant is born with an endowment of iron from the mother. The low birth weight baby has a smaller endowment than that of normal weight, (see Table 2) and is consequently much more likely to become anemic. This endowment is in the form of red cells and in the iron stores which have to last a considerable time.

Table 2   Iron endowment at birth

Infant	Hb. Conc., gm./100 Ml.	Hb. Mass, gm.	Hb. Iron, mg.	Storage Iron, mg.	Tissue Iron, mg.	Total Iron, mg.
Term						
3.3 kg	19.0	55	185	34	23	242
Premature						
1.5 kg	19.0	30	97	15	10	122

Source: Schulman, I., *J. Amer. Med. Assoc.* **175**: 119, 1961.

The production of new red cells virtually ceases during the 6–8 weeks after birth and the concentration of circulating hemoglobin decreases at a rate that is proportional to the short life span of the fetal red cells. The iron from the breakdown of these cells is however not wasted, but retained for use when blood formation resumes.

The diet that the infant receives at this time is usually based on milk, and although human milk contains about three times as much iron as cows milk it is nevertheless a poor source of iron. Infants fed for prolonged periods of time (over 6 months) on milk alone will be unable to meet their iron requirements and they will become increasingly anemic. The anemia must be due to factors other than just the deficiency of dietary iron because the anemia of a baby who has been fed cows milk may be no more severe, as measured by hemoglobin levels, than a baby fed on human milk. For reasons as yet unknown, the breast fed baby responds much more rapidly to iron therapy than the latter.

The supply of iron to the infant must come, therefore, from sources additional to milk. This may be achieved by giving the infant supplementary foods containing iron from the third or fourth month of life onwards. Good sources of iron such as animal foods may not be acceptable or even available, but cereal gruels are usually at hand in most countries, consequently they form the basis of most weaning foods. Although it is doubtful if all of this iron can be utilized by the body, babies fed on cereals are far less liable to develop anemia than those fed on milk alone.[39]

In many countries animal foods are in short supply so the diet may remain predominantly vegetarian. The lack of sufficient animal protein may add to the risk of anemia because it is believed that the presence of animal foods in the diet enhances the absorption of iron in vegetable foods.[40] If there is an overall deficiency of protein in the diet, the protein compound responsible for transporting iron in the blood (*transferrin*) is decreased in quantity and may contribute to the development of iron deficiency anemia. In addition to dietary deficiencies, there are other factors which affect the availability of iron for blood formation and which must be taken into consideration.

Increased demand   For a given level of intake, increased demands for iron may create a relative deficiency of iron. This occurs physiologically in the growing period and during pregnancy, although compensatory increases in the absorption of iron may take place.[41]

Hemorrhage   If there is any loss of blood, extra iron will be required for the repair and restorative processes. These losses may follow accidental or intended trauma such as surgery, obstetrical accidents, or excessive menstrual bleeding. Intestinal bleeding may arise from a variety of causes including inflammation of the intestinal tract in gastroenteritis or dysentery. These are common conditions in infants and children living in unhygienic surroundings. Older persons living in the tropics are frequently troubled by inflammatory conditions of the bowel, such as the chronic ulceration of amebic dysentery.

Deficient clotting of blood   Defects in the coagulating mechanisms of the blood such as hemophilia or vitamin K deficiency are rare, but another form of intestinal bleeding, formerly thought to be uncommon, is now being recognized on an increasing scale. An allergic condition in which the patient has become sensitized to milk protein results in changes in the intestinal epithelium and loss of blood through intestinal hemorrhages.[42]

Malnutrition   Children suffering from protein calorie malnutrition may not be anemic when first seen, but they may become severely anemic after a few weeks of treatment.[43] This is possibly because growth has been restored, for this process itself demands extra iron.

Parasites   Parasites of various forms may cause severe iron deficiency anemia, particularly in tropical areas. *Malaria* is still one of the most important vector borne diseases suffered by man; it can cause severe anemia of an iron deficiency type. Intestinal parasites may cause severe losses of

4*

iron. For example, the liver fluke causes bowel and bladder ulceration (*schistosomiasis*) which may be responsible for iron losses in the amount of 3–5 mg per day.

Hookworm infestations are common in the hot, humid parts of the world, including the southern United States. The species *Necator americanus* is estimated to cause a loss of up to 5 mg per day. The losses due to the species *Ancylostoma duodenale* are even greater, and a load of 100 worms will probably cause anemia in populations whose food does not contain large amounts of absorbable iron. Similarly, the intestinal parasite *Trichuris trichuria*, the whip worm, is likely to induce anemia in children.[44]

Malabsorption can affect the young and the old. Although the causes of malabsorption are not always clear the disturbance appears to be related to the villi of the intestinal tract. Flattening of the villi has been observed in some cases; this undoubtedly results in a reduction of the actual surface over which absorption can take place.[45] Why these changes have taken place is not clear.

Trace elements

A number of nutrients are found in animal tissues in very small quantities; they have been termed *trace elements* or *micronutrients*. Because they are required in small amounts does not mean that they are unimportant. Some of the micronutrients are absolutely essential for the proper function of some enzyme systems.

From a public health point of view the trace element iodine is probably the most important. However, there is a possibility that a deficiency of zinc may have an important bearing on health in certain parts of the world. The dangers of too much fluorine, another trace element, have already been mentioned.

Iodine The thyroid gland responds to deprivation of iodine by cell multiplication and physical enlargement. The enlargement may be diffuse and cause no disability. If the deprivation continues it becomes visible and later a very large goiter may develop which can interfere with swallowing, respiration, and movement of the neck. The diffuse enlargement with a smooth surface consitutes a *simple goiter*. The larger goiters are known as *colloid goiters* because they contain large vesicles filled with colloid material. In long-standing goiters, structural changes may take place culminating in the formation of nodules. On rare occasions such *nodular goiters* may become malignant or produce symptoms of overactivity of the thyroid gland.

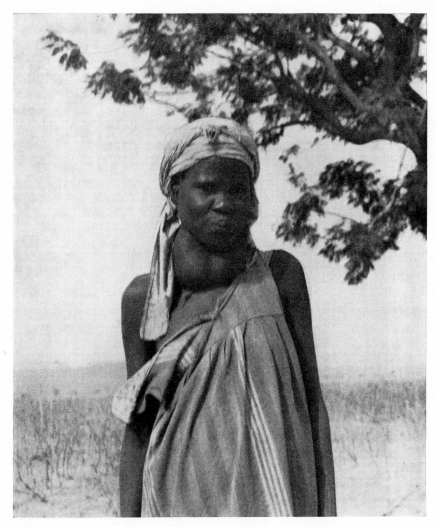

Plate 12   Goiter in a young Sudanese girl (Photograph by Marcel Ganzin, courtesy of the London School of Hygiene and Tropical Medicine, and FAO)

In areas where goiter is endemic, iodine deficiency can cause severe effects known as *cretinism* which is characterised by retarded physical and mental development. Cretinism usually occurs among the offspring of parents who are suffering from goiter. It is possible that the condition is directly caused by iodine deficiency in the mother, since normally functioning thyroid glands have been noted in cretins. This suggests that the damage to the child took place before birth.[46]

The typical *cretin* is partially or completely deaf and because of this, cases of deaf mutism have been attributed to iodine deficiency. There are conflicting views on this as deaf mutism has been noted in population groups where intermarriage of close relatives is practiced; this might indicate a genetic defect as the causal agent.[47]

Retardation of growth has been noted in children with even small goiters and this has been attributed to iodine deficiency, but it must be remembered that where goiter is endemic, diets may also be poor.

There are uncountable millions of persons in the world with goiter the majority of whom suffer no disability, this makes an estimate of its prevalence impossible. It is however endemic in many parts of the world where geological and climatic accidents and events have deprived the soil of iodine. The principal endemic goiter regions in the world are the Alps in Europe, the Himalayas in Asia, the Andes in South America, the Rockies of North America, and the Highland areas of the Philippines and New Guinea. It is also found in the plains around the Great Lakes of North America and in other isolated localities where the water supply is hard. It is more common in females, especially during adolescence and pregnancy.

Seafoods are good sources of iodine but the proximity of the sea does not exclude the possibility of goiter occuring.

There are three arguments supporting the role of iodine in the etiology of goiter. First, it is associated with iodine-free regions in the world. Second, the prevalence of goiter is reduced when iodine becomes available in the diet. Thirdly, the metabolic changes in patients with inadequate thyroid function are commensurate with the known effects of iodine deficiency.

The development of goiter is not simply a matter of iodine deficiency. An adequate intake of iodine has been enjoyed by neighboring populations in the same geographic area; some of the population have contracted goiter, others have not. In some cases the differences have been attributed to hard water, in others to the presence in foodstuffs, of substances antagonistic to the thyroid gland. The consumption of milk from animals fed on these foodstuffs will also lead to the development of goiter in the consumer. The goitrogenic foodstuffs include cabbage leaves, turnips, and the seeds of mustard, rape, and cabbage. The goitrogenic agent has been identified as *thiourea*, a compound now used for controlling overactive thyroid glands.

Zinc   Deficiency of zinc retards growth in children and development of the male genital organs. The recognition of this role is so recent that its global prevalence is still unknown.[48] The disease was first reported in Iran and Egypt.

Zinc is an essential nutrient which is present in the new born infant. The mineral is constantly lost in early infant life; the losses are not made up from breast milk. Despite the assertion that bovine milk contains zinc readily available for absorption there are other reports that a positive zinc balance cannot be maintained in early infant life.[49] At the present time it does not appear certain whether bovine milk has this particular advantage over breast milk. In Iran and Egypt, zinc deficiency has been attributed to the predominance of foods of vegetable origin, such as cereals and legumes, which contain zinc in an unavailable form. The malabsorption caused by the binding of the zinc to other chemical compounds may be aggravated by the presence of excess calcium. The presence of animal protein on the other hand, enhances the absorption of this important trace element.

Much more needs to be learned of the physiological action of zinc and its interrelationships with other nutrients. Because of a possible connection between zinc, protein calorie malnutrition and growth this metal may have public health importance elsewhere in the world.[50]

Protein calorie malnutrition

Of all the diseases so far described none is so widespread as protein calorie malnutrition. This term has been adopted in favor of others such as *nutritional edema* or *dystrophe* since these have clinical orientation but tell little of the etiology of the disease.

While protein is an essential nutrient for growth and the maintainance and repair and tissues, the body gives first priority to the preservation of its energy supply. If the energy intake is inadequate to meet the demands of the body, it will use any nutrient that can be broken down to liberate energy. A diet that is lacking in calories will therefore use any protein that may be present as a source of energy. The relationship between calories and protein is very important and is discussed in further detail in Chapter 3. One other factor of importance is the quality of the protein in the diet, for unless it is of high quality, adequate growth and proper maintenance of body function becomes impossible.

Growth, repair of tissues and organs, and maintenance of body function therefore depends on three factors; first, the provision of adequate quantities of protein, second, the provision of adequate quality protein, and third, the level of the calorie intake.

A diet containing inadequate or poor quality protein, or insufficient calories is of necessity a poor diet and liable to be deficient in other essential nutrients. There is likely to be multiple nutrient deficiencies; this explains

why protein calorie malnutrition is a syndrome with many clinical manifestations. In the interests of achieving a basic understanding of the disease,
the following descriptions of the syndrome have been simplified.

When the main deficiency in the diet is calorie inadequacy, growth stops
and the child is usually thin, undersized, and underweight. Clinically such
a child is described as suffering from *marasmus*. If the diet supplies sufficient
calories but lacks protein, or if the quality of the protein is inadequate,
there is not only growth failure but signs of disturbed body function such
as fluid retention and skin rashes which will be described in detail later.
Because of the adequate calorie intake there may be normal amounts of
subcutaneous fat that may mask underlying muscle wasting. Such a child
is described as having *kwashiorkor*. Between these two extreme syndromes
there are intermediate forms of the disease which may be complicated by
single or multiple deficiencies of other nutrients. Calorie inadequacy is
more liable to affect infants whose mothers have failed to lactate or who
have been fed inadequate amounts of cows milk or milk formulas which are
too dilute. Consequently, marasmus is mainly seen in infants under one
year of age.

Breast milk is usually adequate in quantity and quality for infants up
to 6 or 8 months of age, and proper growth will continue if the child is
weaned on to solid food that provides sufficient calories and protein of good
quality. Unfortunately, in developing countries or impoverished communities
the food that is usually available for weaning children contains inadequate
amounts of protein; frequently it is also inadequate in quality. Because
weaning is often delayed and because it takes time for the signs of deficiency
to develop, kwashiorkor is most prevalent in the second year of life, and
it is often found in even older children. These are generalizations however,
and marasmic children in the older age groups are quite common, and
infants and children in the first year of life may suffer from kwashiorkor.
The reasons for these differences are related to the ecological factors which
influence the diet of the children, and the immediate causal or etiological
factors which precipitate the disease. These are described fully in the next
chapter.

The clinical condition of marasmus has been recognized for many years,
but it has only recently been associated with kwashiorkor and recognized
as part of the *Protein Calorie Malnutrition Syndrome*. The discovery of
kwashiorkor is a relatively recent event which explains why so little attention
has been given to protein calorie malnutrition in the past. The disease was
first described in 1933 by Dr. Cicely Williams, a British pediatrician, who
noticed the disease in children in the Gold Coast, the West African country

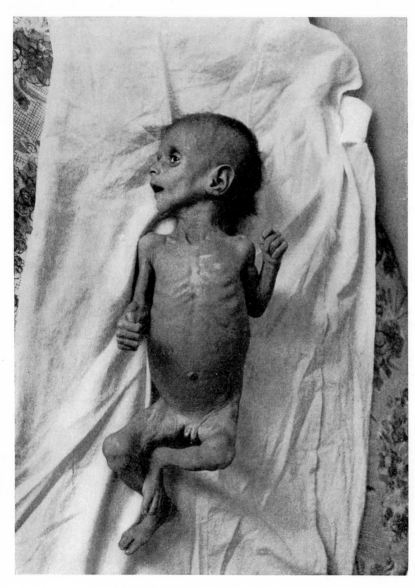

Plate 13 Marasmus (WHO photograph)

now known as Ghana.[51] The word kwashiorkor is derived from the *Ga* language and is said to mean "the sickness of the deprived child".

The discovery of kwashiorkor was of great clinical importance but it came at the peak of the "chemical era" of nutrition and its significance was either ignored or overlooked. The experiences of prisoners of war and detainees during the second World War added to our knowledge of the clinical aspects of starvation and malnutrition. Among these was Cicely Williams, who survived the notorious Changi camp in Singapore.[52] Despite this new knowledge, the important role of protein was still not appreciated. Even in 1949 the agenda of the Joint Expert Committee on Nutrition of the World Health Organization and the Food and Agriculture Organization contained no item under which protein malnutrition could be discussed. By 1956 however, the significance of the disease had been recognized and a considerable amount of information had accumulated on its etiology and treatment, and it was at this time that the concept of the spectrum of protein calorie malnutrition was evolved (see Figure 5).

The manifestations of protein calorie malnutrition may be manifold but certain features of kwashiorkor are present in all cases. These are cessation of growth, wasting of muscles, and overhydration of the body. This latter, while always present, may not be clinically apparent because a considerable amount of water can accumulate in the body before swelling of the dependent parts of the body (*edema*) becomes obvious. Other signs may be present

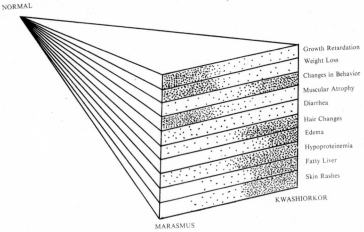

Figure 5   The spectrum of protein calorie malnutrition. (Redrawn from a figure by Behar, M., Viteri, F., Bressani, R., Arroyave, G., Squibb, R. L., and Scrimshaw, N. S. "Principles of treatment and prevention of severe protein calorie malnutrition in children (Kwashiorkor)" *Ann. N. Y. Acad. Sci.* **69**: 954–968, 1958)

but not invariable so. Mental changes such as general indifference, irritability, apathy, and sadness of expression can often be detected very early in the disease. These are important diagnostic signs and a reminder of the close relationship between nutrition, and mental and intellectual development. The marasmic infant may be alert and obviously interested in food in the earlier stages of the disease; later the child becomes fractious and disinterested not only in food but also the environment; there is eventually a loss of appetite. The misery of the child suffering from kwashiorkor may be one of the most distressing aspects of the disease. Frequently the child curls up in the corner and shuns all forms of attention and appears to want nothing but to be left alone to die. Drowsiness is often a feature of the disease. The causation of this encephalopathy is not clear; it was formerly concluded that it was hepatic in origin but in many cases usual signs of severe liver damage, jaundice, and ascites are absent. More recently it has been sug-

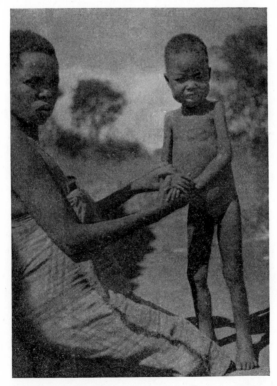

Plate 14   Kwashiorkor in a four year old boy; two younger siblings died from the same disease. The edema, wasting, skin rashes and lesions in the flexure of the elbow are typical of the advanced stages of the disease.

gested that disturbances in sodium metabolism and potassium depletion, may be responsible for the drowsiness.[53] The disease is extremely difficult to treat because of the mental attitude of the patient. The success of treatment may be judged from changes in the degree of apathy. The appearance of a smile is a good prognostic sign.

Many medical textbooks have emphasized the hair changes which may be present. The belief that these must be present before the diagnosis of kwashiorkor can be made has been responsible for much under-reporting of the disease. In several texts, the red hair of advanced kwashiorkor has achieved additional notoriety in the mistaken translation of kwashiorkor as meaning "the red boy". In some cases the hair may be discolored or show abnormal pigmentation, it is frequently thin in appearance and readily pulled out, but these signs are not invariably present. Skin rashes have also been considered a criterion for diagnosis; these may range from minor hyperpigmentation to the more serious flakey paint rash of the legs, and the gross loss of tissue in the flexures of the limbs. However, many cases of kwashiorkor have no skin changes.

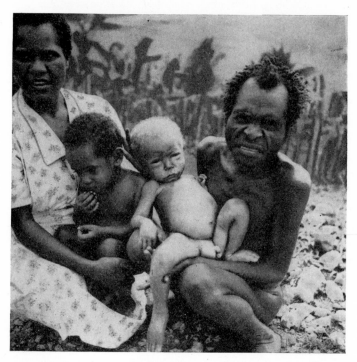

Plate 15   Kwashiorkor. This child has edema and hair changes. The child on the left is a healthy child of the same age (Photograph by Professor H. A. P. C. Oomen)

Diarrhea is another variable feature of the disease. It may be a final terminal event or it may be mild and chronic causing little disability. Frequently its chronicity may be the reason why the mother takes the child to the clinic in the first instance. Personal experience suggests that the nature and severity of the diarrhea is related to the nature of the staple diet. Diarrhea is uncommon in kwashiorkor in the banana eaters of Northern Tanzania but it was nearly always present, mostly severe and sometimes uncontrollable, in the maize, sorghum, and cassava eaters of South West Tanzania. In the Middle East and in the Philippines diarrhea is common, but in these areas infection may be an important part of the etiology of the disease and the respective contribution of the diet and infection cannot always be determined. In the urban areas of Manila, marasmic infants are frequently admitted to hospital as cases of acute gastro-enteritis, but close questioning and examination frequently reveals that the child has been ailing for months and has had numerous bouts of diarrhea. The differentiation of cases of gastro-enteritis complicated by dehydration from marasmic infants is important from the point of view of therapy and is discussed on page 527.

The non-infective diarrhea of protein calorie malnutrition has been attributed to a deficiency of the intestinal digestive enzyme lactose which splits disaccharides into simple sugars. The undigested sugars ferment and cause irritation of the gastro-intestinal tract. It has been noticed that giving a carbohydrate free diet may be followed by a dramatic decrease in the number of stools passed per day. Observations on the secretion of the intestinal juices have confirmed that on recovery, the ability to split and subsequently absorb sugars improves.[54] The pancreatic exocrine secretion is also insufficient in protein calorie malnutrition which means that food material is inadequately digested thereby aggravating the diarrhea still further. Impaired kidney function which disturbs the fluid and electrolyte balance is a further burden to the body.

There are also changes in the chemical composition of the body. Low magnesium levels have been observed during the course of the illness and have been attributed to prolonged losses of magnesium in the diarrhea coupled with a low intake of the mineral in food. (A low intake is especially likely if the staple diet is cassava.) Analyses of organs of children dying from malnutrition have revealed potassium and magnesium depletion of all of the organs.[55] Clinical improvement has been noted in children given magnesium as therapy. This is a further indication that magnesium imbalance is an important feature of kwashiorkor.[56]

It is possible that the electrolyte disturbances are responsible for the cardiac dysfunction that is a feature of severe marasmus and kwashiorkor. In many cases the cardiac output is reduced, the systemic circulation is impaired, and there may be slowing of the pulse.[57] The electrocardiograph abnormalities observed in such cases could be explained by the heart muscle being deprived of potassium.[58,59]

Anemia is a variable feature of the disease, some children are anemic when they first come under medical care. Whether this is a result of protein calorie malnutrition is often not clear because the clinical picture may be complicated by the presence of intestinal parasites, or a recent attack of malaria. Hemoglobin levels may be normal when the child is first examined but during the course of the disease, a severe anemia may develop. An enlarged liver may be found; this finding is not invariable however. A palpable enlargement of the liver is probably indicative of disordered liver function. This may have serious after effects which are described later in this chapter.

The variations of the clinical picture are very great. In order to facilitate the classification of the several types of cases, it has been suggested that the term *marasmus* should be used to describe a child that is less than 60 per cent of its weight for age and which has no edema. *Kwashiorkor* would be used to describe a child with a weight of 60–80 per cent less than that expected for its age and with edema. The term *underweight* would be applied to a child with a weight 60–80 per cent less than expected for its age which had no edema.[60]

The child with clinical signs is in an advanced stage of the disease. The *Iceberg Analogy* draws attention to the larger percentage of cases in early stages of protein calorie malnutrition which are clinically unrecognizable.

The severity of symptoms and signs brings an additional dimension which must be taken into consideration when evaluating the prevalence of kwashiorkor and marasmus. The level of *clinical recognition* will depend on the ability of medical and health personnel to diagnose the disease. In areas served by physicians who have had little experience of protein calorie malnutrition, many cases are missed because the child may not have the classical signs of kwashiorkor, such as red hair and dermatoses. However, with increasing experience, the physician becomes familiar with earlier signs of protein calorie malnutrition and more diagnoses may be expected. Cicely Williams has expressed the opinion that the epidemiology of malnutrition is the epidemiology of the physicians who can recognize the syndrome.[61]

Because of the failure to diagnose early cases, protein calorie malnutrition is very much under-reported. If this syndrome is to be controlled it will be necessary to develop techniques that will assist early diagnosis of cases. While an accurate estimate of the distribution and prevalence of protein calorie malnutrition cannot be made, it is important to realise that it can be found in many diverse situations and countries in widely differing stages of development. Kwashiorkor has been found, for example, in the Bronx in New York, in association with poverty.[62] It has also been reported in the affluent sections of industrialized countries who may be overprotective of their offspring.[63] Socio-cultural malnutrition is now being recognized in the urban "middle class" of developing countries.

The numbers of nutritional surveys which have been completed throughout the world is not considerable but in many of the developing areas of the world the surveys have demonstrated that two-thirds or more of the child population is experiencing less than adequate nutrition, and they are 10 to 40 per cent shorter or lighter in weight than their peers in the highly developed countries.

The prognosis of protein calorie malnutrition   The serious nature of kwashiorkor and marasmus may be judged from studies in Jordan.[64] These revealed that 28.1 per cent of cases admitted to hospital died, with death frequently occuring shortly after admission. Mortality was higher in boys than girls and it was greater in kwashiorkor than marasmus. These are however, the findings in one hospital and in one environment. It is probable that there may be considerable differences in these experiences in other regions of the world. In Jamaica, complete recovery has been noted in survivors of protein calorie malnutrition.[65] Short term observations on hospital patients showed that there was a good recovery over a period of eight weeks.[66] After that time, growth slowed down when the child reached its expected weight for height, a phenomenon that may be due to a decrease in the demand for food. In ideal hospital conditions where therapeutic diets provide ample calories and protein, high rates of growth could not be maintained that would allow the child to "catch up" with its height deficit and achieve its genetic potential. Under home conditions where the protein and calorie intake may be more restricted it may be expected that growth recovery would be even less.

Baganda children in Africa have been followed up after recovery. They were found to be smaller than normal children of the same age and their bone age was some two years less than their chronological age.[67] There is evidence that there may be long term effects on protein metabolism, for children who have been severely malnourished have been found to require more protein than other children raised on an ample diet.[68] The enzyme systems concerned with protein metabolism appear to have been permanently impaired by the period of malnutrition.

Malnutrition and mental development While much attention has focused on the clinical features and high mortality of malnutrition, the cost of survival has been neglected. The permanent physical effects of malnutrition are well known, but only recently has consideration been given to the possibility that intellectual development is affected by childhood malnutrition. In animals fed under optimal conditions of nutrition there is rapid physical growth which is accompanied by rapid motor development. Conversely, there is very good evidence that dietary restrictions interfere with physical growth. At times of maximal growth velocity, inadequacies in the diet will not allow tissues or organs to fulfil their genetic potential and the cells will be reduced in number; nutritional insults which are timed to take place after the period of maximal growth will affect the size of the cells (see page 401). While the brain is similarly affected some growth continues, but in doing so various chemical components accumulate in different amounts. This means that the final weight of a brain from a child who has experienced severe malnutrition may not differ materially from the normal; however, it may differ considerably in chemical composition.

There is also strong evidence that the enzyme systems of the body can be inadequately developed because of malnutrition. On theoretical grounds, it is therefore likely that the function of the brain is disturbed in malnutrition. This theory has supportive evidence from observations made during the experimental deprivation of animals; anatomical and functional changes were noted in the central nervous system. Dogs deprived of protein from the time of weaning onwards, will produce small offspring. If these puppies are raised on low protein diets they may develop an abnormal gait and they are liable to have convulsions; these may be fatal. If however, a normal diet is introduced, the gait returns to normal and the convulsions cease. This experiment indicates that dietary deprivation may affect the second generation; if humans are similarly affected, the dangers of impaired mental development are very real. Observations on deprived humans indicates that there may be damage to brain function. In the acute illness of kwashiorkor there are undoubted behavioral changes; these appear to revert to normal in recovery. The long term effects of protein calorie malnutrition are largely unknown. There is evidence of impaired mental performance that can persist;[69] other studies indicate possible recovery.[70]

The controversy over what are the effects of malnutrition on intellectual development will continue, for the methodology of testing for mental performance is not satisfactory yet. Some of the methods used to evaluate intelligence are not always suitable for use in different cultures so comparisons of studies may not be possible. The environment also has a considerable influence over the intellectual development of infants. Stimulation of the child, affection and reward, encouragement, and the opportunity to learn new skills, will all affect the rate of mental development. The environment of the deprived child suffering from kwashiorkor is itself, not conducive to mental development, nor to concentrating on the tests which are used to evaluate mental development.

Because of these inter-related influences it may not be possible to define the respective roles of the diet and the environment on mental development, but some general conclusions on the effects of malnutrition on mental development can be made. First, there is a loss of learning time. The child is less responsive to his environment while sick, and because of the chronic nature of protein calorie malnutrition several months of learning experience may be lost. Second, there would have been interference with psychomotor development. As learning depends on the successive development of the psychomotor system any delay in development must delay the learning process. It is possible that the final deficiency or disturbance in learning may be quite out of proportion to the actual duration of the interference.

Malnutrition is frequently associated with personality changes such as irritability or apathy, both of which may lead to the child being deprived of potential stimuli.

The timing of the episode of malnutrition may have some important aftereffects. Kwashiorkor is predominantly the disease of developing countries where weaning problems are the main etiological cause of malnutrition. The child is well protected by breast feeding during the critical time of brain growth. Subsequent protein calorie malnutrition, of the kwashiorkor type, therefore affects children mainly after multiplication of brain cells has ceased. Marasmus, on the other hand, is associated with improper formula feeding and it tends to affect infants in early life when the brain cells are still increasing in number. In view of the probability that early malnutrition retards brain growth, the abandonment of breast feeding in favor of inadequate formula feeding will expose an increasing number of children to the risk of inadequate brain growth. The present trend towards formula feeding will have even greater importance if further studies show that recovery of intellectual function does not take place in marasmus.

Dietary deprivation is not of course confined to the developing countries.

Both the full term *immature* baby and the *small for dates* infant that has been born *prematurely* have critical nutrient requirements because the rate of growth of their nervous system is at a peak. Such babies are found in priviledged societies where it is a customary practice to starve low birth weight babies for 48 hours after birth. This practice is potentially harmful and it may help to explain the large pool of mentally retarded children found in highly industrialized countries. It has been estimated, for example, that 3 per cent, or more than 4 million infants born each year in the USA never achieve the intellect of a 12 year old child.[71,72] Prematurity is considered one of the most significant causes of mental retardation, underlining the importance of achievement of adequate nutrition in the fetus and the newly born.

In later childhood, increasing attention is being paid to the disease state *Failure to Thrive* which is characterised by growth failure, secondary to maternal deprivation. The prevalence of this disease is not known, but is affects the affluent as well as the poor. This topic is discussed in further detail in Chapter 5. Too little is known of the permanent effects of this type of nutritional deprivation and its effects on intellectual performance later in life.

Cirrhosis of the liver

Like other tissues, the liver responds to injury by the typical pathological changes which are described as inflammation. As these subside, healing takes place which may involve the development of scar tissue. When the scarring becomes extreme, the morphology of the liver becomes seriously altered, consequently the circulatory and metabolic functions are impaired. The extensive scarring and subsequent formation of nodules is known as *cirrhosis* of the liver.

In addition to infections it is believed, but by no means proven, liver damage can be caused by nutritional factors including undernutrition, overnutrition, and the toxic effects of foods consumed either by accident or design.

Nutrient undernutrition   In protein calorie malnutrition the liver cells become infiltrated with fat; this may become so extreme the organ has the appearance of adipose tissue. In such circumstances many of the cells die and are replaced by collagen fibres, the basis of scar tissue.[73] The end result of this scarring is in doubt, but it seems the repair process may remain static or even disappear. Adult cirrhosis is so common in areas where kwashiorkor is rife it is very tempting to assume a cause and effect relationship, and conclude that the scarring in the infantile liver may progress and become the basis of a cirrhotic liver. It should not be overlooked however, that some other factors, or even a common factor may be responsible for childhood liver scarring and cirrhosis of the liver in adults.

Cirrhosis is a very common sequel to chronic alcoholism and it was formerly thought that the alcohol was having a direct toxic effect on the liver, killing cells which were then being replaced by scar tissue. It is now believed that the condition is the result of nutrient deficiency. In the chronic alcoholic the diet patterns are often poor and the protein intake is frequently low. Deficiency of amino acids in the diet can cause disturbances in the formation of choline which protects the liver from damage by alcohol. Alcoholic fatty degeneration of the liver may progress to cirrhosis and therefore be the sequel to two concurrent events: first, the ingestion of a toxic substance and second, failure to ingest a diet containing nutrients which could counteract the toxic affects of the alcohol.

Nutrient overnutrition Excessive intake of iron can lead to an excess of the pigment *hemosiderin* which is one of the forms in which iron is stored in the body. The accumulation of the hemosiderin can lead to cirrhosis. In those areas of the world where most of the cooking is done in iron cooking pots some of the iron may be incorporated chemically, with nutrients in the food. This can lead to very high iron intakes, even as much as 100 mg per day.[74]

In the more developed parts of the world, high intakes of iron have also been recorded in wine drinkers. It has been suggested that the combination of alcohol and excessive iron intake may combine to facilitate the absorption of the iron into the body.

A rare condition known as *hemochromatosis* which is usually assumed to be an inborn error of iron metabolism, also leads to cirrhosis. This condition is associated with overloading the tissues with iron and the development of cirrhosis and diabetes. The skin is so affected that the disease has been described as *Bronze Diabetes*. The disturbance in the control mechanism that limits the amount of iron absorbed may not be a genetic disorder but a nutritional disorder, for it has been found that some patients have a history of consuming enormous amounts of iron in medicinal tonics.

Toxic substances Many poisons, accidentally ingested, can cause liver damage and ultimate cirrhosis. Some of the organic poisons such as carbon tetrachloride, ethionine, alcohol, and phosphorus are well known. Fortunately ingestion of these poisons is relatively rare. There is evidence that other toxic substances found in food which are potentially cirrhotic, are being consumed inadvertently.

One of the most important is *aflatoxin*, a product of a mold that grows on groundnuts stored in a damp or humid, hot atmosphere.[75] Aflatoxin is a powerful liver poison; it has been recovered from the milk of cows who have been fed on contaminated groundnut meals, and traces have been recovered from peanut butter and maize.[76] It has not been shown that aflatoxin poisoning leads to cirrhosis of the liver in humans, but toxic substances resembling aflatoxin have been recovered from the livers of Indian children suffering from cirrhosis.[77]

Leaves and fruits are consumed as beverages or medicaments in many parts of the world. There is some concern that these may also contain substances which may have toxic effects on the liver. Childhood cirrhosis is common in Jamaica where "bush" teas prepared from species of *Senecio* and *Crotalaria* have been shown to produce a peculiar disease of the liver which may culminate in cirrhosis during childhood. *Cycads*, an ancient family of palm-like trees that represents an evolutionary step from fern to flowering plant, provide emergency food in many tropical countries, for they are able to resist drought and flood. In the preparation of edible starches from cycads, the toxic cycasin is usually washed out, but during the preparation of other foods and medicines a residue of the poison may remain and cause extensive liver damage. A considerable amount of information is now accumulating on naturally occuring toxic agents in food, and the reader is referred to a standard reference.[78]

Cirrhosis is usually been considered a problem of the tropical regions, its prevalence, like most diseases in these parts is conjectural; underreporting must be considerable. A child with severe cirrhosis will develop symptoms that make the parents seek medical attention, if it is available, but the disease may be symptomless for years. In these circumstances it is unlikely that the full extent of the problem will ever be known, and it may only be discovered accidentally. The clinical features of cirrhosis of the liver and its fatal termination are well known but there are other sequelae which are the subject of much speculation. That cirrhosis is prevalent in areas where kwashiorkor is common, is a well established fact, but it may also be significant that primary carcinoma of the liver is common where cirrhosis is found. In Johannesburg, South Africa, a well known focus of protein calorie malnutrition, 52 per cent of all cancers are liver cancers.[79]

It is not sufficient however, to assume that cirrhosis will remain a problem of the impoverished areas of the world and the "skid row" of the cities. It has recently come to light that cirrhosis is a major health problem in at least on large American city. In Baltimore, cirrhosis was the fifth leading cause of death in 1965 for persons aged 25 to 44 years; it was the third leading cause of death in white women and negro men, and the fourth leading cause of death in white men and negro women.[80] The increasing mortality is believed to be the result of an increase in alcohol consumption. If this is so, then this degree of mortality experience gives cause for alarm.

However, it is possible that other toxic substances are being ingested inadvertently; a final an improbable alternative explanation would be that the cirrhosis was the result of infantile malnutrition. The experience in Baltimore emphasise the importance of keeping surveillance of the health and nutritional status of populations and of remembering that the nutritional status of a community is dynamic and ever subject to change.

Favism

Favism is a disease associated with the ingestion of fresh, or uncooked, broad (or *fava*) bean, and characterized by hemolytic anemia. Susceptibility to the disease is believed to be hereditary.

Lathyrism

This is a common disease in the Middle East where certain legumes of the genus *lathyrus* are consumed. Two types of disease have been noted; these are believed to be caused by two distinct and separate toxic substances. One of them affects the nervous system causing paralyses and convulsions; the other appears to interfere with the normal maturation of connective tissue.

Cancrum oris

This disease is also called *noma* and is characterized by a well demarcated gangrene affecting the gums, oral mucosa, and soft tissue of the face. It may be accompanied by extensive destruction of the skin and underlying bone. In typical cases children are recovering from a febrile illness when they complain of a sore mouth. This leads to a reduced food intake and a reluctance even to drink. An early sign of *cancrum oris* may be seen as a gingivitis, frequently in the premolar region. The bone soon becomes exposed and the ulceration spreads rapidly. The external skin may then become involved and the ulceration and destructive process extends to affect all of the layers of the cheeks and lips.

The causation of noma is still the subject of debate, an "anatomical school" claims that the usually well defined areas of the gangrene may be due to the blocking of an artery by a thrombus. This theory cannot answer the clinical observations that there are areas also affected which are served by other arteries, and that the affected area may not always conform to the known distribution of a particular artery. Similar patches of gangrene are sometimes seen elsewhere on the body where they are referred to as *Tropical Ulcers*, which may be extremely extensive and destructive. The tropical ulcers are often associated with the profuse growth of the microorganism known as *Vincents Angina* which are also found in cancrum oris. It has been suggested that an underlying peridontal disease may be the focus of origin of cancrum oris. While the infective nature of the disease cannot be doubted, for it can be transmitted from one child to another, the role of nutrition and infection cannot be ignored, for the disease is usually found in infants and children who are poorly nourished. It is most prevalent in the age groups 2–5 years, a time when protein calorie malnutrition is also prevalent and it also found those countries where malnutrition is rife. It is also interesting to note that the disease was once common in Europe and North America but it has now virtually disappeared. In these countries not only has the general status of nutrition improved, but also standards of hygiene in general, and dental hygiene in particular, have improved.

Malabsorption

This syndrome is characterized by weight loss, anorexia, abdominal distension, muscle wasting, and the passage of bulky, offensive stools. In long standing cases ascites and signs of other nutrient deficiencies appear. These include rarifaction of bone, hemorrhages, anemia, peripheral neuritis, and skin manifestations of deficiencies of nicotinic acid, riboflavin, and vitamin A.

Malabsorption may be due to many factors which may be considered under three headings: factors related to impaired digestion, impaired absorption, and indeterminate causes.

Impaired digestion In chronic pancreatic disease or protein calorie malnutrition there may be a deficiency of the fat splitting enzyme lipase which will cause inadequate lipolysis. Blocking of the bile ducts or hepatitis will prevent bile from entering the intestines and will inhibit the emulsification and digestion of fat.

Impaired absorption Inadequacies in the absorptive surface of the intestinal mucosa may be the result of surgical removal of part of the intestine or it may be caused by part of the small intestine being "by-passed" by an anastomosis between two different part of the intestinal tract. An anastomosis between the stomach and the ileum for example, by-passes the jejunum and represents a considerable loss in absorptive function. The presence of roundworms may also reduce the effective area of the intestinal absorptive surface.

The length of time that the bowel contents are in contact with the intestinal surface is also important; if the diet contains much fibrous material, the bowel contents are moved on too rapidly for proper absorption to take place.

The intestinal mucosa may be lost or damaged in several conditions. It may be, for example, the result of an enteric or disenteric infection or a non-specific ulcerative colitis. These conditions are associated with rapid emptying of the bowel. In protein calorie malnutrition, atrophy of the mucosa aggravates the digestive disturbances caused by the lack of pancreatic enzymes. Biochemical dysfunction of the epithelial cells also inhibits the absorptive function of the mucosa.

The use of antibiotics may affect absorption in two ways. First, they may destroy bacteria, such as the *lactobacillus*, that normally creates a slightly acid medium. This favors the absorption of calcium. The antibiotic *neomycin* has a direct toxic effect on the cells of the mucosa.[81]

Obstruction of the lymphatics by tuberculosis, neoplastic disease, or back pressure from congestive heart disease, will also interfere with the absorption of lipids transported via the lacteals.

Indeterminate causes   These include diseases caused by a deficiency of sugar splitting enzymes. For example, lactase deficiency may be inherited or it may be secondary to a milk protein allergy. In the absence of this enzyme the milk sugar lactose cannot be absorbed, a problem of some importance when milk forms the basis of supplementary feeding programs.

The intestinal mucosa may also be sensitive to wheat gluten; this is the underlying problem in celiac disease. In addition to these conditions steatorrhea of unknown origins have been described.

Because of the multiple causation of the malabsorption syndrome the disease is not rare. As a specific disease it is not a public health problem, but it is possible that mild degrees of malabsorption play a role in the development of protein calorie malnutrition. For example, attacks of infective diarrhea may damage the mucosal cells and impair their absorptive capacity.

Nutrition problems in the industrialized society

The majority of the diseases mentioned so far, have been identified with impoverishment or lack of social, cultural, or economic development. Although advances in development may reduce the prevalence of some health problems there is evidence that they are being replaced by a new pattern of diseases. Several of them are related to nutrition. The victims include people who are neither rich nor poor. They form the majority of the population of highly industrialized countries and the minority in developing countries. The evolution of the middle class is a phenomenon of industrialization. The apparent economic advantages of the city attracts the subsistence-level rural dweller. A life supported by the land is replaced by one dominated by cash and the cost of food and material goods. Food grown and prepared in the home is replaced by food purchased in the market and consumed in restaurants, eating houses, or canteens. In addition to changes in eating habits, psychological and environmental stresses increase. The availability and convenience of automobiles, household appliances, and labor saving devices are reducing energy expenditure to such a degree that overweight is becoming a serious health problem. To overcome this, large sections of the population are practising weight control by restricting their calorie intake. The level of activity is so low however, that in order to avoid weight gain, extreme calorie restriction is necessary. At such low levels of intake it is difficult to meet the requirements for protein and other nutrients. The longterm effects of prolonged weight control have yet to be evaluated.

Nutritional problems in industrialized societies start in infancy. Infant feeding becomes a problem when the mother is under pressure to return to work soon after delivery of her baby. Formula feeding with cows milk is economical and convenient. Weight gain is the accepted measure of growth and hence the effectiveness of the feeding regime. However, weight gain alone is not a true index of growth and a heavy baby may not be growing at a satisfactory rate. Furthermore, it is not known whether a heavy baby is a healthier baby than one of normal weight. Rapid growth in infancy may accelerate the aging process for there is evidence that some "vital molecules" can only be produced during early life.[82] The total endowment of these molecules, which is achieved at the end of the growing period, has to last throughout life. It is possible therefore, that high intakes of food may exhaust them at a faster rate than normal. As they are irreplacable, premature aging may be the consequence. The converse observation that longevity in laboratory animals is promoted by restrictions in nutrient intake supports this theory.

Although a cause and effect relationship has not been established, the widespread use of formula feeding and convenience foods has been accompanied by an increase in certain childhood diseases such as obesity, underweight, anemia, tetany, and milk allergies (see page 116). The legacy of overweight may be carried through childhood into adult life, taking with it the added risks of joint disease, metabolic disturbances such as diabetes, and renal and cardiovascular disease.

Adolescence is frequently a time when a fear of becoming "fat" is very pronounced in the non-obese. Parents, peers, and cosmetic advertising extoll the virtue of slimness and there may even be harsh campaigns against even mild cases of "plumpness".[83] It is not surprising therefore, that chronic malnutrition due to an abnormal pre-occupation with weight is common.

In adult life, stress in highly developed countries influences eating habits. More people are "eating on the move", less time is spent on the preparation and consumption of foods in the home. Convenience foods, whose nutritive value *as consumed* is largely unknown, are being used to an increasing degree. It is still too early to decide whether the consumption of foods containing oxidants, preservatives, antibiotics, pesticide residues, and artificial colorings is harmful. The occasional alarms sounded in the past in relation to agene, artificial sweeteners, (see page 491) and toxins in peanuts, is a reminder that science is fallible.

Degenerative heart disease is the most frequent cause of death in North America, most of Europe, and among the more prosperous segments of populations in many other parts of the world. The increasing dominance of these conditions cannot be explained solely as the result of changes in other causes of mortality, or of age structure of the population. There is little doubt that the mode of life is involved in the etiology of heart disease and from epidemiological studies, the stress of the environment and working conditions, lack of physical exercise, economic status, and nutrition all appear to play some part. The role of nutrition in cardiovascular disease is discussed in detail in Chapter 3. For the present it should be noted that although there is a correlation between diet and cardiovascular disease, it has not yet been shown that any article of diet or nutrient is responsible for the disease state.

Diabetes

Two types of diabetes are recognized.

Diabetes insipidus This disease is caused by infection, tumor, trauma, or congenital disorder that disturbs pituitary function and the secretion of antidiuretic hormone. Normally, the antidiuretic hormone controls the absorption of water from the renal tubule. When it is secreted in inadequate amounts, large quantities of urine are passed which is the main feature of Diabetes insipidus.

Diabetes mellitus This is characterized by multiple disturbances in the metabolic processes of the body. These are directly attributable to an insufficiency in supply of insulin secreted by the *beta* cells of the *Islets of Langerhans* of the pancreas. It is rare in infancy, uncommon in childhood, and most common in adults over 50 years of age. The disease has various stages, the first being characterized by a diminished glucose tolerance, the second by a chemical diabetes. In both stages blood and urine are abnormal under conditions of stress. The stress may by physiological, such as in pregnancy or infection, or artificially induced, as in the glucose tolerance test. Clinical diabetes is the third stage where there are characteristic symptoms such as increased thirst, blurred vision, skin infection, loss of weight, polyuria, and ketosis. This progresses into a chronic diabetic state distinguished by advanced changes in the vessels of the systemic arterial system including the kidney and the retina of the eye. Most cases are genetic in origin but a few may be attributed to pancreatic disease or to disturbances in the endocrine function of the pituitary and adrenal glands. The disease may have an acute onset or it may be more chronic and characterized by vascular disease. It is not known if the primary problem is an insulin inefficiency that is followed by vascular disturbances or alternatively, whether the acute and chronic manifestations of diabetes have a common cause. The current view is that the predisposition to diabetes is inherited and the hyperglycemia occurs when the organism is faced with some extraneous stimuli. Although pregnancy seems to be one stimulus; most other stimuli are undetermined. There is evidence that some environmental or nutritional influences may be involved. It is known, for example, that diabetes in identical twins may occur at different times of life. The prevalence of diabetes also differs in the same ethnic group living in different areas.

Diabetes is frequently found in the obese. It is suggested that man may have been designed originally to convert the small amount of carbohydrate available in prehistoric times into stored fat. Modern agriculture produces large amounts of carbohydrate that are consumed in excess of requirements, consequently excess fat is formed. Perhaps in the former days of continual near-starvation man was protected from diabetes. It has been shown that populations moving from a low calorie intake to a high calorie intake experience an increase in weight, diabetes, and cardiovascular disease. Further support for a relationship between nutrition and diabetes is given by observations on morbidity in countries where fat intakes are high. Diabetes and atherosclerosis are common in populations consuming large quantities of fat. It has also been noted that blood sugar levels are elevated in atherosclerotic populations. There is however no evidence that high intakes of fat cause either diabetes or atherosclerosis. The complexity of the relationships between nutritional status and diabetes is further demonstrated by the fact that starvation of obese diabetics can lead to a restoration of normal glucose tolerance even before much weight is lost.

The extent of diabetes is not known; surveys carried out in many countries have used different criteria for establishing the prevalence of diabetes. Some investigators have based their findings on the presence of sugar in the urine, and others have used glucose tolerance as the screening test. Even when similar tests have been applied, their methodologies have differed so that the result obtained in one survey may not be compared with others, even within the same country. In Britain, the prevalence of diabetes is estimated to be between approximately 2 per cent and 12 per cent of the population. High prevalence rates are quoted for Melanesians living in Northern Australia, North American Indians and the inhabitants of Malta. Very low rates are quoted for Yemenite and Kurdish Jews migrating to Israel, Icelanders and Alaskan Eskimos.

The diseases which are related to nutrition in the affluent society may also be affecting other less privileged groups, but they may not be recognized because they may be succumbing to other diseases at an earlier, or they may not have the health services to detect them.

The survival of man in the affluent society depends on his ability to tolerate the numerous stresses of overcrowding, dissent, economic competition, and the constant struggle to maintain social status. The struggle may be responsible for high mortality rates from cardiovascular disease, but there are sections of the population that combat stress by consuming alcohol. The increasing consumption of alcohol has now created a public health problem in many industrialized countries and may be reflected in the increase in cirrhosis of the liver. Finally, it must be remembered that despite the increasing risks of mortality in middle age, more and more people are surviving these years and contributing to an increasing population of aged persons. Malabsorption and disturbances of calcium metabolism are particular afflictions of the aged; in addition, many old people are continually on the verge of nutrient deficiency because the food sources which supply an adequate and balanced diet are not always available.

The lack of availability may be related to economic status since pensions, and the value of savings, rarely keep pace with price inflation and the cost of living. With increasing urbanization, the neighborhood grocery and food store is disappearing. The elderly may not be sufficiently mobile because of physical handicapping, or because of remoteness of supermarkets, to purchase a proper diet. Sometimes it is difficult for the elderly to cook their own food and many of them have difficulty in masticating fibrous material such as meat and chicken. In these circumstances it is to be expected that anemia, vitamin deficiencies, and protein depletion are common in the "senior citizen".

References

1. A report of the President's Science Advisory Committee. *The World Food Problem*, **2**, p. 6. U. S. Government Printing Office, Washington, D. C., 1967.
2. *Demographic Yearbook*, p. 115, United Nations, New York 1969.
3. Frederiksen, H. "Feedbacks in Economic and Demographic Transition." *Science*, **166**: 837, 1969.
4. Stunkard, A. J. "Environment and Obesity: Recent Advances in Our Understanding of Regulation of Food Intake in Man." *Fed. Proc.* **27**: 1367, 1968.
5. Hirsh, J., Knittle, J. L., Salans, L. B. "Cell Lipid Content and Cell Number in Obese and Non-obese Human Adipose Tissue." *J. Clin. Invest.* **45**: 1023, 1966.
6. Canning, H., Mayer, J. "Obesity—Its Possible Effect on College Acceptance." *New Eng. Jour. Med.* **275**: 1172, 1966.
7. Rauh, J. L., Schumsky, D. A., "Relative Accuracy of Visual Assessment of Juvenile Obesity." *J. Amer. Diet. Ass.* **55**: 459, 1969.
8. Spargo, J. A., Heald, F., Peckos, P. S. "Adolescent Obesity." *Nutrition Today*, Vol. **1**, Number 4, p. 2, 1966.
9. Wilson, R. H. L., Wilson, N. L. "Obesity and Respiratory Stress." *J. Amer. Diet. Ass.* **55**: 465, 1969.
10. Dale, A. E., Lowenburg, M. "Consumption of Vitamin D in Fortified and Natural Foods and in Vitamin Preparations." *J. Pediat.* **70**: 952, 1967.
11. Friedman, W. F., Mills, L. F. "The Relationship Between Vitamin D and the Craniofacial and Dental Anomalies of the Supravalvular Aortic Stenosis Syndrome." *Pediatrics* **43**: 12, 1969.
12. Pierce, W. F. "Hypervitaminosis A." *Illinois Med. J.* **122**: 591, 1962.
13. Di Benedetto, R. J. "Chronic Hypervitaminosis A in an Adult." *J. Amer. Diet. Ass.* **201**: 700, 1967.
14. McLaren, D. S. "Present Knowledge of the Role of Vitamin A in Health and Disease." *Trans. Roy. Soc. Trop. Med. Hyg.* **60**: 441, 1966.
15. Goethe, H., Rinck, G., Gudmundsson, G. "Sickness in German Deep Sea Fishing Industry with Reference to Condition of Dental Bite." *Arch. Gewerpathol. Gewerbehyg.* **17**: 57, 1959.
16. Prior, I. A. M., Evans, J. G., Harvey, H. P. B., Davidson, F., Lindsey, M. "Sodium Intake and Blood Pressure in Two Polynesian Populations." *New Eng. J. Med.* **279**: 515, 1968.
17. Fomon, S. J., Thomas, L. N., Filer, L. J. "Acceptance of Unsalted Strained Foods by Normal Infants." *J. Pediat.* **76**: 243, 1970.
18. Dahl, L. K. "Salt in Processed Baby Foods." *Amer. J. Clin. Nutr.* **21**: 787, 1968.
19. Keys, A., Brozek, J., Henschel, A., Mickelsen, O., Taylor, H. L. *The Biology of Human Starvation*, Vol. **2**, p. 1248, Minneapolis: University of Minnesota Press, 1950.
20. von Muralt, A. Protein Calorie Malnutrition Viewed as a Challenge to Homeostasis. In *Protein Calorie Malnutrition*, p. 3. Ed. von Muralt, A. New York: Springer-Verlag, 1969.
21. Davidson, S., Passmore, R. *Human Nutrition and Dietetics*. Third Ed. p. 354. Baltimore: Williams and Wilkins, 1966.
22. Cravioto, J., DeLicardie, E. R., Birch, H. G. "Nutrition, Growth and Neurointegrative Development. An Experimental and Ecologic Study." *Pediat.* (Supplement) **38**: 319, 1966.

23. Underwood, B. A., Siegel, H., Weisell, R. C., Dolinski, M. "Liver Stores of Vitamin A in a Normal Population Dying Suddenly or Rapidly from Unnatural Causes in New York City." *Amer. J. Clin. Nutr.* **23:** 1037, 1970.

24. Latham, M. C. "Nutritional Aetiology of a Neuropathy Found in Tanganyika." *Brit. J. Nutr.* **18:** 129, 1964.

25. Haddock, D. R. W., Ebrahim, G. J., Kapur, B. B. "Atoxic Neurological Syndrome Found in Tanganyika." *Brit. Med. J.* Part 2, p. 1442, 1962.

26. Haddock, D. R. W. "Neurological Signs in African Patients Without Overt Neurological Disease." *E. Afr. Med. J.* **40:** 601, 1963.

27. Hanafy, M. M., Konbar, A. A., Zeitoun, M. M., Hassan, A. I. "Gastric and Pancreatic Secretions in Pellagra in Egyptian Children." *J. Trop. Med. Hyg.* **71:** 125, 1968.

28. Terris, M. *Goldberger on Pellagra.* Louisiana Press, 1963.

29. Gopalan, C. "Possible Role for Dietary Leucine in the Pathogenesis of Pellagra." *The Lancet,* **1:** 197, 1969.

30. Henderson, J. G., Strachan, R. W., Beck, J. S., Dawson, A. A. "The Antigastric Antibody Test as a Screening Procedure for Vitamin B_{12} Deficiency in Psychiatric Practice." *The Lancet* **2:** 809, 1966.

31. Hood, J., Hodges, R. E. "Ocular Lesions in Scurvy." *Amer. J. Clin Nutr.* **22:** 559, 1969.

32. Schaefer, A. Report to the Senate Select Committee on Nutrition and Human Needs, April 1970.

33. LeBovit, C. "U. S. Diets and Enrichment." *J. Agr. Food Chem.* **16:** 153, 1968.

34. Pelletier, O. "Vitamin C Status of Cigarette Smokers and Nonsmokers." *Amer. J. Clin. Nutr.* **23:** 520, 1970.

35, Smith, R. W., Rizek, J., Frame, B. "Determinants of Serum Anti-Rachitic Activity." Special Reference to involutional osteoporosis *Amer. J. Clin. Nutr.* **14:** 98, 1964.

36. "Rickets in Greece." *Nutr. Rev.* **27:** 51, 1969.

37. *Nutritional Anemias.* Technical Report Series No. 405, p. 9. World Health Organization, Geneva, 1968.

38. Myers, A. M., Saunders, C. R. G., Chalmers, D. G. "The Haemoglobin Level of Fit Elderly People." *The Lancet* **2:** 261, 1968.

39. Jacobs, A., Greenman, D. A. "Availability of Food Iron." *Brit. Med. J.* **1:** 673, 1969.

40. Layrisse, M., Martinez, C., Roche, M. "Effect of the Interaction of Various Foods on Iron Absorption. "*Amer. J. Clin Nutr.* **21:** 1175, 1968.

41. Apte, S. V., Iyengar, L. "Absorption of Dietary Iron in Pregnancy." *Amer. J. Clin. Nutr.* **23:** 73, 1970.

42. Gerrard, J. W., Lubos, M. C., Hardy, L. W., Holmlund, B. A., Webster, D. "Milk Allergy. Clinical Picture and Familial Incidence." *Canad. Med. Ass.* J. **97:** 780, 1967.

43. Adams, E. B. "Anemia Associated with Kwashiorkor." *Amer. J. Clin. Nutr.* **22:** 1634, 1969.

44. *Nutritional Anemias.* Technical Report Series No. 405, p. 18. World Health Organization, Geneva, 1968.

45. Sprinz, H., Sribhibhadh, R., Gangarosa, E. J., Benyajati, C., Kundel, D., Halstead, S. "Biopsy of Small Bowel of Thai People. With special reference to recovery from Asiatic cholera and to an intestinal malabsorption syndrome." *Amer. J. Clin. Path.* **38:** 43, 1962.

46. Stanbury, J. B., Querido, A. "Genetic and Environmental Factors in Cretinism: A Classification." *J. Clin. Endocr.* **16:** 1522, 1956.

47. Clements, F. W. Personal Communication.
48. Prasad, A. S., Schulert, A. R., Miale, A., Farid, Z., Sandstead, H. H. "Zinc and Iron Deficiencies in Male Subjects with Dwarfism and Hypogonadism but Without Ancylostomiasis, Schistosomiasis or Severe Anemia." *Amer. J. Clin. Nutr.* **12**: 437, 1963.
49. Oberleas, D., Prasad, A. S. "Adequacy of Trace Minerals in Bovine Milk for Human Consumption." *Amer. J. Clin. Nutr.* **22**: 196, 1969.
50. Oberleas, D., Prasad, A. S. "Growth as Affected by Zinc and Protein Nutrition." *Amer. J. Clin. Nutr.* **22**: 1304, 1969.
51. Williams, C. D. "Nutritional Disease of Childhood Associated with Maize Diets." *Arch. Dis. Childh.* **8**: 423, 1933.
52. Dally, A., *Cicely: The Story of a Doctor.* London: Victor Gollancz, 1968.
53. Balmer, S., Howells, G., Wharton, B. "The Acute Encephalopathy of Kwashiorkor." *Develop. Med. Child Neurol.* **10**: 766, 1968.
54. James, W. P. T. "Intestinal Absorption in Protein Calorie Malnutrition." *The Lancet* **1**: 333, 1968.
55. Alleyne, G. A. O., Halliday, D., Waterlow, J. C., Nichols, B. L. "Chemical Composition of Organs of Children Who Died From Malnutrition." *Brit. J. Nutr.* **23**: 783, 1969.
56. Cadell, J. L. "Studies in Protein Calorie Malnutrition." *New Eng. J. Med.* **276**: 535, 1967.
57. Alleyne, G. A. O. "Cardiac Function in Severely Malnourished Jamaican Children." *Clin. Sci.* **30**: 553, 1966.
58. Horsfall, P. A. L., Waldmann, E. "Electrocardiographic Changes in Kwashiorkor and Marasmus." *Cent. Afr. J. Med.* **14**: 170, 1968.
59. Khalil, M., El Khateeb, S., Kassem, S., Ellozy, M., Gabr, Y., Elwaseef, A. "Electrocardiographic Studies in Kwashiorkor." *J. Trop. Med. Hyg.* **72**: 291, 1969.
60. "Classification of Infantile Malnutrition." *The Lancet* **2**: 302, 1970.
61. Williams, C. D. Malnutrition and Mortality in the Pre-School Child. In *Pre-school Child Malnutrition.* p. 3, Publication 1282. National Academy of Sciences. Washington, D. C. 1966.
62. Taitz, L. S., Finberg, L. "Kwashiorkor in the Bronx." *Amer. J. Dis. Child.* **112**: 76, 1966.
63. Shappley, B. G., Williams, T. E., McLemore, B., Donaldson, M. H. "Kwashiorkor with Psychologic Etiology." *Clin. Ped.* **8**: 709, 1969.
64. McLaren, D. S., Shirajian, E., Loshkajian, H., Shadarevian, S. "Short-term Prognosis in Protein-Calorie Malnutrition." *Amer. J. Clin. Nutr.* **22**: 863, 1969.
65. Garrow, J. S., Pike, M. C. "The Long Term Prognosis of Severe Infantile Malnutrition." *The Lancet* **1**: 1, 1967.
66. Ashworth, A. "Growth Rates in Children Recovering from Protein Calorie Malnutrition." *Brit. J. Nutr.* **23**: 835, 1969.
67. Krueger, R. H. "Some Long Term Effects of Severe Malnutrition in Early Life." *The Lancet* **2**: 514, 1969.
68. Chow, B. F., Blackwell, R. R., Blackwell, B., Hou, T. Y., Anilane, J. J., Sherwin, R. W. "Maternal Nutrition and Metabolism of the Offspring, Studies in Rats and Man." *Amer. J. Public Health* **58**: 668, 1968.
69. Champakan, S., Srikantia, S. G., Gopalan, C. "Kwashiorkor and Mental Development." *Amer. J. Clin. Nutr.* **21**: 844, 1968.

70. Cravioto, J., Robles, B. "Evaluation of Adaptive and Motor Behaviour During Rehabilitation from Kwashiorkor." *Amer. J. Orthopsychiat.* **35:** 449, 1965.
71. Clifford, S. H. "High Risk Pregnancy." *New Eng. J. Med.* **271:** 243, 1964.
72. Masland, R. L., Sarason, S. B., Gladwin, T. *Mental Subnormality: Biological, Psychological and Cultural Factors*, p. 3. New York: Basic Books, 1958.
73. Trowell, H. C., Davies, J. N. P., Dean, R. F. A. *Kwashiorkor in Children* p. 136. London: Arnold, 1954.
74. Davidson, S., Passmore, R. *Human Nutrition and Dietetics.* 3rd. Ed. p. 166. Baltimore: Williams and Wilkins, 1966.
75. Allcroft, R., Carnaghan, R. B. A., Sargeant, K., O'Kelly, J. "A Toxic Factor in Brazilian Groundnut Meal." *Vet. Rec.* **73:** 428, 1961.
76. Miller, J. A. Tumorigenic and Carcinogenic Natural Products. In *Toxicants Occuring Naturally in Food*, p. 28. Publication 1354. National Academy of Sciences, Washington, D. C. 1966.
77. Yadgiri, B., Reddy, V., Tulpule, P. G., Srikantia, S. G., Gopalan, C. "Aflatoxin and Indian Childhood Cirrhosis." *Amer. J. Clin. Nutr.* **23:** 94, 1970.
78. *Toxicants Occuring Naturally in Food.* Publication 1534. National Academy of Sciences. Washington, D. C. 1966.
79. Boyd, W. *Textbook of Pathology*, p. 873, 8th Ed. Lea and Febiger, 1970.
80. Kuller, L. H., Kramer, K., Fisher, R. "Changing Trends in Cirrhosis and Fatty Liver Mortality." *Amer. J. Public Health* **59:** 1124, 1969.
81. "Malabsorption Due to Neomycin." *Nutr. Rev.* **27:** 102, 1969.
82. Strehler, B. L. "Molecular Biology of Aging." *Die Naturwissenschaften* **56:** 57, 1969.
83. Bruch, H. "Psychosomatic Aspects of Malnutrition During Adolescence." *Postgrad. Med.* **47:** 98, No. 5, 1970.

CHAPTER 2

The Ecology and Etiology of Malnutrition

The ecology of malnutrition

In this chapter, it will be assumed that *ecology* is concerned with the relationships between the environment and the organism, (in this case, the community). *Etiology* will be assumed to be the study of the causation of malnutrition in individuals.

The termination of all nutritional processes is the metabolic machine of the cell. For proper and efficient metabolism, nutrients of precisely the right quality, and in the correct quantities, must be presented to the cell at the most appropriate time. If these demands are not met, unused or partly used nutrients in the form of metabolites can accumulate and cause harm. A chain of events must be completed in an orderly fashion if the cell is to function properly; each stage in the chain is dependent on a previous event.

If nutrients are to be utilized in the cell, they must be transported there. The presence of nutrients for transport assumes they have been freed from the food by the digestive process and absorbed efficiently into the body. The presence of nutrients in the food presupposes there has been an adequate and proper intake of food. The proper intake of food, in turn, is dependent on the availability of foods as sources of nutrients.

Food availability

The land and the people   The availability of food depends first on the quantity and quality of land and its use, and second on the quantity and the characteristics of the population. Figure 6 shows some of the interrelationships of factors which influence the intake of food. It can be seen, for example, that the greater the population the more pressure there will be on the land; if productivity per unit area is not increased then the *per capita* availability of food must diminish.

Absolute numbers alone do not count, for the character of the population largely determines what food is available and what will be consumed.

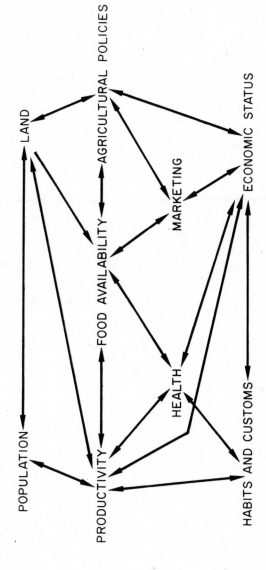

Figure 6   The inter-relationship of factors influencing the intake of food

A population composed mainly of young children has different demands in comparison to a population whose numbers are more evenly distributed throughout the various age groups. The quality of the land must be taken into consideration also, for the geography, geology, topography and climate all influence productivity. Many parts of the world, such as the polar areas, the subarctic tundra, the deserts and semi-deserts are unproductive. Other areas apparently ideal for agricultural use may be supporting its populations in a most precarious fashion because the topography promotes erosion, or because it is subject to sea water tidal refluxes which build up salinity in the soil. The rainfall may be adequate when evaluated on an annual basis, but it may be inequitably distributed throughout the year because of local features of geography. If the land does not drain properly, an exceptionally heavy rainfall may precipitate flooding or it may convert good agricultural land into a swamp. The presence of favorable or unfavorable topographical or climatic features alone does not determine the potential productivity of the area. The outcome is largely dependent on the inhabitants of the area and their ability to adapt.

Adaptation The Kalahari bushmen have learned how to exploit natural water supplies for the preservation of their own life.[1] Despite a hand to mouth existence, and limited food resources, the Kung bushmen have adapted to their environment. They have succeeded in developing a way of life that seems complex and wasteful of energy but it ensures their survival. The bushmen are highly selective in their food habits, and their hunting and collection of food seem individualized. Nevertheless they have learned to pool their resources and families succeed in obtaining a wide variety of foods comprising a nutritionally acceptable diet.[2]

Some cultures have exploited naturally occurring accidents of nature. The lakes forming the Tonle Sap area of Cambodia are inundated annually by back pressure from the Mekong river when it becomes swollen with monsoon rains. The inundation drives fish into areas that are normally forest or farmland. The flood provides an enormous reserve of fish that the Cambodians have learned to harvest and which is now vital to their well being.[3] Factors, other than climate may force a population to adapt, for example warfare and civil strife are important motivators.

The *Matengo* tribe of southwest Tanzania foiled the genocidal raids of the *Ngoni* by fleeing to the highlands where they developed an ingenious pit system of agriculture that allowed the successful cultivation of steep slopes.[4,5] The pits protect the hills from erosion and produce high yields of crops. The availability of foods to the *Matengo* would be drastically

6*

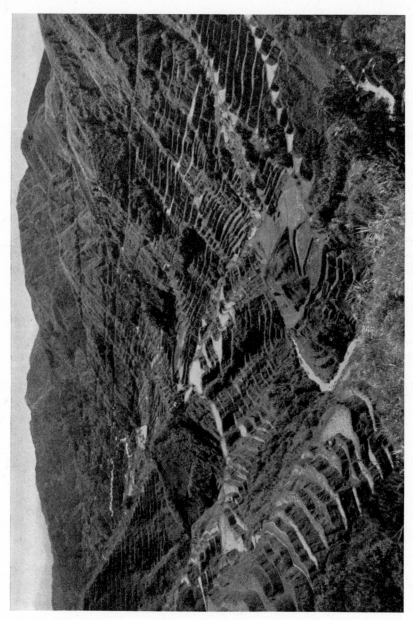

Plate 16   Rice terraces in Ifugao in Mountain Province, Luzon, Phillipines (FAO photograph by P. A. Pittet)

reduced if, for any reason, this type of agriculture was changed. A similar adaptation by the *Ifugao* tribesmen of the Philippines in response to population pressures has led to the use of terraces in the rice fields.

In other societies, where adaptation for survival is not so critical other clearly defined and interrelated factors greatly influence the existing security of living conditions. These factors determine whether development, including the improvement of food supplies and nutritional status, will take place.[6]

Under-utilization of land and labor   In countries with surplus land, much may remain unutilized because of limitations imposed by primitive farming techniques or by natural hazards such as the *tsetse* fly, or inadequate rainfall. Although accurate figures are not available, about 27 per cent of Africa (excluding South Africa) is potentially usable for agriculture. This means that there are, on average, about 20 acres of land per person capable of producing food. The average area in use is only about eight acres.

Under-utilization of labor   Seasonal patterns of rainfall limit the productive agriculture in many parts of Africa to 120 days per year. The labor employed during this time is characterized by low levels of productivity. The lure of higher incomes attracts potential agricultural labor to rapidly growing urban centers. Here they add to the high rates of unemployment that already adversely affect agricultural, and industrial development.

The majority of African farmers cultivate small holdings and they have limited technical skills. Their use of purchased implements and aids to cultivate is limited and they are content, for the most part, to use family labor. Although output tends to increase with the amount of labor committed, prod uctivity still remains low in many developing countries. The United States has only about six to seven per cent of its labor force in agriculture but it produces large surpluses. Japan has only about 22 per cent of its labor force in agriculture and is barely able to feed itself. Despite the high percentage of effort devoted to agriculture, industrialization is nevertheless developing and throwing an additional strain on the primary producer.

Migration of labor   The development of industrialization in predominantly agricultural countries attracts workers from the rural areas, with the result that agriculturally productive areas are frequently deprived of essential farm workers. Migration for work in these circumstances may be undesirable. In other situations, for example when the rains have failed, it may be a life saving measure. Migration for work on a permanent or temporary basis, is perhaps an immediate solution to impoverishment, but dependence on labor as a saleable commodity can be catastrophic if the labor market situation deteriorates. In Songea, it was shown that the effect of migration was felt by the women who were left to complete heavy work tasks which are normally the responsibility of the men; treefelling and other essential preludes to cultivating new land was beyond their physical capabilities.

Influence of energy expenditure in relation to work   Increasing industrialization in urban areas frequently results in a wide geographical separation of home and work. Public transport systems do not always develop at the same pace so workers may be required to walk or cycle several miles from their homes to their place of work. In a study in Dar es Salaam in Tanzania, out of a total factory work force of 47, 39 of the employees walked to work, 5 cycled and only 3 used a bus service. Of the 39 who walked, 9 of them walked over 8 miles each, travelling to and from work.[7] This extra energy expenditure may tip a marginal calorie balance to the negative side.

Farmers are usually required to carry their produce to market. In the simplest of societies this is carried by hand, on the shoulders or back, or on the head. With increasing development, hand carts may be used to facilitate this task. If the terrain is suitable, and if endemic animal diseases permit them, pack animals may be used to replace the human labor. For the farmer who is forced to use his own muscle power, any device that economizes in energy expenditure may be critical in preserving positive energy balances. The introduction of the pneumatic tire and ball-bearings as part of an industrializing process may be an important factor in conserving energy expenditure and preventing malnutrition. A study of ergonomics may be therefore an essential part of a study of the ecology of malnutrition.

Ethnic, religious, cultural and family customs and habits may have a profound influence on productivity and the availability of food to an individual or a population. Food availability is related to economic status, this in turn is related to customs and habits and productivity; some examples of these interrelationships will be examined.

Food habits   One of the characteristics of man is his remarkable attitude, belief and superstition regarding food.

The earliest forerunners of *homo sapiens* spent most of their life foraging for food, resting between the foraging expeditions, and moving from one food source to another. They were probably vegetarian at this stage but later they acquired hunting skills, and started to consume small animals. Feeding would be indiscriminate and the pattern of intake would depend on the food supplies, the environment and climate, tools, hunting methods and the ability for men to make collective efforts. With the discovery of fire and the acquisition of greater skills including cultivation of crops more choices of food would become available. The choice of food would increase as families and groups shared their resources.

Patterns of consumption would emerge, eventually depending not only on taste but also on the availability of food and fuel, and the ability of the groups to hunt and cultivate. Man has no physiological or inborn urge to maintain proper nutrition and he relies on taste to determine his food choices. Taste is variable however and cannot be relied on to ensure that the diet will meet the nutrient requirements. Food preferences seem inexplicable but the fact that the name of the staple may be the local word for food indicates how important is the choice of the staple to the community.

Factors such a floods, droughts and epidemics influence the supplies of preferred food; these events might be expected to have great importance and become tied to religious beliefs. A catastrophe like a flood might coincide with the trial of a new food. If the latter causes a gastric upset it might be linked to the catastrophe and become *taboo*. Thereafter it might become part of the folklore of local food beliefs. The origins of taboos are not understood. With no instinct guiding food choices, and in the presence of strong feelings towards food, it is to be expected that food habits would be susceptible to every kind of superstition, wrong inference, and inexplicable prejudice.

Some habits are related to religious beliefs and are very widespread, crossing both cultural and international boundaries. Fasting of a prolonged nature is practised by the majority of the 400 million Moslems throughout the world, and by 12–14 million Ethiopians who observe the fasts of the *Ethiopian Orthodox Church*.[8] In the 28 day annual Moslem fast of *Ramadhan*, there is a total abstension from food and liquids between sunrise and sunset. In the strictest sects of this religion, even the saliva must not be swallowed. Pregnant and lactating women are exempt, but their normal life is inevitably disrupted by the need to prepare food late into the night. When the religion is practised in northern climates where the days are long, there is considerable discomfort and fatigue. The fast undoubtedly throws additional stress on the manual worker.

The *Ethiopian Orthodox* fast is potentially much more dangerous to health. Lay people are required to fast on 110 to 150 occasions each year; for the devout there are approximately 220 fasting days to be observed. On fasting days, fish, but no other animal foods, may be consumed and the main source of food is vegetable in origin. Sickness is no reason for exemption, but sometimes pregnant and lactating women are allowed to eat animal foods. They are not however, permitted to eat beans, a good source of protein in the predominantly vegetable diet of the Ethiopians. Children under the age of eight are completely exempt from the fasting rules but over that age they may be compelled to conform to customs. Unlike adults, children do not have to wait until noon time of the day following the fast, before normal eating can be resumed. During fast days, and over fasting periods the food markets are inactive. This often means that those persons exempt are unable to purchase animal foods so they may have to subsist on vegetables.

While religious fasts are international in extent, local habits based on superstition and beliefs may limit the choice of food and the scope of the diet. In addition to these local influences on diet there are other habits which are very personal. These habits may affect an individual, or small groups of individuals, and may be more related to the emotion of craving.

Habits based on superstition or beliefs may be protective to the society and developed through simple logic. For example, many East African tribes insist that the male head of the household has first choice of the food, served in a communal bowl or dish. The father, therefore has the best opportunity to satisfy his appetite. He is also at liberty to take the most tasty portions of the meal; this may be the most nutritious such as muscle meat or offal. The eldest son has the next choice and he is followed by other sons and daughters. The last to take a share is the mother who may be hand-feeding a small child; she may be lactating or pregnant and therefore responsible for supplying her developing fetus with nutrients. The food is actually offered to the family in the reverse order to that dictated by nutrient priorities.

Many of the societies practising this custom believe that the male is the provider for, and the protector of, the household. They believe that it is liable to disaster if he is weak. In the African bush, this is a reasonable supposition when tribal warfare and predatory animals add to the risks of precarious subsistence-level farming. In these circumstances, it is good sense and justifiable to ensure that the head of the household and his heir are offered preferential treatment.

The *Tsembaga* of New Guinea provide another example of food habits protecting the community. In this society, domesticated pigs are not normally eaten but during warfare or when injury or serious illness threatens the well-being of the community, a ritual slaughter of the pigs takes place. This immediately makes large amounts of high quality protein available for consumption.[9]

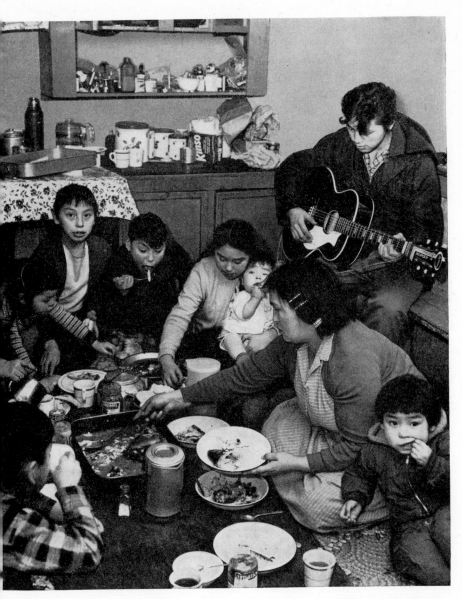

Plate 17   Communal feeding in an Eskimo family in Canada (WHO photograph by Paul Almasy)

Other food habits may protect the individual or perhaps a particularly vulnerable group of individuals. The consumption of beer made from *eleusine* millet is restricted to the pregnant women of some East African tribes. This is an excellent source of calcium (see page 141) which could help to meet the nutritional needs of pregnancy.

Other food taboos appear to be completely irrational and may be based on a superstition of obscure origin or belief relating to food and its function. In many societies, there is a division of edible items into *food* and *non food*. Within a single village inhabited by members of different tribes it has been observed that fish was highly regarded as a *food* by one tribal group yet completely disregarded by another.

Such beliefs are not confined to developing countries, for frogs and snails, highly esteemed in France, are classified as *non food* by the majority of the population of the British Isles. In the same country, for inexplicable reasons, Welsh miners will eat cheese while miners from the North of England will not.

Taboos may be associated with physiological states or with certain age groups. Young children and infants may be denied fish in the belief that they are the cause of "worms". Pregnant and lactating women may also be expected to avoid certain foods as they are believed to lead to fetal abnormality or premature delivery.

Some foods may only be consumed on *feast days* or national celebrations. The roasting of oxen in England and sucking pigs in Polynesia, and the *barrio fiesta* of the Philippines are examples of customs that make a food available to the underprivileged.

Foods may be forbidden because they have an association with illness; fish for example, is believed to cause leprosy, convulsions and menstrual disorders.[10] In illness all foods may be forbidden; starvation therapy is applied by mothers in cases of febrile illness or gastroenteritis and it may hasten the onset of protein calorie malnutrition. Rice in the Far East, and plantains in Buganda, are considered *super foods*, while elsewhere other foods have become associated with prestige and status. This is extremely common in towns and cities where newcomers, migrating from rural areas, who have been accustomed to coarse whole meal flours abandon their staple and eat white bread. They may place a self-imposed ban on their traditional foods which then lose prestige, or may even have a negative prestige value. The rejection of beans as a food, because they are identified with the poor, is a well known phenomenon of urbanization.[11]

In Europe, venison and game birds such as pheasant and grouse are associated with the elite and the financially affluent.

It is quite common for food to be related to local concepts of body function.[12] In India, foods are classified according to whether they are *heating* or *cooling* to the body. In England, spleen is rarely eaten; this taboo can be traced back to the humoral theories of Galen who postulated that the spleen was the site of a melancholic tumor. Foods may also have magic properties according to local folk lore. These include the beliefs of many athletes that eating large quantities of undercooked steak helps to build muscle and improves muscle strength.

An individual craving, or obsessional desire for unusual and inappropriate food is more difficult to understand. In some cases there may be an instinctive drive to consume a particular food, or other substance containing a nutrient needed by the body. The cravings are grouped into three categories, a craving for a specific food, craving for edible earths (*geophagia*) and cravings for non food materials (*pica*).

Food cravings Pregnant women are renowned for developing a craving for some accustomed article of diet, or perhaps a food that has never been consumed before. Apart from providing extra calories, there does not seem to be any instinctive physiological bases for the choice. On nutritional grounds, it is difficult to justify the consumption of 4 pounds of cornstarch per week by a pregnant female in the USA.[13]

On the other hand there is some evidence that the practice may be harmful; in some cases parotid gland enlargement and *gastroliths* have been reported in cornstarch eaters.

Geophagia The eating of earth is reported from many places usually it occurs in proverty stricken populations where the nutritional status is less than optimal, however, the habit is not limited to the poor.[14]

Where geophagia is practised it is customary to find that a particular river bed, or clay pit on a river bank, may be selected in preference to other sites. In Africa, women may walk several miles through the bush to collect *edible earth* although the selected place does not appear to differ in soil composition from the surrounding area. The earth, mixed in with a bean or green leaf relish, is often consumed by the whole family. While this practice does not imply that everyone in the family has a craving, it may be an expression of concern by the mother for her family. Although geophagia is usually identified with women, men and children also indulge in the habit. The cause is unclear, but the craving may be so strong that sometimes symptoms resembling drug withdrawal appear if an attempt is made to break the custom. Geophagia may be a means to achieve satiety in areas where hunger and undernutrition exists. It has also been suggested that the trait is a carry over from childhood, when exploratory examination of the floor of the hut may have led the child to put some earth in its mouth, thereby establishing a habit that is continued into older life.

Clay eating This is not without harm for it is associated with iron deficiency anemia, potassium deficiency, and in some parts of the Middle East it is believed to be responsible for zinc deficiency in children. Absence of gastric hydrochloric acid has also been found in clay eaters in the United States and Iran. *In vitro*, it has been shown that clay can remove potassium cations from both aqueous media and serum. If this exchange also takes place *in vivo* it may be responsible for iron deficiency anemia too. The cause of the zinc deficiency has not been established but preliminary laboratory investigations suggest that a similar cation exchange mechanism may be responsible.

Pica This is a common habit in children and adults. Many children between the ages of two and four years will eat dirt, plaster, wood or coal. The cause is obscure and does not appear to be related to dietary deficiency, but it is commonly observed in children suffering from hookworm anemia.

The habit of picking up objects and placing them in the mouth usually starts in the second year of life, and it may continue for years; in some cases it is used to attract attention. Pica is usually innocuous, but 250,000 children were estimated to have suffered from lead poisoning in 1968, mostly as a result of children gnawing painted surfaces.[15]

Family influences on food availability

Family size When a family is barely subsisting, additional mouths to feed may reduce the per capita availability of food to a danger level. Gopalan[16] estimates that 62 per cent of all nutritional deficiency states encountered in Indian children are encountered in birth orders of four and above.

Family stability Family structure, and traditional social customs associated with marriage, are important determinants of food availability and food intake patterns. For example, illegitimacy is an accepted part of life in the Caribbean, and is associated with family units whose head is the mother or grandmother.[17] Biological fathers play only a minor role in caring for their young children and may assume little responsibility for providing for them. The burden falls on the mother and grandmother and it may have serious consequences so far as rearing and feeding the child are concerned.

Social and cultural influences When an agrarian community moves towards the city, the established patterns of living are disrupted and new patterns are adopted. One of the features of the new life is a decline in breast feeding, a rise in the use of cows milk fed by bottle, and a tendency to purchase manufactured or expensive imported foods.

There are several reasons for the changes. First, there may be difficulty in continuing breast feeding because the mother may have to go out to work, to supplement the family income. She may come under the persuasive influence of commercial enterprises that over emphasize the advantages of their product as a convenient method of feeding infants. There is a tendency for new arrivals in the cities to mimic their social superiors who may have adopted formula feeding already. They may be influenced by friends, neighbors, or even misguided health and nutrition educators who may be advocating infant feeding practices which are really only practicable in a far more sophisticated environment.

The use of an expensive formula places an extra burden on the family budget; in the interests of economy the formula is diluted. When the milk is prepared in poor kitchen facilities lacking adequate hygiene, a chain of events is started that usually ends in the infant suffering from diarrhea and eventually marasmus.

Later in the life of the infant, inadequate amounts of proprietary weaning foods may be the cause of kwashiorkor. The pernicious nature of the demand for sophisticated foods is exemplified in the Caribbean, where mothers living on the edge of poverty will purchase a jar of strained banana at twenty or thirty times the cost of the raw product growing in their own gardens.

The problems of deficiencies, growth retardation and overt malnutrition are not restricted to the poor. The relatively well-to-do are caught up in the urbanization pattern. They may abandon breast feeding and employ nursemaids to feed formulae to their babies; the end result may be the same as in the poor household.

A type of malnutrition is found that is not caused by lack of food materials or abject poverty. It has been termed *sociocultural* malnutrition.[18] The disease becomes evident in children after they contract a minor upper respiratory infection, or gastro-intestinal trouble. They have enjoyed normal development up to that point. The height achievement of these children may be satisfactory but their weight is usually retarded. The diet patterns of children suffering from sociocultural malnutrition are characteristic. Breast feeding is treated with nonchalance by parents; milk formulae tend to be used improperly. There is a dependence on milk, juices, and fruits which become major components of the diet, at the expense of meat dishes and vegetables. There is usually excessive consumption of expensive and highly advertised foodstuffs such as ice cream and carbonated beverages.

Economic levels

Economic considerations may be an important cause of improper nutrition. The impoverished may be unable to purchase sufficient food. The subsistence farmer may be unable to grow sufficient food, or he may be forced to sell a quota of a vital food. This may leave him unable to meet the needs of himself and family.

Increasing the economic levels of a population or a community may not, on the other hand, be followed by an improvement in nutritional status. New-found financial resources may be diverted towards the purchase of material goods carrying social status. The net result may be an actual reduction in food purchasing power.

When a community does not grow its own food, the food must be purchased directly by cash, or indirectly through barter. Some communities in developing countries rely entirely on cash crops and cottage industries for the purchase of the essentials of life. Their welfare is very much dependant on market prices.

Many of the commodities grown for cash such as coffee, cocoa, rubber, sisal and tobacco are liable to wide price fluctuations, depending on the state of the world markets. A fall in the price of sisal or rubber, in London or New York, can greatly reduce the availability of food in a remote African village or Malaysian *Kampong*. The value of cocoa exports from Ghana fell from an average of 204.3 million dollars between 1963 and 1965, to 163.0 million dollars in 1966.[19] The effect of such falls on the purchasing power of the Ghanian farmer must be considerable. Because of the lack of diversification of agriculture, most farmers can do little but continue to grow their crops, and hope for a change in fortunes.

Apart from these purely economic reasons, there are some fundamental and important facts pertaining to subsistence production by farm households. Food purchases, or subsistence production, are known to be the basic determinants of the pattern of food consumption and consequently the nutritive quality of the diets. The pattern of food consumption is also influenced strongly by population increases in the sections of the community that are dependant on purchased foods. It may be seen that the extra demands of the enlarged population will necessitate an expansion, and improvement, of the food marketing system, the development of better methods of food processing, and more sophisticated transport and storage facilities.

Economic considerations frequently determine the agricultural policies of a country. When agricultural and economic considerations are predominant, the majority of the efforts may be directed towards production of non-food commodities for cash or trade on a national or international level. In many countries, agricultural and food production policies often conflict. Even if they are in alignment, there may be no relation between the food production policy and the nutritional needs of the population.

The food intake of the subsistence level farmer is determined largely by the food he grows. Therefore his nutrient intake may depend on local agricultural practises and policies within his village group as well as the practises and policies of his national government. In turn, these latter policies may be influenced by international events. For these reasons, changes or deterioration in international relations, may have considerable nutritional implications. The Vietnamese, Cambodian, Egyptian, and Israeli farmers are contemporary witnesses of this situation.

Marketing Food may be present in abundance on a national scale but inadequate marketing and distributing facilities may deprive local areas of an important food. Simultaneously a neighboring area may be experiencing a surfeit of the same food.

Some years ago in the highland areas of the Pare Mountains of Tanzania, coffee was grown as a cash crop, and vegetables were grown for home consumption. At one time the people of that region were experiencing difficulty in obtaining adequate supplies of foods of animal origin. In the plains some 4,000 feet below the coffee farming area, a pastoral tribe with large resources of livestock was suffering from xeropthalmia, (caused by a lack of dark green vegetables). The geographical separation of these two groups was no more than a mile and the problems of each group were capable of solution by the resources of the other. It took a considerable amount of persuasion and tact to build a road between the two groups and to establish marketing and trade facilities for the sale and exchange of vegetables and meat.

The establishment of markets on a cooperative basis may be an essential first step towards commercial development in rural areas. In time however, trade and profit are likely to become the prime considerations. When this happens, overproduction can lead to dumping of foods in an effort to maintain profits, and commodity prices can be fixed by unscrupulous merchants and traders.

One of the marketing problems of the urban ghetto of Detroit in the USA is the disparity in the cost of food commodities sold in the city food shops and markets, compared with the cost of food in the suburban areas. The price of the same brand of evaporated milk was 31 per cent higher in the small grocery of the "Inner City" than in the suburban supermarket chain; a 16 oz can of Pork and Beans cost 79 per cent more in the Inner City. In independant stores, in areas where the population was earning on average more than $ 12,000 per year, a selected shopping list of food cost $ 12.81. In the Inner City, where the population was earning less than $ 4,000 per year, the same selected shopping list cost $ 14.50.

The quality of food offered for sale is often inferior in the Inner City. Damaged cans, partially filled bottles, meat and bacon with excessive fat, may have to be accepted by the poor as no alternative source of supply may be available.[20]

Food storage and processing

Food Storage   At the subsistence farming level, food storage is on a small scale but nevertheless storage losses are probably considerable. Unfortunately, a scientific estimate of the extent is impossible for practical reasons. In peasant farms the current crop is stored in, or around the house, for use during the year. A proportion is always kept as a reserve for seed for the following year. If the harvest is good, some will be kept as a reserve to be used during the times of natural catastrophes, such as drought or unseasonal rain. When food production is a means of livelihood, and where it is produced for export to other areas, the quality of grain and food storage is important not only from the economic viewpoint, but also as a means of increasing the amount of food which will be available to other populations.

Food storage losses are considerable in all parts of the world. Seven and a half per cent of the maize stored in the USA between 1951 and 1960 was lost at a total cost of US $ 373 million (see Table 3). It was estimated that losses in India amounted to 25 per cent of all grains and in West Africa, 41 per cent of the sorghum and rice crop was lost (see Table 4).

The losses occur in a wide variety of ways; insect pests take a toll in the home and on the farm (see Table 5). In warehouses, inadequate vermin-proofing may allow considerable depredation and spoilage by rats. Birds may also gain access to domestic and commercial stores. Many warehouses fail to protect the crops during the rainy season and losses occur because of sprouting, mold, and damp. Some conditions of storage are known to encourage the development of toxic substances in the food. The dangers of aflatoxin in ground nuts stored in a damp climate have been described in the previous chapter (see page 67 and 144).

Diet patterns may be modified because of difficulties in storage. A certain food may be cheap, readily available and acceptable, but if it is liable to

Table 3 Estimates of losses in storage in the United States, average 1951–60

	Quantity %	Loss in Quality %	Value Million U.S. $
Wheat	4.0	0.1	127
Rye	1.2	0.1	1
Barley	3.5	0.1	16
Oats	1.0	0.1	8
Maize	7.5	0.2	373
Sorghum, grain	5.4	0.2	22
Rice	2.5	0.1	5
Total cereals			552
All crops			1,042

Source: U. S. D. A. Agric. Handbook, No. **291**, p. 69 Washington, D. C., 1965.

Table 4 Estimates of grain losses in different countries

Country	Material	Percentage Loss
Nigeria	Sorghum	46
India	All grains	25
	Field loss	15
	Storage loss	
	Handling and processing loss	7
	Other losses	3
Sierra Leone	Rice	41
	Maize	14
Tropical Africa	All crops (storage and handling)	30

Reproduced from CERES, The F. A. O. Magazine, No. **5**, Sept.–Oct. 1969.

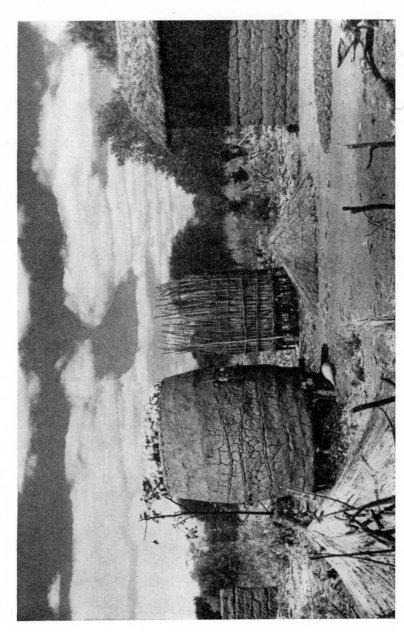

Plate 18 Mud and wattle silos for storing grain in an East African homestead. Although this method of storage is not very effective against rodents, it is an improvement on haphazard storage on the floor or among the roof timbers of huts (FAO photograph)

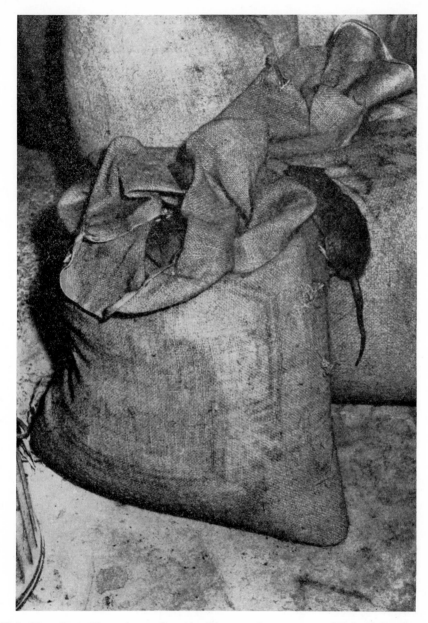

Plate 19   Rats. The progeny of a pair of rats can be as many as 900 in 12 months. They can be responsible for huge losses of grain products

Table 5 Estimates of losses in stored food grain in India

Cause of Loss	Wheat %	Rice %	Jowar %	Bajra %	Maize %	Millets %	Pulses %	Total million tons
Rodents	2.5	2.5	2.5	2.5	2.5	2.5	2.5	2.0
Birds	0.5	1.0	1.0	1.0	0.5	2.0	0.9	0.7
Insects	3.0	2.0	2.0	1.0	3.0	0.5	2.5	2.0
Moisture	0.5	0.5	2.0	0.5	0.5	0.5	0.7	0.5
Total	6.5	6.0	7.5	5.0	6.5	5.5	6.6	5.2

Source: India, Ministry of Food, Agriculture, Community Development and Co-operation, New Delhi. (In) State of Food and Agriculture, 1968, p. 118, F. A. O. Rome.

rapid spoilage it is unlikely to become part of the diet. Conversely, a food which keeps well in a hot climate may be nutritionally inferior but is readily adopted by the population. Refined cereal flours owe much of their popularity to their apparent resistance to insect spoilage. The failure of insects to use these flours as a food medium is usually a reflection of its nutrient quality which will not meet the requirements for growth of the insect larvae.

Food processing   Even the most primitive societies practice some form of food processing. Fruit, vegetables and meat may be dried or partly cooked and stored. Pickling and salting is a widespread practice. The ability to process foods so that spoilage is prevented is an advantage in any community, but the introduction of new methods of processing and preserving food may not be acceptable unless the raw product is approved according to local customs, beliefs and attitudes. Many foods are being made available and are being consumed although the raw product would not, itself, be acceptable. The best example of this is provided by fermented foods such as the Javanese *ontjom* prepared from ground nut press cake, and *bongkrek* from coconut press cake that would be virtually inedible raw.[21]

Because of the economic and nutritional advantages of processing and storing food, more and more attention is being given to food technology. Legislation is frequently introduced to avoid the use of harmful technical procedures, and nutritional and economic exploitation of the consumer. The laws may control the methodology or the materials used, as well as the quality of the final product. It is obviously prudent to ensure that the water supply to the processing plant is safe, that harmful coloring agents are not incorporated in food, and that the indiscriminate use of antibiotics and hormones is halted.

The more sophisticated countries usually draft the first regulations. When a developing country decides to control food processing, existing laws are usually adopted or adapted. However, the legislation may be inappropriate or unenforceable. If the regulating standards are too high, or too strict, there may be other unfortunate effects, including the deprivation of the population of a perfectly safe and wholesome food. Although the processing of milk into a cheese may ensure a perfectly safe food product, legislation may prohibit the use of milk having a bacterial count in excess of certain reference standards.

Preservation of food by freezing is an excellent example of a technological process meeting the needs of the public and the producer. The former wants a constant supply of food all the year round, and the latter demands some marketing system to absorb surplus production when the market is saturated with seasonal gluts.

Freeze drying and irradiation of foods are newer techniques. The long term effects of this type of preservation of food have yet to be assessed. Present knowledge of these processes indicates that their effect on nutritive value is not greater than the losses caused by conventional cooking processes.[22]

There is evidence however, that domestic refrigeration may cause harmful changes in certain vegetables. Under refrigeration, the nitrates in fresh spinach may be reduced to nitrites within one to four days. The consumption of nitrites can cause *methemoglobinemia*, a condition which interferes with oxygen transport of the blood. In young infants this condition can be dangerous.[23]

Nutrient utilization

Although an adequate intake of food may be achieved according to dietary recommendations, the nutrients present in the food may not be utilized by the body. The reasons for this are many and varied; some of these will be discussed in further detail.

Characteristics of the food and diet   The nutrient composition of food can be altered during processing and cooking. Some methods of cooking and processing not only improve digestibility but they may also alter the chemical composition of the food, and enhance the potential utilization of the nutrients. The cooking of vegetables for example, helps to break down the cellulose envelope of the cells and free the contained nutrients. Some carbohydrates in foodstuffs are unavailable but cooking may alter their chemical composition and make them available. *Camas* bulbs (*Quamassia esculentia*) are consumed by the *Flathead Indians* of North America; an analysis of the raw bulb reveals that the high carbohydrate content is attributable to *inulin* which cannot be utilized by humans. On first consideration, it would appear that the nutritive value of Camas is very poor but studies have revealed that the pitroasting of the bulb produces steam and an acidic smoke capable of converting unavailable inulin into readily available *fructose*.[24]

Food Mixtures   Some mixtures of food are essential for the proper absorption and utilization of nutrients. Vitamin A is a fat soluble vitamin, so unless a source of fat is also present in the diet the absorption and utilization of vitamin A, or its carotene precursor, may be inhibited. This is an example of mixtures of foods enhancing the utilization of nutrients, other mixtures can inhibit their absorption. This phenomenon is well illustrated by the case of wheat and rice which contain *phytates*. These chemical compounds form insoluble salts with iron and calcium in other food sources. In geophagia, the properties of the clay may inhibit iron and zinc absorption.

The antagonistic and synergistic actions of food mixtures are not fully understood. Iron from vegetable foods such as wheat, maize, spinach and black gram are poorly absorbed when consumed alone, but when veal is combined with a meal of maize the absorption of the iron in the maize is greatly enhanced.[25]

Malabsorption The multiple causation of the malabsorption syndrome has been discussed in Chapter 1. The following will re-emphasize those causes of malabsorption relating to food or malnutrition. The physical nature of the intestinal content can cause rapid evacuation of the bowel contents so there is less time for the absorbtive process to be complete. The bran of cereals used by food manufacturers in breakfast preparations adds bulk to the stool thereby encouraging intestinal motility. Rye bread and maize cause considerable *intestinal hustle*, the latter may be one of the reasons why maize eaters are particularly prone to nicotinic acid deficiency. Intestinal bacteria may break down complex indigestible carbohydrates thereby freeing less complex substances which may then be digested and absorbed.[26] This important function may be affected by antibiotics present in the food or taken therapeutically.

Other pathologic conditions *Diphyllobothrium latum* is a parasite of sea fish that can be transmitted to man. The tape worm utilizes vitamin B_{12} of the host, eventually the diversion of the vitamin to the fish may cause a deficiency in the host who may develop megaloblastic anemia.

Protein calorie malnutrition in early infancy may cause a reduced efficiency in the utilization of protein. Children who have been severely malnourished have been found to require more protein for growth than others raised on an ample diet.[27]

The enzyme systems of cells are liable to be changed by genetic modification. Although mutation is rare it can result in an inability to metabolize a particular nutrient. In some cases the gradual accumulation of the unused nutrient may have harmful effects on the body. *Phenylketonuria* is one of a number of diseases classified under the term *Inborn Errors of Metabolism*.[28] In phenylketonuria the body is unable to metabolize *phenylalanine*; the nutrient accumulates in the blood and is associated with mental retardation and growth failure.

The deficiency of one nutrient may interfere with the utilization of another. Protein lack can lead to a deficiency of the protein complex that transports iron in the blood. Anemia ensues because the iron can not be taken to the blood forming tissues.

The etiology of malnutrition

The first part of this chapter has been devoted to the remote factors influencing the nutritional status of the community. The more immediate *causal* or *etiological* factors which precipitate malnutrition in the community will now be examined.

Figure 7 summarizes in schematic form the etiology of protein calorie malnutrition, it will be seen that many of the ecological factors are also involved in the immediate cause of malnutrition. In most developing countries the etiology is relatively simple and has been aptly described by The President of the Republic of Tanzania, Julius K. Nyerere as "Poverty, Ignorance, Prejudice and Disease".

Infant feeding practices in developing countries

"Poverty, Ignorance, Prejudice and Disease" are very closely associated with infant feeding habits. Much of the morbidity and mortality experience of infants and pre-school age children is directly attributable to inadequate and improper feeding in infancy and during weaning.

Figure 8 summarizes the two main patterns of infant feeding practices. These determine whether a malnourished child will suffer from marasmus or kwashiorkor. In developing countries infants are traditionally fed at the breast. This supplies milk perfectly adequate to meet the demands of growth until the infant reaches six months of age.

From this time onwards however, he must receive protein from other sources. The gradual change from a liquid diet to foods which are predominantly solid is known as the weaning process. For this to be successful the infant must be provided with food which is acceptable in taste, easy to chew and free from contaminants, pathogenic bacteria and parasites. It must provide ample calories and it must provide protein that is both sufficient in quantity and quality. Finally, the food must comply with the traditional beliefs of the family and society. Because of these criteria, the provision of a suitable weaning food is no easy task. In some ways it is remarkable that infants in developing countries ever succeed in obtaining a satisfactory food.

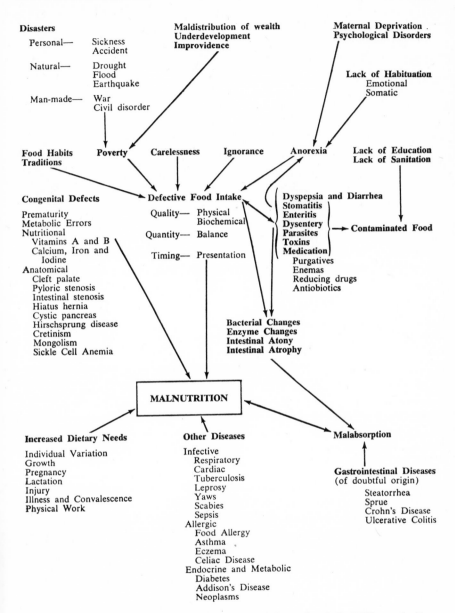

Figure 7 The etiology of malnutrition (Original figure by C. D. Williams, in Proceedings Western Hemisphere Nutrition Congress, p. 20, 1965). Reproduced with the permission of the American Medical Association

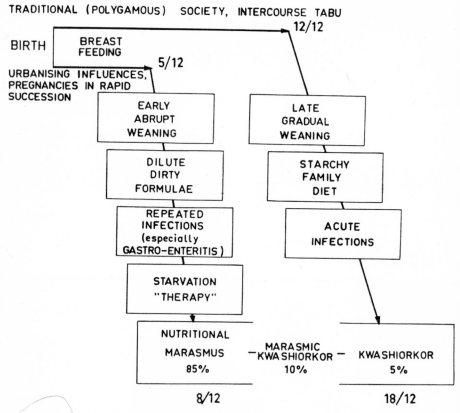

TRADITIONAL (POLYGAMOUS)   SOCIETY, INTERCOURSE TABU

Figure 8   Infant feeding patterns. Paths leading from early weaning to nutritional marasmus and from protracted breast feeding to kwashiorkor. Numbers represent approximate age in months. Percentages of types of malnutrition are based on figures for Jordan but are typical for many other countries (Figure reproduced from Lancet August 27, 1966, by kind permission of Professor D. S. McLaren)

Breast feeding continues into the second year of life or even later in many societies which means that the infant is weaned very gradually. Usually the child is introduced to a cereal gruel in the second half of the first year of life. In some cultures the food may be fed with some force, a practice that may seem brutal; it may however, be a nutritionally sound procedure.

The semi-liquid gruel is usually replaced by more solid food such as rice or doughs made from sorghum, maize, or cassava. The best of these foods contain only about eight per cent of protein of limited biological value. These doughs are bulky and filling. Table 6 shows the amount of cooked staple a two year old child would have to consume to meet his daily requirements.

Table 6 Quantity of cooked cereals required to meet the calorie requirements of a two year old child

Food	Amount (kgs)
Maize gruel	1.53
Maize dough	1.60
Sorghum	1.59
Rice	1.10

Regardless of the cereal fed the amount to be consumed is formidable; the forced feeding already noted may help the child to meet his nutrient needs. The situation with respect to the protein intake is more serious. If the protein requirement of a two year old child is 30 grams, the 1.1 kgs of rice that he would have to consume to meet his calorie requirement would only supply about 22 grams of protein. The child will be replete before he can achieve his calorie requirement so the protein will be used as a source of energy and will not be available for growth.

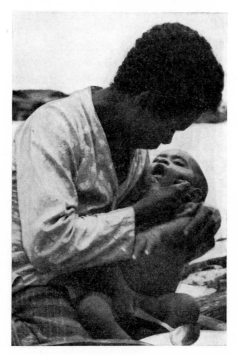

Plate 20   Mouth feeding in New Guinea. This may help the child to achieve an adequate calorie intake (Photograph by Professor H. A. P. C. Oomen)

The biological value of cereals is so poor, other sources of protein must be ingested if an adequate intake of amino acids is to be achieved. Good quality protein like meat or fish is often in short supply. Legumes could make a useful contribution to the diet but many mothers lack the necessary knowledge and facilities to prepare digestible and acceptable dishes from beans and peas. The main source of protein may therefore be the staple cereal.

Food consumption habits are changing in rural societies and in developing countries. In some areas, staple cereals such as sorghum are being abandoned in favor of maize which is nutritionally inferior. It is also being noticed that communities whose staple is maize are now beginning to consume more and more starchy foods. Because of the inadequacies of cereal and starchy staples, feeding of breast milk should continue as a supplement. It has been noted that as much as 357 grams of milk may be secreted over a period of 24 hours by women in their second year of lactation.[29] Supplementation of the diet with such quantities of breast milk may be sufficient to maintain life, if not growth, in children. Any factor depriving the child of breast milk as a supplement may be responsible for precipitating protein calorie malnutrition. Unfortunately the events which may deprive the child of a breast milk supplement are numerous.

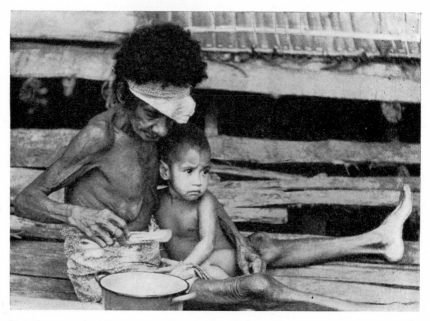

Plate 21   Infant feeding practices in New Guinea. This child is being fed sago by his grandmother. Protein calorie malnutrition is inevitable unless the diet is supplemented with some high quality protein (Photograph by Professor H. A. P. C. Oomen)

In many societies breast feeding must stop when the mother becomes pregnant. In the same cultures pregnancy is controlled by a taboo on intercourse for a period of a year or more after delivery. When the society makes contact with the more advanced population groups the intercourse taboo is soon abandoned but the habit of stopping breast feeding when pregnancy intervenes is maintained. Consequently many young children are left without the breast milk supplement which is so vital to their well being.

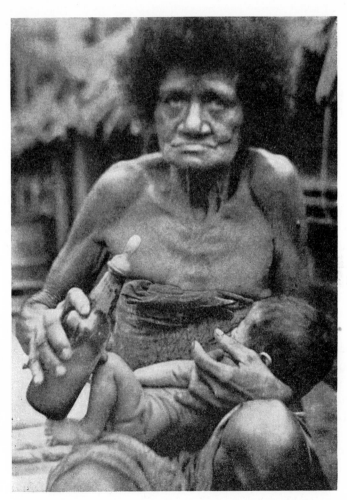

Plate 22   Infant feeding in New Guinea. The risks of bottle feeding in these circumstances are all too apparent (Photograph by Professor H. A. P. C. Oomen)

In some populations children are placed in the care of grandparents, not only are the new guardians unlikely to supply a breast milk supplement but they may be unable to ensure a proper dietary intake. Children in such circumstances are very liable to become malnourished.

The deprivation of the breast milk to the child may be brought about on purpose by misguided nutrition education. The "expert" text books, and doctors trained by these books from highly industrialized countries, are very likely to prescribe the feeding regime of the sophisticated societies; this invariably recommends cessation of breast feeding around the sixth month. In a developing country such advice could be catastrophic unless an adequate substitute for breast milk is made available. In the urban areas of the developing countries these substitutes are costly and in many cases the mother may not be able to afford them. Furthermore she may not know how to prepare weaning foods made from inexpensive local sources of protein.

During the early months of life when the child is dependent entirely on the mothers supply of breast milk, he is relatively protected from pathogenic organisms. As the society develops, and formula feeding is adopted, the risks of feeding cows milk formulae, contaminated with pathogenic organisms is very great and marasmus may be the end result (see Figure 8). Infection is inevitable in infancy, but breast feeding at least helps to delay the first attack. This is usually contracted when infected gruel, water, or some other material which may have been picked up off the ground, is ingested.

The added stress of infection in states of marginal nutrition is extremely critical and will be discussed in greater detail.

Nutrition and infection

Retarded growth and development, and high death and morbidity rates in children, are characteristic of the impoverished and deprived populations of the world. The infant and the preschool child are the most affected, but the total death and illness which these children suffer cannot be explained by their diet alone. It is well known that many of the deaths which occur in the malnourished are precipitated by infections. Some infective agents cause little harm in well-nourished populations but in the poorly-nourished they may have very serious effects on health. In 1962 the mortality rate for measles ranged from 0.1 to 0.5 per 100,000 population in western Europe but in Mexico it was 85 times greater, in Guatemala it was 268 times greater.

The virulence of the measles virus is virtually the same in England as it is in Guatemala. Differences in the mortality experience cannot be attributed to the better medical care in England for the availability of antibiotics and better health facilities has not lowered mortality significantly. The nutritional status of populations in developing countries where measles mortality rates are high is usually poor, whereas the nutritional status of highly industrialized populations is usually good. Studies in Guatemala and Africa for example, have shown a high correlation between the severity of measles and the degree of malnutrition.[30,31] In a study in the state of Michigan, U. S. A., over half of the children under 5 years of age dying from measles were found to have severe deficits in height and weight that was not related to genetic factors. It is possible that the underlying cause may have been improper nutrition.[32]

Diarrhea and dysentery are the most common infections of early childhood in developing countries and they are especially important between the fourth and twenty-fourth months of life. Because of its association with the weaning process it has become known as *weanling diarrhea*. The prevalence of weanling diarrhea is low in children while they are breast fed, but it increases as soon as other foods are introduced. This leaves little doubt that weaning, rather than age, is the etiological agent (see Table 7).

Table 7   Cases of acute diarrheal disease among wholly breast-fed children, By quarter years, in three Guatemalan highland villages, 1959–62

Age (Months)	All children breast-fed	Breastmilk only Number	%	Cases of acute diarrheal disease among children breast-fed only	Incidence (cases per 100 wholly breast-fed children per year)
0–2	294	284	97	51	72
3–5	290	239	82	100	167
6–8	288	95	33	45	190
9–11	280	13	5	7	215
12–14	261	3	1	3	400
15–17	221	0	0	0	0
TOTAL		634		206	130

Source: Scrimshaw, N. S., Taylor, C. E., Gordon, J. E., Wld. Hlth. Org. Monograph No. 57, p. 252, 1968.

Studies in Guatemala have shown that the most severely malnourished children have more attacks of diarrhea than normal children and the attacks are more severe.[33]

The episodes of diarrhea are rarely single and the number of attacks that a child may suffer may increase through the second six months and second year of life (see Table 8).

Table 8   Attack rate of acute diarrheal disease in four Guatemalan villages, 1956–59

Age-group	Number of persons	Cases of diarrhea	Attack rate (cases/year/100 persons)
0–5 months	92	43	46.7
6–11 months	79	87	110.1
1 year	135	162	120.0
2 years	122	129	105.7
3 years	119	66	55.5
4–6 years	406	86	21.2
7–14 years	839	69	8.2
15+ years	2,390	109	4.6
All ages	4,182	751	18.0

Source: Scrimshaw, N. S., Taylor, C. E., Gordon, J. E. Wld. Hlth. Org., Monograph No. **57**, p. 241, 1968.

The beneficial effect of a better diet on mortality experience has also been demonstrated. In Guatemala, the preschool children who were participating in a supplementary feeding program suffered no deaths from diarrhea over a five year period, while other preschool children in surrounding villages who did not receive nutritional supplements continued to experience high mortality. The overall death rate in the population was also significantly reduced.

The infective organism may be from the dysentery, salmonella or coliform group of bacteria but entero-viruses and protozoa may also be involved. Many of the organisms are of low pathogenicity and may be introduced into the child through a symptomless carrier. Because of the debilitation of the child by malnutrition, invasion of the body tissues takes place; this is followed by further deterioration and the appearance of clinical signs of disease.

It is possible that the micro-organisms of the intestinal tract range from those that are completely harmless to those that are pathogenic. In malnutrition the dividing line between these two types is shifted to one side therefore organisms which are normally non-pathogenic become invasive or cause diarrhea.

There is considerable epidemiological, clinical and experimental evidence of the importance of nutritional factors in tuberculosis. While the virtual disappearance of tuberculosis in some countries can be attributed to the use of antibiotics, it should be remembered that tuberculosis was declining in the United Kingdom before antibiotics were discovered. There was a sharp decrease when the average diet in England improved during the second world war. In Holland, during the famine of 1945, a relationship was shown between the decline in the quality and quantity of food and the increase in tuberculosis.

In the marginally nourished, an infection may precipitate overt deficiency diseases such as xerophthalmia, scurvy, beri-beri, pellagra and protein calorie malnutrition. Communicable diseases are far more common in developing countries than in the highly industrialized parts of the world and the constant presence of infections, and the repeated exposure of children to them, is one of the principle reasons why the prevalence rates for protein calorie malnutrition are so high. Gastroenteritis, whooping cough, rubella, mumps and chicken pox have their greatest incidence in the first two years of life, a time when the diet is lacking in calories and protein of adequate quality.

It is not only micro-organisms which may precipitate overt disease in malnourished children. Parasites have also been associated with this phenomena and it is possible that normally harmless inhabitants of the body may become pathogenic in hosts debilitated by malnutrition. *Pneumocystis carinii* is an organism normally found in animals but it is capable of being transmitted to humans, where it may cause pneumonia. The disease has been recognized for some thirty years; it has a predilection for low birth-weight and debilitated infants. Personal observation of an outbreak of *Pneumocystis* pneumonia in an orphanage in Iran suggested that it was the undernourished who were particularly at risk. Other parasites may also have some synergism with nutrition. The malaria parasites for example, may interfere with fetal growth for it has been found that the average weight of babies born of mothers with infected placentae were significantly lower than those born of healthy mothers.[34] There is also evidence that growth is retarded in infants who have very heavy round worm infections and it would seem reasonable to assume that an intestine packed with worms could interfere with the digestion and absorption of nutrients. Certain helminths such as *Giardia lamblia* have a specific inhibiting effect on the absorption of vitamin A. Some parasites also migrate through the body, in doing so they may cause systemic effects accompanied by a rise in fever and destruction of tissues. The invasion of parasites undoubtedly places an additional stress on the body which in the malnourished state may tip the balance and precipitate overt malnutrition.

The role of nutrition in preventing infection has not been thoroughly explored. However Schneider[35] has made some interesting observations regarding the presence of a *Salmonella Resistance Factor* or *Pacifarin* which appears to be present in cereal grains, barley sprouts and dried green and black tea. In Schneider's experiments a linear relationship was established between the concentration of pacifarin and the survival rate of an experimental population of rats exposed to Salmonella infection. It is believed that pacifarin may be produced by the bacillus *Aerobacter* which sometimes contaminates cereals. The chemistry of pacifarin is not fully understood, it is neither a vitamin nor is it an antibiotic; it has remarkable effects in minute doses, for 200–400 parts per billion will increase survivorship in infected animals from 10–90 per cent. It has been proposed that pacifarin should be classified as an ecological ectocrine which is defined as a substance biosynthesized by one species and which exerts an effect on the function of another via the external medium.

The effect of infection on nutrition   One of the first effects of infection is a loss of appetite. If fever or diarrhea is present, the mother and the physician may deprive the patient of solid food completely, or at best, they may give the child a soft or liquid starchy diet. In the Philippines a thin rice gruel (*lugao*) is frequently the only food offered to febrile children, or those with diarrhea. Diets such as this are virtually protein free and their continued consumption will eventually lead to protein calorie malnutrition.

The onset of the fever places an extra strain on the resources of the body, and usually more nitrogen is lost than normal. The negative nitrogen balance should be compensated by an increase in the nitrogen intake and would be achieved by consuming extra protein of good quality. Because of the loss of appetite, the diet, or the starvation therapy, protein intake is likely to be minimal or even at the zero level.

It is not only the infective agent that can place the body in negative nitrogen balance for this undesirable state of affairs has been noticed after immunization with vaccines such as measles and yellow fever. In children from impoverished or deprived populations, the tissues are usually depleted before infection so recurrent infections will soon have very serious effects unless the protein stores are repleted during convalescence.

Effect of malnutrition on infection   The first line of the body defences lie in the anatomical barriers and physiological secretions which protect delicate membranes. The integrity of the skin and mucous membranes, and the presence of nasal and mouth secretions, and tears to bathe the eyes, must play a significant part in warding off infection. However, these protective mechanisms may be nonfunctioning in deficiency states. For example, the precorneal film is lost in vitamin A infections, and dryness of the eye may be a feature of riboflavin and vitamin A deficiency. The intestinal tract is inflamed in nicotinic acid deficiency, and the integrity of the skin is frequently lost in pellagra and protein calorie malnutrition. Nutrient deficiency can therefore facilitate the entry of micro-organisms into the body. The reduced healing properties of tissues in the malnourished may facilitate the spread of infection and promote septicemia.

Once entrance to the body has been gained, the humoral and tissue defense mechanisms resist the further multiplication of the infective organism, and invasion of the tissues. In malnutrition these defenses are weakened or may not even be present. For example, children suffering from protein calorie malnutrition have been found to have an impaired capacity to form antibodies to yellow fever, and typhoid vaccine.[36] On repletion of the body with protein, the capacity for antibody formation returns.[37] Other nutrient deficiencies, notably those of nicotinic acid and pyridoxine, may also interfere with antibody formation in humans. Animal experimentation suggest that antibody formation may be inhibited by a wider range of nutrient deficiencies including tryptophan, vitamins A and D, ascorbic acid, thiamine, riboflavin, nicotinic acid, pyridoxine, pantothenic acid, folic acid and vitamin B_{12}.

The circulating leucocytes of the blood and the sedentary cells of the reticulo-endothelial system in the liver and the spleen are normally able to ingest microorganisms and remove them from the circulation. In malnutrition this facility may be lost. The general systemic response of the body may also be inhibited. Normally the invasion of the body by pathogenic organisms is followed by a rise in body temperature. This is a reflection of increased metabolic activity associated with the mobilization of body defenses. The temperature rise itself may change a favorable environment to unfavorable; in malnourished individuals the ability to produce pyrexia may be lacking.

While there is little doubt concerning the synergism between nutrition and infection, the respective contributory factors cannot be evaluated. Poverty, poor housing and poor environmental conditions that cause, or aggravate malnutrition, or facilitate the transmission of infections are all interrelated. Programs aimed at improving nutritional status and the control of communicable disease frequently ignore these interrelationships. This may account for the continued high mortality experiences in the urban slums.

8*

Infant feeding practices in industrialized countries

Both marasmus and kwashiorkor are rare in industrialized countries, nevertheless, infant feeding practices have been adopted which may be hazardous to health.

One of the most frequent hazards of formula feeding is overfeeding.[38] This is especially likely to happen in societies where weight, in infants, is considered a desirable attribute. The prevalence and dangers of overweight in infancy have already been described. Dependance on milk as the only source of nutrients beyond six months of age is inevitably accompanied by iron deficiency anemia. There is also a risk of calorie overfeeding, but even before this, the baby fed cows milk may face several nutritional problems.

Calcium absorption is impaired in formula fed babies and is attributed to the characteristics of the fatty acids in cows milk (see page 126). The malabsorption can be severe; if there is a considerable fall in serum calcium levels the infant may develop convulsions, a condition known as hypocalcemia or *neonatal tetany*. A recent increase in this disease has been reported and associated with the practice of feeding infants large quantities of undiluted milk. The lowering of the calcium levels is probably related to the high phosphorus content of cows milk. The relationship between calcium and phosphorus in the blood is such that the sum of their ions is a constant and may be expressed by the formula $Ca^{++} \times HPO^{4--} = K$. Therefore, if calcium enters the blood stream, phosphate ions have to be reduced. Conversely, if phosphate ions increase, the calcium level in the blood is decreased. As the phosphate in cows milk is absorbed preferentially over calcium, the blood phosphate levels rise at the expense of calcium. This theory is supported by studies that have revealed high phosphate levels in the blood of formula fed infants suffering from neonatal tetany. A reduction in the phosphate content of the milk is followed by a rise in calcium levels. This phenomenon has been utilized in the preparation of *adapted milks* which are now being prepared on a commercial scale.[39]

There is now some concern over increasing reports of milk intolerance in infants due to deficiencies of *lactase*, the enzyme which breaks down milk sugar.[40] Formerly, it had been assumed that the deficiency was genetic in origin, this may be true in some, but not all cases. In mammals, other than man, it has been noted that lactase is only secreted during the suckling period; after weaning the enzyme disappears. In humans, similar physiological events may take place, consequently in societies where breast feeding is neither replaced nor supplemented by cows milk, the enzyme may disappear after weaning. Later in life, when cows milk is provided as a snack or as the basis of a protein supplement, lactase may not be available to digest milk sugar and digestive upsets follow.

A true allergy to milk protein also occurs in infants. The exact mechanism of its development is not fully understood but during the early days of infant life, it is believed that the intestinal epithelium is permeable to large protein molecules. This permeability facilitates the entry of antibodies and other protein material in the colostrum into the body. If cows milk is offered shortly after birth, the milk protein may also enter the tissues and stimulate antibody formation. The resultant allergic response between the milk in the diet and the protein-sensitized mucosa, produces cramps and diarrhea. This latter symptom may be caused by the allergic reaction destroying lactase, since many cases of milk allergy exhibit lactose intolerance. The symptoms and signs of lactose intolerance subside when the milk protein is removed from the diet.[41]

High titres of antibodies to the protein of cows milk have been noted in infants fed cowsmilk.[42] The titres may be indicative of a hypersensitivity of the infant to milk protein and may be responsible for causing *cot (crib) death*. This is a term given to normal healthy infants who are found dead in their cots; usually there are no pathological lesions to indicate the cause of death. Experimentally, it is possible to cause sudden death in animals sensitized to milk protein. Death has followed the introduction of small quantities of cows milk into the respiratory tract of anesthetized guinea pigs that had been previously sensitized to milk protein. The same results have followed the introduction of milk protein, and the stomach contents of infants found dead in their cots.[43]

Problems in the weaning period   In highly industrialized countries, it is customary to introduce solid foods much earlier in life and it is now quite common for a child to be offered an iron-enriched cereal food a month or so, after delivery. The availability of proprietary baby foods has facilitated the adoption of this practice. The introduction of cereals into the feeding regime is soon followed by a variety of strained meats, vegetables, fruits, and meat and vegetable soups. The addition of these foods is generally considered to be advantageous and it can not be denied they help to make up the deficiency of iron in cows milk. However, processed baby foods (with the exception of fruits) may contain up to one hundred times as much salt as the natural product.[44] The daily sodium chloride requirements for salt are small. Human milk contains little sodium and there seems to be no justification on physiological, biochemical, physical, or psychological grounds for including salt in the food. The reason for its inclusion is related to the tastes of the mother since infants will accept unsalted food readily.[45]

The infant kidney already has problems excreting the solutes in cows milk that are in excess of human milk. While the infant may be able to handle salt loads if there is an adequate water intake, heat stress or restriction of fluid intake may cause harm. The long-term effects of high salt intakes have yet to be assessed. There is evidence that hypertension is related to high salt intake in animals and humans. Furthermore, the disease has been induced experimentally in rats fed baby foods with a high salt content.

The availability of foods fortified with vitamin D has led to some concern that the cumulative effects of consuming such foods may be causing vitamin D toxemia (see page 24).

The potential hazards of modern infant feeding practises are not recognized widely. There is a great need for scientific studies to evaluate growth in formula-fed babies, and the long term effects of feeding cows milk formulae and processed baby foods.

Feeding the low birthweight baby   A low birthweight baby has a weight at birth of 2500 grams or less.[46] The baby may be underweight for two reasons. First the pregnancy may have been interrupted before the expected date; such a child is the victim of *prematurity*. Alternatively the fetus may have been suffering from intrauterine malnutrition; even though the pregnancy may progress to full term, the baby would still be immature. Whether the baby has a low birthweight because of *prematurity* or *immaturity* he has special feeding problems.

During fetal life, glucose is passed from the mother to the fetus; any glucose present in the fetus in excess of immediate requirements is stored in the liver and heart, as glycogen. There is a considerable fall in glycogen levels in both of these organs during the anoxic periods of parturition.

After delivery, the demand for oxygen by the infant brain is very high. Because of the special metabolism of the brain the energy needs of this tissue can only be met by metabolizing glucose. Since the blood sugar levels of new born babies are low, the demand is met by converting liver glycogen and fat into glucose. The low birthweight baby who has suffered from intra-uterine growth failure has a relatively large brain and a small liver; the demand for glucose is therefore high but the supply of liver glycogen is limited. The premature baby, on the other hand, has a brain which is more proportionate to his liver but being premature he may not have had time to build up adequate stores of glycogen. The low birthweight baby, whether immature or premature, may therefore have inadequate glycogen supplies and very low blood sugar levels. This condition of hypoglycemia is dangerous for it can cause brain damage.

If the low birthweight infant has been subjected to an abnormal delivery, the situation will be even more serious because the liver and heart glycogen levels may be almost completely exhausted (see Table 9). The need for glucose is apparent yet it has been the custom for many years to starve new born babies for up to 48 hours. This is now believed to be harmful; in a study in Britain, the highest incidence of physical handicaps in children were found in those who had the most rigorous starvation.[47] It has also been found that the introduction of liberal breast feeding to low birthweight babies immediately after delivery, has lessened the time taken to regain birthweight, and lowered the incidence of neurological defects.

Table 9   Glycogen depletion in organs following delivery (per gram of tissue)

	After Normal Delivery	After Abnormal Delivery
Liver	30–70 mgs	7 mgs
Heart	20–40 mgs	2 mgs

Source: *Pediatrics* **39**: 594, 1967.

The limited capacity of the newborn baby for food and liquid and his poor renal function, provided the main reasons for starving the new born infant. Progress in growth was evaluated by weight, and as weight gain was greater when low birthweight babies were fed high-protein, low-fat formulae, this regime was adopted as a routine. Subsequently it was shown that the high protein diet was placing an additional load on the kidney which was harming the immature organ. It was also recognized that the apparent kidney infections of low birthweight babies, fed a high protein diet, were caused by renal failure. High protein feeding has now been abandoned and feeding with breast milk, and formulae of normal protein content, is now the vogue. Postnatal starvation is still practised and carries risks of hypoglycemia and possible interference with the growth of brain and nervous tissue. The low birthweight baby with hypoglycemia is especially at risk and must be detected as soon as possible so that he may be given emergency treatment. For this reason screening of blood glucose levels is advocated for all twins and babies whose weight is below the 25th percentile for weight.

Foods as sources of nutrients

So far, only the patterns of food intake have been discussed; it is now necessary to examine the role of foods as sources of nutrients. Special attention will be given to some of the foods that play a particularly important role in the diet.

Neither a botanical, nor a zoological classification of food materials, is satisfactory to the nutrition worker. Foods in a particular botanical genus or species, do not always have the same nutritional significance. Some foods of a given genus may be unacceptable on cultural grounds, while closely related species may be highly esteemed. For example, the *Allium* genus includes onion which is very acceptable to most people but it also includes garlic which is viewed with disfavor by others. Over the centuries, terms have been applied to food stuffs that may be both ambiguous in meaning and uninformative of their nutrient content. The term "vegetables" may be applied to leaves such as cabbage, roots (carrots), bulbs (onions), or pods, such as string beans. Other terms are given to food materials and they may infer inedibility, for example, *stems* or *shoots*.

The following classification is based on the nutrient composition of foodstuffs. On this basis the foods may be considered in three groups, *foodstuffs of animal origin*, *foodstuffs of vegetable origin*, and *miscellaneous foodstuffs*.

Foodstuffs of animal origin

Milk and milk products

Human milk Mammalian females, including humans, are equipped with glands that secrete milk to feed the young. Milk is usually considered the sole natural food for the first few months of life. There can be no doubt survival of the human race formerly depended on the supply of breast milk, until the cow, the ass and other animals became domesticated.

Wet nurses were widely used as a source of milk for infants. By the middle of the eighteenth century the low standards of morality of wet nurses, the enormous spread of vice in the *Industrial Revolution* and the very high infant mortality had raised, in England, the possibility of using animal milks for infant feeding.[48] The research of Liebig in the middle of the nineteenth century not only drew attention to the chemistry of nutrition but also it led to the development of an artificial food for infants based on cows milk.[49] This artificial food was the forerunner of proprietary preparations that are used for infant feeding throughout the world. For reasons, largely unknown, the artificial formulae have replaced breast feeding in most industrialized countries.

Despite the adoption of cows milk as an infant food, whole populations still depend on breast milk for rearing infants. Climatic vagaries and animal diseases such as *trypanosomiasis* prevent cattle from being reared in many developing countries. In other countries, taboos based on religious grounds or superstition, may prohibit the consumption of cows milk.

It would seem logical to assume that a mammalian species produces milk that is suited more to the needs of its own species, than to the needs of others. If this premise is accepted, it infers the composition of human milk is suited best to the nutritional needs of human infants, and the milk of cows is best suited to the nutritional needs of calves. The process of feeding offspring is not, however, entirely confined to furnishing nutrients. In the human, as well as other animals, the breast-feeding process brings a close relationship between the mother and the child which seems beneficial to the development of the infant.

Nutritionists have been too concerned about the quantitative aspects of diets and nutrients, in consequence the quality of the intake has been neglected. When the composition of breast milk is examined, considerable variations in the quality of the milk are observed in individuals and during lactation. In adequately fed populations, the quantity of the secretion can vary but on poor dietary intakes a fairly constant output of milk can be maintained (see Table 10). The constancy of the volume and the fact that growth was being maintained indicates that the quality of the milk must have change during lactation.

Table 10 Weights of babies and 24 hour milk yield in 14 poor Indian women

Weeks of lactation	Mean weight of infants g	Mean milk output (g/24 hours)
1	2778	454
2	2920	476
3	3119	479
4	3260	496
6	3714	499
10	4196	473
12	4394	471
16	4820	527
20	5538	454
24	5755	516

Source: Gopalan, C., *J. Trop. Ped.* **4**: 87, 1958.

The identification of changes in composition is difficult because the several phases of lactation make the collection of representative samples almost impossible. Nevertheless, certain changes have been described and are believed to be typical of human lactation. Human milk contains some sixty nutrients, the most important of these, and their concentration in human milk, are described in Table 11. This tabulation provides only an overall picture of the composition of milk since there are variations in composition between individuals. The same individual may produce milk of different quality from one lactation to another. Furthermore there are variations throughout lactation, during the day, and even during a single feed.

During the first few days, the mammary gland secretes *colostrum*; the colostrum is replaced by *transitional* milk. After a period of time varying between 2 weeks and 2 months, the milk becomes *mature* milk.

The newborn baby has special needs; these may be reflected in the unique composition of colostrum. The first secretion of the mammary gland contains globulins which provide the newborn with antibodies; it also provides a culture medium for the flora of the intestinal tract. The content of vitamin A,

Table 11   Composition of mature human milk. (Mean values per 100 ml of whole milk)

Calories	71
Protein	1.2 g
Casein	0.4 g
Lactalbumin	0.3 g
Lactoglobulin	0.2 g
Whey protein	0.6 g
Fat	3.8 g
Lactose	7.0 g
Calcium	33 mg
Phosphorus	15 mg
Sodium	15 mg
Potassium	55 mg
Iron	0.15 mg
Vitamin A (as retinol)	16 µg
Carotenes (as retinol)	16 µg
Vitamin D	0.42 i.u.
Ascorbic acid	4.3 mg
Riboflavin	42 µg
Thiamine	16 µg
Nicotinic acid	172 µg

Source: Macy, I. G., Kelly, H. J., (in) *Milk: The Mammary Gland and Its Secretion.* Vol. **2**, pp. 275–277. Academic Press, London, 1961.

vitamin E, and other nutrients essential for growth, is higher in colostrum than either transitional or mature milk.

The protein contents of human milk remains constant even under stress. Despite undernutrition, disease, psychological stress, or a very heavy work output, the human female still manages to maintain a protein concentration in her milk that does not usually fall much below 0.9 grams per 100 ml. Slight variations are observed, but they may be due to the samples being taken at different times in lactation.

It has been noted in British women, that the protein content was as high as 1.4 grams per 100 ml during the first two weeks of lactation.[50] It then fell to 1.0 grams per 100 ml between third and sixth weeks of lactation. After this, there was a further fall to 0.91 grams per 100 ml of milk. In contrast to protein, the fat in human milk is subject to considerable variation. During a single feed, the fat content of the milk may rise from 0.45 to 6.25 grams per 100 ml of milk.[51] The late appearance of fat in the feed is probably due to the globules tending to adhere to the cells lining the milk ducts. The reluctance of the fat to leave the gland emphasizes the need to empty the breast completely at each feed. In addition to the variation during a feed, the fat secretion increases between 6 a.m. and 10 a.m. and declines during the rest of the day. Throughout lactation the variations in fat content are considerable, but as the milk matures the average fat content rises from 2.0 to 5.0 grams per 100 ml of milk.

Lactose levels rise during the first week of lactation. Initially there may be considerable day to day variation, but after about one month the level is stabilized, and there may be only a minor decline in concentration over the whole feed.

Minerals are of concern chiefly because breast milk contains minimal amounts of iron. Unless utilizable iron is made available from other dietary sources, anemia is inevitable, if breast feeding continues for more than six months.

Sodium levels in milk maintain osmotic stability, consequently breast milk neither hydrates, nor dehydrates, the infant tissues.

Vitamin A and carotene levels in colostrum are high. This helps to adjust the low blood concentrations of vitamin A and carotenes of the newborn baby.

Calcium, phosphorus and vitamin D are present in small amounts in human milk, nevertheless rickets is a rare disease in breastfed babies. It is believed that the high lactose concentration may enhance the absorption of the calcium. Vitamin D adequacy may be achieved by exposure of the infant skin to ultra-violet radiation.

Thiamine levels in breast milk are low; nevertheless infantile beri beri is only seen when the mothers intake has been inadequate. The intake of thiamine in the breast fed infant is much lower than that recommended but as ill effects are relatively rare, it would seem that the recommendations include a wide safety margin. Riboflavin is present in the colostrum and it increases during the first weeks of lactation, therefore the infant is well endowed with this vitamin.

Nicotinic acid is present in colostrum in higher concentrations than transitional or mature milks. There is little evidence that breast fed infants suffer from nicotinic acid deficiency. It has been noticed that the intake of maize and the nicotinic acid content of milk are inversely related. Mothers in South Africa consuming maize as a staple, had low levels of nicotinic acid in their milk whereas urban mothers on an omniverous diet had higher levels. However, even the maize-eating mothers had a higher concentration of nicotinic acid in their milk than levels found in cows milk.[52]

Vitamin C is present in high concentrations in the colostrum, the actual level being dependent on the maternal diet. Subsequent milk, in the transitional and mature phases, has lower concentrations but it is still adequate for the nutrition of the infant.

Water comprises approximately 87 per cent of human milk. It is essential to life and the role of breast milk in supplying this nutrient should not be overlooked. Water not only plays a major role in cellular metabolism but it also contributes to the temperature regulating mechanism of the infant body.

Humans appear to be able to produce milk that is subject to great variations in composition. However, there also appears to be an ability to maintain certain minimal nutrient concentrations in the milk despite a variety of stresses and adverse influences. There is little doubt that the quality and quantity of the milk supply is largely independant of the diet and nutritional state of the mother.[53,54] It would seem reasonable to assume that the characteristics of the milk secretion and composition are related to the nutrient needs of the infant.

Cows milk In view of the great differences between humans and cows, differences in composition of the two milks are to be expected. These are summarized in Table 12. Equal volumes of human milk are almost isocaloric. Cows milk contains, however, more protein, calcium, phosphorus, sodium, potassium, vitamin D, riboflavin and thiamine. It contains less lactose, iron, ascorbic acid, and nicotinic acid than human milk. It has been customary to dilute cows milk with water until the protein concentration of the two milks is approximately equal. The deficiency in calories is made up with sugar. This simplest of *modified* milks is an isocaloric product of equal protein value. It still differs in several ways from human milk, for example, it contains less lactose, ascorbic acid, vitamin A, iron, and nicotinic acid.

To compensate for these deficiencies, nutrients are added to the milk with the object of making the milk formula comparable with human milk. While these attempts to *humanize* milk may succeed quantitatively, there are still differences in the quality of the two milks. The protein in cows milk differs from human milk in several ways. The casein in both milks is similar chemically, but cows milk casein provides 80 per cent of the total protein, whereas human milk casein provides only 40 per cent of the total protein. This has some practical importance when the physical properties of the two caseins are compared. The curd formed by the casein in cows milk is much denser that the curd of human milk protein. The curd of

Table 12 Constituents of human milk compared with cows milk. Mean values per 100 ml of whole milk

Constituent	Human milk	Cows milk
Calories	71	69
Protein	1.2 g	3.3 g
Casein	0.4 g	2.8 g
Lactalbumin	0.3 g	0.4 g
Lactoglobulin	0.2 g	0.2 g
Whey protein	0.6 g	0.6 g
Fat	3.8 g	3.7 g
Lactose	7.0 g	4.8 g
Calcium	33 mg	125 mg
Phosphorus	15 mg	96 mg
Sodium	15 mg	58 mg
Potassium	55 mg	138 mg
Iron	0.15 mg	0.10 mg
Vitamin A (as retinol)	16 μg	10 μg
Carotenes (as retinol)	16 μg	22 μg
Vitamin D	0.42 i.u.	2.36 i.u.
Ascorbic acid	4.3 mg	1.6 mg
Riboflavine	42.6 μg	157.0 μg
Thiamine	16 μg	42 μg
Nicotinic acid	172 μg	85 μg

Source: Macy, I. G., Kelly, H, J., (in) *Milk: The Mammary Gland and Its Secretion*. Vol. **2**, pp. 275–277. Academic Press, London, 1961.

untreated cows milk is indigestible, consequently a high proportion of the total protein may not be available to the infant. The highly digestible whey of cows milk contains only 20 per cent of the total milk protein.

A large proportion of the calcium and phosphorus in cows milk may be bound up in the casein, so these minerals may not be available. Heat treatment which makes the curd digestible is now an established part of the technology of preparing milk formulae. Since some amino acids and vitamins such as thiamine and vitamin C are destroyed by heat, the nutritive value of the milk is adversely affected.[55]

The fat in modified cows milk is not only lower in concentration than human milk, but its physical characteristics also differ. In order to make the fat in cows milk similar to human milk, some manufacturers substitute butter fat with a mixture that resembles the fat of breast milk, in droplet size, degree of saturation, and fatty acid composition. Despite these additional modifications, difficulties in absorbing the fat and calcium have still been experienced by some babies.[56]

There are two possible explanations for malabsorption of fat of non-human origin. Human fat may be more readily absorbed because of its unusual glyceride structure. Alternatively the intestine of the young infant may be too immature and therefore unable to absorb non-human fat, as efficiently as the fat in human milk.

The mineral content of cows milk is more than three times greater than human milk. Even when it is diluted, cows milk remains more concentrated than either colostrum, transitional or mature milk. The infant kidney is limited in its ability to concentrate urine, hence the electrolyte load induced by the consumption of cows milk, and the water balance of the infant, are very important.

The quantity of water excreted in the urine depends on the intake of water, the water produced by metabolic processes, and the water lost through the skin and lungs. If a child is fed undiluted cows milk and then subjected to heat stress (which is quite likely, if he is heavily clothed and kept in heated rooms), it is possible that the limits of physiological concentration of urine may be reached. It has been shown however that if the formula is diluted to a concentration equivalent to human milk, the infant kidney is able to concentrate the urine adequately despite heat stress.[57] Manufacturers have continued in their attempts to *humanize* cows milk. A typical product of modern technology uses whey, with added casein from dried skimmed milk, so that the ratio of lactalbumin to casein is the same as that in human milk. Lactose is added and excess electrolytes removed. The fatty acid composition and droplet size of human milk is copied to the limits of existing knowledge. Vitamins which may have been destroyed by heat treatment are replaced, or added in excess of the quantities normally found in human milk. Similarly, minerals such as iron may be added in the belief that the quantities in human milk are marginal for proper nutrition.

The technical problems in preparing these humanized milks are matched by the difficulties of evaluating them. The achievement of rapid growth is often assumed to be an index of good nutrition. There is no evidence to show that the fastest growing baby is the healthiest baby, nor is it certain that the biggest baby, or the baby who stores most nigrogen, or calcium, has a greater advantage. Growth rates can be determined from increases in body length, but they are difficult to measure accurately over short intervals of time.

The habit of feeding cows milk to infants is well established. In many highly industrialized countries, cows milk is the only source of food for the majority of infants during the first few months of life. Convenience and social pressures have been given as the main reasons for the change. In the United States, it is claimed formula feeding is less costly than breast feeding.[58]

This claim assumes the lactating mother needs a supplementary diet to meet the additional nutrient requirements of lactation. The cost of this supplement is considerably more than the cost of infant formulae based on cows milk, modified cows milk, or evaporated milk. It has also been assumed lactating mothers require vitamin supplements throughout lactation.

In developing countries milk formulae are relatively expensive, local foods to supplement the diets of lactating women are cheaper. If the lactating mother is consuming an adequate mixed diet, vitamin supplementation may not be necessary, except in areas where vitamin A, D, and C deficiencies are prevalent.

Modified milks The food industry has provided a wide variety of foods for feeding infants to meet the increasing demand for milk formulae. In the United States, more cows milk is consumed by infants during their first year of life than all other types of milk or milk substitutes. Throughout most of the world, the choice of preparation lies between fresh cows milk, evaporated milk, premodified milk, or *ready-to-use* formulae. In highly industrialized countries milk is usually pasteurized or sterilized; it may be homogenized and it may be fortified with vitamin D. In many countries, raw milk of good quality and free from pathogenic organisms, is not available. For these reasons, most milks are subjected to heat treatment, these processes include pasteurization, boiling, or sterilization. The milk may be bottled, put in cartons, marketed as a concentrated liquid or in the form of a dry powder. The high butterfat content of milks may be reduced by separating off some of the fat, leaving a residual percentage of two to three per cent. Such products are known as *low-fat* milks.

Concentrated liquid milks These are prepared by heat treatment in vacuum pans which removes the water from the milk. Evaporated milk is concentrated until about half of the original volume of water is removed; it is then homogenized, cooled, canned, and sterilized. Most evaporated milk is fortified with vitamin D.

In the preparation of condensed milk, raw milk and dried milk are mixed and evaporated to one quarter volume. Sweetened condensed milk contains up to 42 per cent of sugar added to the mixture prior to evaporation. At this high concentration, sugar acts as a preservative; condensed milk therefore keeps well and does not freeze in cold climates. Typical analyses of evaporated and condensed milks are given in Table 13. The high carbohydrate content of condensed milk places a considerable load on the infant kidney function, because of this, condensed milk is considered unsuitable for infants.

Evaporated milk can be the basis of a safe, adequate, infant food, but because of its cost, or because mothers may not know how to prepare a proper formula, there is a tendency for the milk to be over-diluted. Naturally, the dilute formula fails to supply the required nutrients.

Table 13 Nutrient composition of raw and processed milks

Food	(Values per 100 g) Protein	Fat	Carbohydrate	Sodium	Calcium
	g	g	g	mg	mg
Milk, fresh Whole	3.4	3.7	4.8	50	120
Milk, fresh Skimmed	3.5	0.2	5.1	52	124
Milk, condensed Unsweetened	7.8	8.4	12.3	161	290
Milk, condensed Sweetened	8.2	12.0	56.0	143	344
Evaporated milk (Dilute 1 : 1)	3.5	3.8	4.8	59	126

Sources: McCance, R. A., Widdowson, R. M., Special Report Series No. 297. Third Impression. H. M. S. O. 1969. Composition of Foods Agriculture Handbook No. 8, U. S. D. A. 1963.

Dehydrated milk The water in raw milk which amounts to 87 per cent of its total composition, is removed under vacuum. Dried whole milk prepared in this way may be reconstituted with water and fed to infants. It is frequently transported on a large scale as a powder and may be mixed with water at a central distributing point as *reconstituted* milk.

During the preparation of skimmed milk, all the butter fat is removed before drying and it is therefore deficient in fatty acids and the fat soluble vitamins. Although the vitamins are sometimes replaced, skimmed milk is still deficient in calories and unsuitable for feeding infants. It has a very useful function however in providing the growing infant and child with a protein supplement. It forms the basis of many supplementary weaning foods and as the immediate therapy for protein calorie malnutrition.

Premodified milks are marketed in powder form and are diluted with water before feeding. The various proprietary brands differ in the content of sugar, minerals, fat, iron, vitamin C and vitamin A, but most are fortified with vitamin D so that the diluted formula, when fed at the required level, will meet the minimum daily requirement for this vitamin. The variation in composition of these milks (see Table 14) is an indication of the dis-

Table 14 Approximate analyses of commonly used infant formulas

Standard formulas	Normal dilution	Cal/ Oz.	Percentage Fat	Protein	CHO	Per qt. Normal dilution Units A	Units D	mg C	mg Iron
Baker's									
Infant formula	1 : 1	20	3.3	2.2	7.0	2500	400	50	7.5
Bremil	1 : 1	20	3.5	1.5	7.0	2500	400	50	Trace
Carnalac	1 : 1	20	2.7	2.4	8.2	1035	400	80	Trace
Cow's Milk									
(undiluted)	—	20	4.1	3.5	5.0	946	38	17	Trace
Enfamil	1 : 1	20	3.7	1.5	7.0	1500	400	50	1.4
Evaporated 1 : 2	1 : 2	15	2.7	2.4	3.4	800	265	—	Trace
Formil	1 : 1	20	3.5	1.65	7.0	2500	400	50	Trace
Human Milk	—	20	3.8	1.25	7.0	1419	95	40	Trace
Lactum	1 : 1	20	2.8	2.7	7.8	400	400	2	Trace
Modilac	1 : 1	20	2.7	2.15	7.7	1500	400	45	10
Optimil	1 : 1	20	3.8	1.47	7.2	2500	400	80	8
Purevap	1 : 2	20	2.6	2.3	8.0	800	400	—	Trace
Similac	1 : 1	20	3.4	1.7	6.6	2500	400	50	Trace
SMA S-26	1 : 1	20	3.6	1.5	7.2	2500	400	50	7.5

Source: *Handbook of Infant Formulas*. J. B. Roerig Division, Chas. Pfizer. New York, 1967.

parity of views on what is considered adequate food for the growth, development, and maintenance of health, of the infant.

Ready-made formulae are prepared by manufacturers for use nationally or on a more local scale. Hospitals for example, may produce ready-to-use formulae for use in the maternity and pediatric wards. The ready-to use formulae in disposable packages are undoubtedly convenient, but the extra cost of packaging adds considerably to the price.

Imitation and filled milks   In recent years, foodstuffs packaged in a similar manner to those containing milk products and ostensibly serving as replacements for fresh milk have appeared on the market. For the most part they are cheaper than fresh milk and it is inevitable that the public will be attracted by their low price. Although common sense suggests that the nutritive value of such foodstuffs should be examined carefully if they are to be the basis of an infant feeding regime, very little information is available on their effects on growth and health. The foodstuffs fall into two categories, *Filled Milk* and *Imitation Milk*.

Filled milk is prepared in two ways, the first uses fluid skim milk with added vegetable fat, and the second uses dried skimmed milk with added water, vegetable fat, and protein supplied by either milk casein or soya. Vitamins may be added in both processes.

Imitation milk is a white liquid consisting of vegetable fat, water, protein, sugar and other non-dairy ingredients. Imitation milk has better keeping qualities than fresh milk but it has a lower calorie content. The protein is usually soya protein, with or without casein; vitamin A and D may be added. The nutritive value of these foods depends mainly on the quality of the protein and fat used in its preparation.

Imitation milk contains only one per cent of protein, if this is provided by soya protein its biological value will not be as high as cows milk because of a deficiency of methionine. In view of the low concentration and doubtful quality of the protein, imitation milks should not be used for infant feeding.

Coconut oil is used mainly in the manufacture of filled milk. It is saturated highly, however, and it also contains lauric acid, both of these two chemical properties are associated with the development of high blood cholesterol levels.

In addition to this, coconut oil also lacks linoleic acid, an essential fatty acid. It would therefore seem unwise to use filled milk based on coconut oil alone. The nutritional inadequacies of coconut oil have been recognized by some manufacturers, who supplement the fat in filled milk with other vegetable oils. Ground nut oil, and cotton seed oil are widely used in industry.

Other dairy products In many countries, milk is soured by the bacterial breakdown of the sugar present in milk, lactic acid is formed. Souring may also be achieved by artificial agents such as *rennet*. Souring takes about 24 hours to complete; at the end of this time, the sour milk, or *yogurt*, contains all the protein, fat, and calcium, of whole milk. In hot climates, where contamination of milk and water supplies with pathogenic organisms is likely, yogurt is a much safer food product than raw milk. There are many different preparations of yogurt, depending on whether cows, goats, sheep, or buffalo, supply the milk.

The temperature at which souring takes place, also affects the character of the product. Mares milk fermented in a warm atmosphere contains a small amount of alcohol and is known as *koumiss* in Russia, and Central Asia.

Cheese is made from milk that has been clotted by rennet, or curdled by bacteria or acids. The clot, or curd, contains most of the protein in the milk and it entangles fat and other nutrients. The curd is then removed from the whey, and pressed into a cake and allowed to "ripen" by fermentation. The type of microorganism used, determines the particular flavor of the cheese.

The introduction of molds during the ripening process, provides the cheese with its characteristic coloration.

The amount of pressure applied to express the whey, determines its physical characteristics. Light pressure produces a soft cheese, whereas heavy pressure will produce a hard cheese.

Other differences in quality may be attributed to the fat content of the milk. Some cheeses use skimmed milk, while others use milk with added cream.

Meat Carcase meat is usually considered as muscle. However, most "cuts" of meat, even when prepared by professional butchers, contain connective tissue (gristle) and fat. The quantity of fat on any animal depends on several factors, including its diet prior to death. It is well known that some animals are "fattened" prior to slaughter. Since a cold environment encourages the deposition of fat, cattle reared in temperate zones have more carcase fat than those raised in the tropics. Selective breeding has also produced breeds which have fat deposited between the groups of muscles in addition to the subcutaneous fat. This *marbling* is associated with "tenderness" and is considered a sign of excellence in North America. In some breeds of African and Indian domesticated cattle, fat is deposited between the muscle fibrils but is not visible to the naked eye.

For these reasons the calorie value of carcase meat varies and estimations of the energy content of meat are subject to large errors. The protein has a high biological value, and is in the range of 16–24 per cent of the total weight of the raw meat. In addition to providing calories and protein, meat is also a source of minerals and vitamins of the B group. Cooked meat loses water and shrinks, consequently it has more food value for a given weight than raw meat.

Since man first started to hunt animals, and eat meat, he has been faced with the problems of preserving the surplus for his future use. The discovery of fire and roasting flesh no doubt allowed primitive man to stretch his supplies further. Smoking of the meat followed, but its adoption depended on the availability of fuel. Several other processes enabled him to store meat for prolonged periods.

Freezing of meat in the arctic wastes is a well known method of food preservation and is practised by Eskimos, the North American Indians and the inhabitants of Northern Europe. Frost drying of reindeer meat is in reality a freeze dried product involving the evaporation of water from the frozen meat. In the preparation of *pemmican*, meat is embedded in fat. In Latin America, fat is also used to seal jars filled with roasted meat.

Drying of meat, either in the sun or by fire, is another effective method of preserving meat. In South Africa, the former method is used in the preparation of *biltong*; in Brazil the dried meat is known as *xarqui* from which the term *jerky* is derived.

Many centuries ago, the Chinese discovered how to pickle meat in salt. In Europe the use of salt and *saltpeter* has reached a high degree of sophistication and is used to preserve pork, bacon and ham.

Fermentation is also used in Europe to prepare *summer sausages* and *salami*. The distinctive flavors of these foods is provided by cultures of micro organisms.

Mammalian organs   Heart, liver, pancreas, kidney, brain, and intestines are highly edible foods. The nutritive value of each varies, but in general they all provide high quality protein, minerals and vitamins of the B group.

Heart is denser than skeletal muscle, it contains vitamin A and considerable amounts of thiamine, riboflavin and nicotinic acid. Since heart muscle is less digestible than some of the skeletal muscle, nutrients may not be available for utilization by the body. Liver has very little connective tissue and it is consequently easily digested. In addition to providing high quality protein, liver also contains more vitamins than skeletal muscle; it is especially rich in vitamin A, riboflavin, and iron. Kidneys are also good sources of high quality protein, iron, vitamin A, and the vitamins of the B group. Pancreas is extremely cellular and digestible. It is also a source of nucleic acids so it should not be consumed by sufferers of gout who are unable to metabolize purine, a product of nucleic acid breakdown. Brain contains large amounts of lipids including phospolipids. It is digested quickly, but it is not absorbed readily; brain is not such a valuable food as the raw composition would suggest. Intestines and the stomach are easily digested and well absorbed; they are a good source of high quality protein. Since the stomach is treated with lime during preparation the calcium content is greatly increased.

Birds The breast of non flying birds is tender and digestible but their legs are tough. The legs of flying birds on the other hand, are far more tender than the walking, wading, or swimming birds. The nutrient content of bird flesh does not differ materially from that of mammalian flesh. The aquatic birds tend to have more fat than terrestial species, consequently the total calorie content of duck and goose flesh is higher than chickens or guinea fowl.

Fish Variations in the composition of fish flesh are caused by differences in the fat content. Even within a species there are annual and seasonal variations which may be a response to changes in water temperature. The fish of colder waters develop more fat than those of tropical seas. Some fresh water fish survive prolonged drought by burying themselves in the mud, they have a very high fat content prior to *estivation*. The eel may have 17 per cent of its carcase weight in the form of fat.

On average, fish flesh is comprised of approximately 10 per cent of protein but the actual percentage composition depends on the form in which the fish is consumed. The protein has a high biological value. Smoking and drying increases the protein content considerably; the nutritive value also depends on whether the bones are consumed. When small fish are consumed whole, the bones add considerably to the calcium content of the diet. This is especially important in cereal eaters who may have an inadequate intake of calcium. The fish oils of certain fish, namely cod, halibut, and shark, are rich sources of vitamins A and D. The roe of fish contains 20–25 per cent of protein, rich in nucleic acids.

The keeping quality of fish is not good, and a variety of processes have been developed which prevent spoilage. Freezing, drying, and pickling in brine, are the usual methods of preserving fish in temperate and colder climates.

In the warmer areas of the world, drying is usually accompanied by fermentation. This is carried to the extreme in the preparation of *nuoc-mam* in Vietnam. The final result of this fermentation process being a colorless fish hydrolysate, loaded with water soluble amino acids.

Where spoilage is rapid, because of high environmental temperatures, fish is roasted and preserved in fat, in a like manner to meat. The addition of salt to fish, inhibits the growth of pathogenic organisms. The salted fish heads of the Eskimo, and the herrings and trout of Scandinavia which appear to have decomposed, are quite wholesome. The preservation of fresh fish in brine was known to the Romans who added vinegar as an aid in the preparation of *garum*. This practice still exists in the specialized Italian cooking of the present day.

The curing of fish with smoke is universal but in Northern England this process has been developed further. The smoke of aromatic woods is used to cure herrings, the process being known as *kippering*.

Crustaceans   These have large indigestible muscle fibres, the flesh has a relatively low calorie content. Nevertheless, shrimps, prawns, and lobsters are a valuable source of protein for populations subsisting on predominantly vegetable diets of poor biological value.

Shellfish   Oysters, clams, and mussels, contain more protein than some marine fish. The edible parts contain about eight per cent protein and four per cent carbohydrate which is mainly in the form of glycogen. The edible parts are readily digested when eaten raw, the digestibility decreases with cooking. Shellfish are a good source of iron, iodine and copper. Oysters are frequently found near sources of excreta, consequently they may be responsible for the transmission of enteric disease. Other marine foods such as cuttlefish, squid, octopus and the sea cucumber are eaten with relish by some peoples around the world, to others, these foods are unacceptable. Very little is known of their nutritive value and the availability of their protein and iodine content.

Insects, grubs, snails and small animals   These are consumed by many groups throughout the world. In Africa, locusts and white ants are fried and eaten; the "lake flies" of the large lakes are made into cakes and are considered a delicacy by local tribes. The sago grub may make a significant contribution to the diet of some New Guinea tribes.[59] In Europe the snail has a limited acceptability. The consumption of small animals such as rabbits, guinea pigs, rats, and other vermin, depends on the attitudes prevailing in the culture. Some animals, like dogs, are highly regarded as food by many Asian populations, yet the thought of using this food source would arouse strong feelings of revulsion in most European countries.

The contribution of protein, calories, and other nutrients from insects, to marginal diets is unknown. It has been reported frequently that some communities live on very low intakes of protein. It is very difficult, however, to make an accurate record of the intakes of food in populations with haphazard eating habits that include casual gleaning. It is easy to overlook the random consumption of insects, grubs, and other bizarre foods that may convert a marginal diet into one adequate in quantity and quality.

Eggs   Chicken eggs provide protein of high quality; they also provide vitamin A, riboflavin, nicotinic acid, thiamine, calcium, and iron. They do not, however, contain ascorbic acid. Eggs of other birds have virtually the same composition. Modern technology has succeeded in drying eggs in order to absorb surplus production. Dried egg is not highly regarded as a food but it is used in the baking industry. Outbreaks of *salmonella* food poisoning have been reported from time to time. It is believed the pathogens are able to pass though the egg apparatus of the hen into the egg. If the egg is inadequately treated by heat during the drying process, transmission of the disease becomes possible.

In addition to the customary household preparation of eggs by boiling or frying, there are other methods of preparing eggs. The Chinese have devised a novel method of preserving eggs by a chemical process that takes about four weeks to complete. Because of their appearance, eggs prepared in this way are known as "1000 year old eggs". In the Philippines, duck eggs are incubated for a period of 17 days before being eaten. The embryonic food is known as *balut* and is eaten as a snack; its biological value must be high.

Foodstuffs of vegetable origin

Cereals   These include wheat, barley, oats, rice, maize (corn), millet, and sorghum. They form the staple diets for most populations; the health and life of many millions of people depend on regular crops. The failure of cereal grops because of droughts, floods, locust plagues, and plant disease has been the cause of many of the major famines of the world.

The climate and topography of the land determines to a large extent the type of cereal grown. Wheat is found in the more temperate regions, but it is also cultivated in the highlands of equatorial areas. Rice is found predominantly where there is a high rainfall. Maize is the only cereal originating from the Americas; it is now widely cultivated in Europe, Africa, Asia, and the Pacific.

Cereals provide a cheap and concentrated source of energy, they are also a valuable source of protein. Six to thirteen per cent of the grain is protein but it has a limited biological value; mixtures of cereals tend to overcome this problem and provide the body with a reasonable balance of amino acids. Whole grains are good sources of minerals and vitamins of the B group; during milling and cooking the nutritive value of the grain may be reduced considerably (see Figure 9).

The bran is comprised mainly of cellulose, a material useless as a human food. This outer layer is removed therefore, either by handpounding or by machine-milling the grain. During this process some of the other parts of the cereal grain are removed also, including the aleurone layer, the germ,

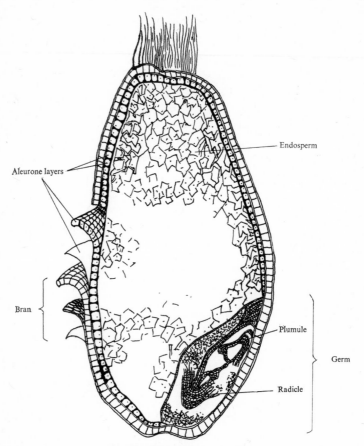

Figure 9   Diagrammatic section of a typical cereal grain

and the endosperm. All of these parts are rich in nutrients. In a typical grain such as wheat, the aleurone layer contains riboflavin and nicotinic acid, the germ contains protein, fats, thiamine, riboflavin, nicotinic acid and minerals. The endosperm contains carbohydrates and a little protein and fat. Thiamine, riboflavin, and nicotinic acid are water soluble. Considerable losses of these nutrients can occur of the processing requires the grain to be soaked in water which is discarded afterwards. The more the grain is milled, the greater is the loss of the aleurone layer and the germ. Highly milled cereals therefore contain much less protein and vitamins than lightly milled products. The degree of milling also affects the utilization of the nutrients. Lightly milled cereals are far less digestible than highly milled grains (see Table 15). A coarse grain may have a high nutrient content but because it is indigestible, the nutrients may not be as readily available as the more highly milled product. This has considerable significance in evaluating the nutritive value of cereals *as consumed*. The depreciation of the nutritive value of cereals during milling has prompted experimentation with *fortification* or enrichment of cereal grains, with added nutrients (see page 485).

In order to meet the world demand for cereals, plant geneticists have been breeding high yielding varieties. Although the protein content of the grains may be increased by selective breeding, the essential amino acids may not be increased proportionately.

Table 15   Digestibility of wheat flours

Wheat flour % extraction	Digestibility
75 (refined white flour)	97.0
85	93.9
90	91.5
95	88.7
100 (whole meal)	86.3

Source: Nicholls, L., Sinclair, H. M., Jelliffe, D. B. *Tropical Nutrition and Dietetics*, p. 187, 4th Ed. Bailliere Tindall and Cox, London 1961.

Wheat   More wheat is grown than any other cereal, almost all of it is converted into flour. The whole grain may be soaked and boiled, it has been used in this way in remote parts of Europe where it constituted a considerable part of the daily intake of food.

Wheat flour is used in the preparation of bread, either unleavened or leavened. In recent years, bread made from pure white flour has much greater prestige than whole meal (brown) bread. Because of this, many communities are depriving themselves of much needed nutrients. By careful milling, a white flour of acceptable appearance and with a high nutritive value can be prepared. In England, during the second world war, millers and scientists collaborated to produce a *National Flour* with an extraction rate of 82 per cent, most of the nutrients were retained however. Since that time, the trend in many countries has been to disregard nutritional qualities and produce a flour highly acceptable from the point of view of keeping qualities, baking qualities, and appearance. The use of chemicals to achieve these objectives is now commonplace. Some years ago the chemical *agene* was added to bread, subsequently it was found to be toxic. It is hoped that this experience will keep governments alert to the potential dangers of such practises.

Elsewhere in the world, wheat is used in other ways. In India and Pakistan, whole meal wheat flour (*atta*) is made into *chappaties*. In Chinese cultures, it forms the basis of *noodles*, and in South East Europe, wheat is consumed in the form of pastas such as spaghetti, macaroni, and vermicelli. Biscuits, *pizzas*, cakes, and pastries, are also made from wheat flour and they are being consumed in increasing amounts in many countries. As the trend is to use highly refined flour, this practise could have adverse effects on public health.

Rice Rice is cultivated on a large scale in many Asian, African, and American countries. The breeding of high-yield varieties of rice, appeared at first, to be one answer to the world food shortage. There are indications, however, that new varieties may be susceptible to disease; ultimate benefits may depend on breeding resistant varieties.

Many strains of rice are cultivated to meet the individual tastes of populations, some of whom prefer a glutinous rice, while others may prefer a long grained rice which is so dry the grains tend to separate. Rice is usually consumed as a grain but rice flour is also used in the preparation of gruels and cakes.

In the past, the milling and polishing of rice has been responsible for beri beri, a disease that has caused widespread morbidity and mortality in Asia. The disease is being controlled in two ways. In the first method, the grain is soaked and boiled prior to milling, a process known as *parboiling*. Formerly this procedure was used only on a household scale but now much of the commercial milling of rice is parboiled by steam. While the grain is being soaked and heated, the water soluble vitamins, thiamine and riboflavin, are distributed more evenly throughout the endosperm so that much of these nutrients are conserved after milling and polishing is completed.The effectiveness of this technique is shown in Table 16. The nutritive value of polished rice may be restored by enrichment of the grain. Premixes of vitamins are added to the milled rice, therefore the final product should have a nutritive value equivalent to the raw product. After cooking, the rice may have a patchy yellow coloration caused by the addition of riboflavin; this frequently detracts from its acceptability. It must also be remembered however, that the thiamine still left in, or on, the grain after parboiling or enrichment, is also liable to be lost during washing and cooking.

Table 16 Thiamine content of milled rice

Percentage of bran removed	Thiamine content in milled product from raw rice	from parboiled rice
0	3.5	2.5
6	2.6	2.5
8	2.3	2.5
12	1.6	2.4
15	0.9	2.3
20	0.5	2.2

Source: Nicholls, L., Sinclair, H. M., Jelliffe, D. B., *Tropical Nutrition and Dietetics*, p. 200. 4th Ed. Bailliere Tindall and Cox. London 1961.

Maize This cereal is also known as corn in many parts of the world. In highly industrialized countries it is frequently considered an animal food, but it provides a staple for large sections of the world populations. It has achieved popularity because it can grow in adverse conditions of soil and climate.

Plant geneticists have also influenced maize production by breeding strains of grain of varying shape, size and color. Some of the yellow and red varieties contain more carotenes, (the precursors of vitamin A), than the white variety. They have been introduced from the United States and elsewhere, to developing countries in an effort to meet local food demands and to promote international good will. Unfortunately, it has been overlooked that the color of the grain is culturally important. Consequently, many populations have refused to accept red and yellow varieties of corn.

Where the introduction of these strains has taken place other effects have been noted. New strains of red and yellow maize which have been planted by accident or design in proximity to domestic crops of white corn have genetically "tainted" the latter, causing considerable concern to both cultivators and consumers whose food preferences have been insulted. The main nutritional shortcoming of maize is that it is deficient in nicotinic acid, consequently pellagra is prevalent among populations who use maize as a staple.

Maize can be prepared in a variety of ways. The grain may be cracked and boiled, or it may be cracked, soaked and allowed to ferment. It may be hand or machine milled dry, or it may be soaked and pounded. The flour may be mixed with boiling water to form a gruel or dough of varying consistencies.

In Mexico, the grain is soaked in lime water, heated, and allowed to stand for a day or so, it is then ground and made into flat cakes and cooked quickly. This method of preparation greatly increases the calcium content of the maize. The use of an iron plate may also increase its iron content. Soaking in lime water, and heating also probably distributes the vitamins throughout the grain and helps to maintain the vitamin content of the flour.

In the industrialized parts of the world, maize flour is used as a basis for cakes and puddings. Unfortunately in the impoverished parts of these countries, highly refined flour, which is little more than starch, is cheap and it is consequently being used on an increasing scale as a staple food for adults and children.

Because of the high oil content of maize, and the association of the consumption of saturated fatty acids with cardiovascular disease, consumer demand for oils containing unsaturated fatty acids has increased. The high unsaturated fat content of maize has provided an incentive for increasing the commercial extraction of corn oil from maize. What effect this will have on the availability of highly refined maize flour or starch is conjectural but it is conceivable that these products may become cheaper, and more available to the poor.

Maize also forms the basis of native beers in many parts of the world. While the social ill effects of alcoholism are not challenged, it must be remembered that the alcohol and other nutrients may contribute as much as 500 calories per pint of beer.[60] Beer may be important in ensuring the success of essential communal work efforts such as clearing the bush or felling trees. The fermentation of the beers may also add to the nutritive value of the diet, because beer prepared from sprouting grains contains large amounts of vitamin C. The vitamin B content is also usually increased and may provide a much needed supplement to the diet.

Millets Several millets are consumed by humans throughout Africa, America and Asia. Attitudes toward these cereals varies, in Europe sorghum is used for feeding pet birds. In North America the stalk is crushed and used as a syrup, and the cereal grain is frequently considered to be fit only for consumption by cattle, but in Africa and Asia whole populations depend on it as a staple food. Attempts have been made to produce varieties that are resistant both to drought and to the ravages of birds. Some varieties have been bred which are indeed too bitter for birds but they also tend to be unacceptable to humans. Sorghum flour is frequently discolored which also detracts from its acceptability.

Because of the higher yields of maize, and its ability to grow in more unfavorable circumstances, the use of sorghum is decreasing. This is unfortunate because sorghum contains more calcium and nicotinic acid than maize. Pellagra frequently appears in areas where maize replaces sorghum as a staple food. It is usually consumed as a thin gruel or as a dough, but sorghum beer is a popular beverage. Like maize beer it contains more vitamins than the raw cereal because of the natural enrichment brought about by sprouting and fermentation.

Bulrush millet (*Pennisetum*) and *Finger Millet* (*Eleusine*) are also consumed in India and Africa. Millet is likely to ripen rapidly and then dehisce so that much of the harvest may be lost. Beers are prepared from both varieties but among certain East African tribes the Eleusine millet is reserved for the preparation of beer for consumption only by pregnant women. It is interesting to note that the Eleusine grain contains approximately 20 times as much calcium as other cereal grains and could therefore be a most valuable contribution to the diet of the gravid female.

Oats This cereal has a husk that can only be separated from the kernel with difficulty. Because of this, it usually contains a high percentage of fibre. The cereal has a high content of protein and fat but its calcium is probably not available because of the coincidental presence of phytin, with which it forms an insoluble compound. A staple diet based on oats should include another source of calcium to compensate for any possible deficiency in the availability of the calcium in the oats.

Rye This is a cereal of the cooler climates where it may be consumed as black bread, but because of its poor digestibility much of the nutritive value of this food may be lost.

Starchy roots and fruits

Foods from this group are of importance because of their calorie content; they are widely and increasingly used as staples. Some of them, like cassava in the tropics, and the potato in Europe, are very cheap sources of energy.

They are easy to grow and give good yields. Others like plantain, provide a very poor return for cost.

The Irish (or Common) Potato   The potato was introduced from South America into Europe where it is now the staple food in most countries in that region. It is also grown in the cooler mountainous parts of the tropics. The potato has saved many countries from famine but too much dependence on this food has led to national catastrophes such as the *Irish Potato Famine* of the 19th Century, when over one million lives were estimated to be lost. Such disasters are not confined however to potatoes; they are a constant hazard when only one crop is grown.

In England, potatoes replaced bread as a staple in the middle of the early nineteenth century. The change was probably precipitated by the industrial revolution that brought not only urban development but also problems of distributing and processing cereal grains. This same phenomenon is being observed in many parts of the developing world. Not only have cereals of good nutritional value (*sorghum*) been replaced by those having lesser value (such as *maize*) but even maize is now being replaced by *cassava*. This trend is undoubtedly associated with the higher yields of cassava and maize compared with other crops. Although there is no question that the foods in this group are nutritionally inferior to cereals, they make a significant contribution to the diet. Despite the small vitamin content of many of the roots and tubers, so much is consumed that they provide adequate amounts of some of the essential nutrients. This is especially important to the manual worker who may not be able to afford to pay the price of more expensive sources of these vitamins.

While potato has a protein content of two percent some of this is in a form which is unavailable to the human body. Potatoes are also a very important source of vitamin C. The actual quantity of the vitamin available at the time of consumption varies according to the losses during storage and cooking. Because of the large quantities eaten, these losses are offset and the total intake is usually sufficient to prevent scurvy.

Sweet potatoes   A number of varieties of sweet potatoes are suitable for consumption; their protein content is low although the biological value is reasonably high. Some of the varieties contain the yellow or red pigments of carotenes; they are also a good source of vitamin C. The leaves of the sweet potato are edible so that the consumption of the whole plant makes a very useful contribution to the intakes of both vitamin A and C.

Yams   These are perennial climbing plants, the wild varieties contain poisonous substances, but selective cultivation has produced a tuber that is a good energy source and safe to eat. They also provide protein and small amounts of vitamins of the *B* group as well as vitamin C.

Cassava (Manioc) This is a shrub which originated in South America, but it is widely cultivated in Africa, Asia and the Pacific Region where it is propagated with remarkable ease from cuttings. It was introduced in many places as a famine and cash crop, for the processed root can be manufactured commercially into starch and tapioca. Cassava has enormous yields and the crop is rarely lost because of adverse climatic conditions. The root can also be harvested throughout the year which is a great advantage. Cassava has become firmly entrenched as a staple; because of this and its lack of protein and other nutrients, it is responsible for widespread deficiency disease.

The outer coats of the root are a source of *hydrogen cyanide* but after peeling and washing, the root is relatively safe and can be dried, roasted, boiled, or pounded, into a flour. It is a popular food because it 'fills the stomach', but it requires supplementation with other nutrients, including good quality protein, before it can be considered a safe staple food for growing children.

The leaves of cassava are also eaten, the leaf protein probably makes a valuable contribution to the biological value of the total protein intake. Little is known of the relationship between the nutritive value and the physical state, and age of the leaf, but the African housewife takes great care in selecting leaves of a particular size, color and texture.

Plantain and bananas The plantain is usually cooked before eating and the banana is usually consumed raw. The unripe plantain may be dried, pounded and made into a flour, and the ripe plantain is normally boiled or steamed. The carbohydrate in these fruits provides a good source of calories, but the protein value is low. Consequently when used as a staple the fruit needs supplementation with good protein. The ripe banana provides a convenient introductory weaning food because it is easily prepared. Banana is practically uncontaminated with micro-organisms when eaten straight from its pod and it is easily digested. Banana is, however, totally inadequate as a protein source for growth or even maintainance of body function. For unknown reasons, banana eaters are far less liable to diarrhea when suffering from protein calorie malnutrition, than cereal eaters.

Legumes, pulses, nuts and seeds

In diets that are almost entirely vegetable in origin, this group is of the greatest nutritional importance. Most of the foods in this group contain useful amounts of protein of good biological value. A very good intake of good quality protein can be achieved when the diet is composed of a mixture of cereals and foods such as beans and peas. Many diets in impoverished areas are based on legumes and pulses but they have little status. A desire for sophistication may motivate people to abandon the basically sound nutritional practice of eating legumes and adopt other nutritionally inadequate, but prestigious foods. A diet based on an intake of cereal and beans, with small amounts of meat or fish will have a greater nutritional value than a diet based on white bread (that the family can ill afford) supplemented infrequently, by small amounts of animal protein.

The term *legume* is usually applied to beans and peas in the *fresh* state; in the *dry* state they are known as *pulses*.

Dried pulses may contain as much as 20 per cent of protein. Most pulses are poor sources of fat, with the exception of the soya bean and the ground nut (peanut) which may contain up to 40 per cent of fat. Beans and peas are good sources of calcium and vitamins of the B complex, some also contain carotenes. The vitamin C content of pulses is poor, unless the seed is allowed to sprout, when considerable quantities of this vitamin are generated.

Because of their high protein content and other nutritive advantages, legumes have been advocated as an answer to protein calorie nalnutrition. However, they tend to be indigestible, in addition much of the carbohydrate is unavailable. The carbohydrate is broken down in the intestines and may cause flatulence. In young children who need a protein source during the weaning period, beans and peas could provide an answer to the protein deficiencies which are a feature of weaning. Even in this age group legume preparations are frequently unacceptable to the young. There is a great need for further information relating to the availability of the nutrients in legumes, their digestibility, and legume dishes that will promote growth and still be acceptable as a weaning food.

Soya beans and ground nuts   Both have assumed commercial importance because of their high oil content. The protein residue, a byproduct of the vegetable oil industry has been used in the past as the basis of animal feeds. Recently, attention has focused on the use of soya and ground nuts as a source of protein for human consumption. Infant foods based on ground nut flour received a serious setback with the discovery that the nuts may acquire dangerous toxins during storage (see page 96 and 97). The biological value of the protein in ground nuts is also limited by deficiencies of the amino acids methionine and lysine.

The outlook for soya is much more favorable but the bean requires special preparation to overcome some undesirable properties. These include failure of the bean to soften during cooking, so it remains hard and indigestible. Soya beans also contain a substance which inhibits the action of trypsin, a digestive enzyme that breaks up protein. It is unfortunate also that the trypsin inhibitor and other substances impart a bitter flavor to the bean. These problems can be overcome by grinding the bean into a flour and heating it, to destroy the trypsin inhibiting factor. Such procedures are a routine part of the commercial preparation of soya beans. In the domestic household, the soya bean is usually consumed as a fermented food, the preparation of which overcomes the difficulties mentioned above. Reports of the fermentation of soya date back to 2000 B. C. in China. During the fermentation process, molds and micro-organisms are used to make the beans accessible to the digestive juices.

Tofu is a Japanese food resembling cottage cheese. In the first stage of preparation the beans are milled, soaked, and the fluid expressed. This is known as soya 'milk'. Calcium salts are then added which brings its calcium content up to approximately twice as much as that of cows milk. Tofu can be further treated by a mold, the final product is known as *sufu*.

Miso is a preparation utilizing the fungus *Aspergillus oryzae* and other micro-organisms normally found in association with the rice grain. The rice fungus requires phosphorus and calcium, this is provided by the addition of a vegetable ash to the culture medium. These elements are incorporated in the final product which also includes alcohols and lactic acid produced during fermentation.

Soya sauce is the product of prolonged fermentation of soya beans but its salt content is so high it can only be consumed in small quantities.

Dhals These are peas, they are extremely indigestible until their tough outer coat is removed; in bringing this about, the seed is usually split into two parts and then polished. Yellow dhal is usually made from pigeon pea but several other varieties resembling pigeon pea may be harvested and used. Sometimes the *lathyrus* pea is inadvertently included among the dhals. If they are ingested, *lathyrism* may ensue (see page 69).

Pea flour is prepared from seeds that are first soaked and dried. This process loosens the outer shells and is frequently carried out by the sun which may reduce the riboflavin content of the flour. Pea flour has poor keeping qualities in hot climates.

Some members of the pea family are known as grams. Green gram and black gram are important legumes in many diet regimes. Green gram may be allowed to sprout and used as a vegetable, black gram pods are similarly used. The gram seeds must be softened by soaking and boiling, they may then be split like dhals. A paste may be prepared from the ground gram, the paste is then squeezed dry, boiled again and finally dried. The gram flour may be baked into flat cakes.

Some beans are consumed in the pod, these include the kidney bean, scarlet runner bean and the cow pea. Others such as the lima bean, chickpea, sword bean, velvet bean, garden pea, and broad bean, are used in a wide variety of foods throughout the world.

Oil seeds and nuts   The vegetable sources most commonly used for the production of oil are, the soya bean, ground nut, the seeds of cotton, rape, sesame and sunflower, maize and wheat germ. The possibility of using the protein residues of these seeds is currently being explored. The problems and nutritional deficiencies of the soya bean and the ground nut have been discussed already. Sesame protein has been successfully used in *laubina*, a vegetable protein mixture developed in the American University of Beirut.

Laubina and other oil seed residues left after oil extraction, are the basis of supplementary foods used in the prevention of protein calorie malnutrition. This subject is discussed in Chapter 6.

Cotton seed has the disadvantage of containing gossypol, a toxic substance that inhibits the action of the digestive enzymes pepsin and trypsin. Sunflower protein is deficient in the amino acids, lysine and iso-leucine.

The palm family provide fruits such as dates, feculas like sago, vegetables such as the palm cabbage, as well as sugars, sweet saps and alcoholic beverages, but the family is used mainly for the production of coconuts. The coconut kernel contains 30–45 per cent of oil, four to five per cent nitrogenous matter and 30–35 per cent of carbohydrate, but little of the latter is available for utilization by the human body. The nitrogenous matter too is not all protein, nevertheless it is receiving considerable attention from the food industry who have hopes of producing a product that may be used for feeding infants. This is important in developing countries having immense copra industries and a problem of childhood malnutrition.

Coconut oil contains very little unsaturated fatty acids and it also lacks vitamin A which further detracts from its nutritive value. Coconut is used as a source of oil in the preparation of 'filled milk' (see page 130). Coconut milk is prepared from the kernel of the nut and is not to be confused with the watery fluid in the cavity of the coconut. The milk is prepared by grating the fresh kernel, water is added and the mixture is squeezed, the resultant emulsion has the appearance of cows milk. Coconut milk contains about

80 per cent of the oil but the fibrous indigestible material in the kernel is almost eliminated, and it is therefore much more digestible. Grated coconut is also used in various food preparations; since the nutrients may not be available its food value is questionable.

Red palm oil This is a very important oil seed. Formerly cultivation was confined to West Africa, but it is now being grown on an increasing scale in other parts of Africa and Malaysia where the oil is being used as an alternative to rubber as a cash crop. The oil palm nut provides two kinds of oil in about equal proportions. The first comes from the pulp, it is rich in carotenes and may contain 24–28 mgs of β carotenes per 100 gm of oil. The second is found in the kernel and is much lighter in color and a less valuable source of carotenes.

Vegetables These may be conveniently classified into *Leafy* vegetables or *Mixed* vegetables comprising a variety of sources such as roots, tubers, pods or shoots.

Leafy vegetables may be further sub-divided into two groups according to their carotene content, the first being known as *Dark Green* vegetables and the second as *Pale* leafy vegetables.

Dark green leafy vegetables These have a very high carotene and vitamin C content. As much as 7.8 mgs of carotene per 100 grams, and 100 mg of ascorbic acid per 100 grams may be found in some leaves. Dark green leafy vegetables include the amaranth species, broccoli, mustard and cress, spinach, cassava and sweet potato leaves, turnip greens, watercress, parsley and mint. Dark green leaves may contain large amounts of iron but the availability of the mineral is not known. On a raw basis the protein content of dark green leaves is not high, but the amino acid composition may make a significant contribution to the biological value of protein from other sources. In many parts of the world it is customary for cassava leaves to be consumed as a side dish, or relish.

In the recent Biafran war, cassava leaves were a large part of the diet of many West Africans.[61] An analysis of the leaves has shown that they contained 30–40 per cent of protein an a *dry-matter* basis. The biological value of the protein was low, however, because of methionine deficiency. This indicates that methionine should be made available from other sources, if cassava leaves constitute a major part of the diet.

A large assortment of leaves is consumed by populations throughout the world. Some populations go to great lengths to obtain a regular supply of fresh leaves. In Central Tanzania *xeropthalmia* is common among the inhabitants of the semi-desert. However the women of one tribe have

10*

learned how to protect the health of themselves and their families by gathering minute green shoots which grow in very small depressions in the sandy earth. Despite the dry climate, sufficient dew collects in the depressions to allow seeds to germinate. The women can collect enough shoots to maintain an adequate vitamin A status in the community.

The ability to preserve dark green leaves for use during the long dry seasons of the tropics, or the long winters of Europe and North America often determines whether a population will maintain adequate vitamin A and C status.

Pale leafy vegetables These include cabbage, lettuce, brussels sprouts, cauliflower, bamboo shoots and palm cabbage.

The carotene content of pale leaves may range from zero to 0.6 mg per 100 gram of leaf. The vitamin C content of this group of vegetables also tends to be lower than the green leaves but the difference is not as great as the carotene content.

Mixed vegetables Carrots, turnips, artichokes, asparagus, onions, beetroot, celery, leeks, marrow, tomatoes, cucumber, squash and pumpkins okra, beans and peas in the pod, are included in this group. These are generally good sources of vitamin C and carotene. The vitamin C content of raw vegetables varies, even within varieties of the same species. The vitamin levels also may fall during storage (see page 96 and 389).

The nutritive value of all vegetables is dependent on the method of preparation. Some of the carotenes, for example, may not be freed unless the cell envelope is ruptured during processing and cooking. These precursors of vitamin A are fat soluble, so their absorption depends on the availability of fat, or oil, in the diet. Vitamin C is water soluble, and readily destroyed by heat and exposure to air. Because of these properties, there may be considerable losses of the vitamin during cooking, especially when the water, in which the vegetables are cooked, is thrown away.

Fruits These are important sources of vitamin C, carotenes, minerals, and vitamins of the *B* complex. There is however, a very large variation in the contribution of nutrients made by the different types of fruits. They may be considered in three groups, citrus fruit, berries, and other miscellaneous fruits.

Citrus fruits have a high ascorbic acid content; this group includes the orange, lemon, lime, grapefruit, tangerine, and *calamansi*.

The *berry* group includes the *drupes* such as the peach, apricot, West Indian cherry, and the small berries like the raspberry, blackberry, strawberry, gooseberry, blueberry, and bilberry. Some of these fruits contain protein and minerals, as well as calories in the form of readily available sugars. Some of these fruits are dried, in this state, their nutrient value is much higher.

The *miscellaneous* fruits include apples, pears, pineapples, papaya, mango, bananas, and avocado. They are generally good sources of vitamin C, some contain small amounts of protein. The fruits in this group contribute very little to the vitamin B intake of persons consuming a good mixed diet, but in the marginally nourished, fruit may contain sufficient vitamins of the *B* complex, to maintain health. In impoverished communities a liberal intake of fruits may be important. Fruits contain cellulose which may adversely affect digestibility and the availability of nutrients. The fibrous material in some fruits may irritate the bowel and precipitate diarrhea; this could have serious consequencies in the protein deprived child. Usually the sugars in fruits are readily assimilated, and are not likely to precipitate a fermentative diarrhea.

Fungi and yeasts   There is considerable variation in the acceptance of fungi as food. On the continent of Europe, a wide variety of fungi is consumed, but in Britain, the attitude is much more conservative. Some African tribes have a fear of consuming any sort of fungus, while others consider them a delicacy. There is a tendency for the latter groups to be indiscriminate in their selection, sometimes with dire results. They contain about three per cent of protein, and small amounts of carbohydrate, and fat. Their dietary value is enhanced if they are fried in oil, or fat; as a *relish* they make other foods more acceptable.

Miscellaneous foodstuffs

Fats and oils   These are important because they are a rich source of calories, and a source of *essential fatty acids*; some oils also contain fat soluble vitamins. Fats and oils may be considered under three headings, vegetable oils, marine oils, and animal fat.

Vegetable Oils   The oil seeds and nuts, already described, provide cotton seed, sesame, groundnut, soya, sunflower, red palm and coconut oil. Of these, only red palm oil contributes carotenes.

Vegetable oils are used in the preparation of margarine which has the nutritional advantage of containing unsaturated fatty acids. The process of hydrogenation hardens the product, but it also saturates some of the oils.

Marine oils   The livers of several fish are excellent sources of vitamin A and vitamin D. The best known marine oils are codliver oil, halibut liver oil and shark liver oil. These oils are used extensively in welfare programs in Europe to control rickets.

Animal fats   Pigfat is used as *lard* in cooking; beef *dripping* is used for frying. In the Middle East fat from lamb, sheep, or goats, is incorporated in many dishes. The most important source of animal fats is the dairy industry; here the fat is separated from the milk solids and converted into butter. Good butter may contain up to 1.2 μg of retinol per 100 g; this level may be much lower in winter when fresh grass is unavailable to the cattle. It is doubtful whether butter has any nutritional advantage over margarine since the latter product has vitamin A added.[62]

In Asia, butter fat is clarified by heating, *ghee* prepared in this way, has a variable vitamin content, depending on the method of processing. If care is not exercised, up to 50 per cent of the vitamin A content may be lost.

It is unusual for carcase fat to be consumed as a food, by itself but the skin and blubber of the *narwhal* are left by Eskimos for periods of several years in the frozen arctic ground. Fermentation prevents the fat from becoming rancid. Fat is also the basis of *pemmican*, a food originated by the *Cree* Indians of North America.

Algae and sea-weeds   *Sea-weeds* are consumed in many countries of the world, but they are not good sources of protein; in addition their carbohydrate is indigestible. However, they have a rich content of minerals, and they may be important sources of iodine, copper, and iron.

Feculas and syrups   *Sago* is prepared from the trunk of the sago palm where it exists as a starch, in the pith of the trunk. The pith is removed in chips and washed; the starch is recovered from the watery suspension by sedimentation. The sago may be roasted or made into a flour. The nutrient value of sago lies in its calorie content; sago contains only about 0.5 per cent of protein and traces of other nutrients.

Arrowroot also provides a starchy fecula, devoid of protein.

Honey contains readily available sugars, but very little protein and only traces of other nutrients. In regions where the calorie intake is marginal, honey is an important food, supplementing the energy intake.

Sugar cane contains a juice which is the main supply of sucrose. In the manufacturing process, the juice is concentrated and the sugar is crystallized out. The thick syrup is separated from the sugar and is known as *molasses*. The sugar is usually refined while the molasses, or *treacle*, containing sugars, minerals, and pectins, is used as an animal food, or manufactured into rum. Clarified molasses may be eaten with bread, or added to gruels, and milk beverages. Raw sugar cane is consumed as a snack, providing valuable calories for children receiving an inadequate diet.

Condiments and spices   These are frequently part of the culture of populations. They are important because they help to make monotonous food appetizing. Many condiments have a carminative effect which lessens the flatulence that is a consequence of a predominantly vegetarian diet.

Beverages   *Tea* contains *caffeine*, tannins and an essential oil that provides the characteristic aroma.

Coffee contains less caffeine and tannin than tea; it acquires the aroma during the roasting process, when pungent oils are liberated from the coffee bean.

Cocoa contains caffeine, and the drug *theobromine*.

Maté is prepared from the leaves of *Ilex paraguayensis*, a shrub resembling holly. Widely consumed in Latin America it contains caffeine and tannins.

Alcoholic beverages are produced by the fermentation of sugars by yeasts. Beer and wines are the end result of fermentation; spirits and liquors are made by distilling the fermented products. The alcohol content varies from three to five per cent for beers, through a range of 10 to 15 per cent for wines to 45 to 50 per cent for spirits and strong liquors.

Toddy is the fermented sap of palm trees, a similar product is prepared from the sap of *bamboo*. Native beers are made from millets, and other grains, which have been allowed to sprout before fermentation. Many of the beers are not clarified, the whole unfiltered liquid contains valuable minerals such as calcium, and iron, as well as vitamin C and the vitamins of the *B* complex. The clarification of native beer, and the trend towards an increased consumption of prestigious imported beers, may be depriving populations of a cheap, and readily available, source of nutrients. In the past, the nutrient supplementation offered by beer may have been helping to ensure nutritional adequacy.

The role of animal and vegetable foods in the diet

There is a wide belief that animal foods are superior to vegetable foods, this belief is especially prevalent with respect to protein. Increasing emphasis has been placed on animal food production in recent years, because of the prevalence of protein calorie malnutrition in developing countries. The whole question of quantity and quality of protein production, and the respective values of animal and vegetable food production has to be considered in relation to local conditions.

Because foodstuffs can be grown intensively in highly organized countries, this does not mean that the methodology can be, or even should be, copied in developing countries.

In the developing countries the usual protein sources, cereal grains, roots, tubers, plantains, bananas, and sago contain too little protein. There are two solutions to this problem, first total productivity of existing crops can be increased, and second the production of foods containing better quality protein can be encouraged.

Increasing the production of foods with a low concentration of protein, will not be effective because the physical bulk of the food produces satiety before the protein requirements of the body can be met. It has been suggested that total food production may be increased by cultivating hybrid strains of seeds, and by the intensive use of fertilizers. It is argued that benefits will inevitably accrue to the general population if the total food production of a country increases. However the tempting arguments that cash from crops will be available for the purchase of good quality food (perhaps, even imported), may not be supported by practice.

The Green Revolution which followed the introduction of high yielding rice has had some serious setbacks.[63] The shortness of the stalk of some of the highest yielding varieties is a serious disadvantage if the paddy fields undergo exceptional flooding. Some varieties are susceptible to disease. It has also been reported that the benefits which are supposed to go to the needy may, in fact, be giving benefit to a few influential families.[64] There is perhaps, more resistance and critical appraisal of these new products by small farmers, who are becoming increasingly skeptical of new ideas. At a subsistence level a new farming method represents a gamble; on the one hand it may bring some material benefit, but on the other it may prove to be a catastrophe if the method fails. The loss of a crop to the subsistence farmer is sure to bring illness to the family, and possibly death. In Nigeria, it was pointed out recently, that a new hybrid maize required more care, cultivation, and fertilizer than the traditional variety. Not only was more energy required to grow the hybrid but more capital outlay is required for the fertilizer. The amount of cash required for this, would be beyond the financial resources of most farmers. Finally, the local method of preparing the maize for cooking, would probably result in the loss of the extra water-soluble nutrients that the hybrid was to supply.[65]

In addition to cultivating more food, it has been suggested that fossil carbon might be used as a food source. The carbon in oil, and natural gas, can be utilized by certain micro-organisms; the multiplication of the cells represents a crop that can be harvested. The process is sophisticated and costly, and unlikely to bring benefit to developing countries for some years. It should also be noted that this technology is not creating new carbon for human use, but only converting carbon that is already present.

Much of the land in the wet tropic areas cannot be used for animal production, but many other regions in developing countries do have a potential and could be exploited. Animal foods have the desired concentration of protein, and in general, it is of high biological value. It is argued that much land is unsuitable for arable farming and it should be used, therefore, for grazing and browzing by ruminants. This hypothesis is reasonably sound, but it should be remembered that the efficiency of food conversion depends, essentially, on the type of food that the animal eats. If the ruminant is consuming food that man cannot eat, then browzing and grazing is justified. If however, the animal is eating food which humans can use, or if it is consuming food growing on land that could be used for human food, then the efficiency of converting this vegetable food needs closer examination.

"It is the ratio of the amount of human food that is produced by an average population of animals (not just one animal at the peak of its productivity), to the amount that would have been produced by the alternative method of use. Animals considered in this way, seldom return as much as a tenth of what they eat."[66] The author of the above quotation compares a grazing animal with nine men in a boat, five of them fishing and four throwing the fish back into the sea. These fish are not wasted because the five men can catch them all over again, but it would be difficult to persuade the five that their colleagues were usefully employed. It is therefore extravagant to use arable land for grazing, browzing, or the production of animal feed.

The world food production problem is serious. It will not be solved however, by the simple application of successful agricultural principles of the western world, to the developing countries which have different problems in their agriculture, different resources, and people with different attitudes.

References

1. Allan, W. *The African Husbandman*, p. 258. London: Oliver and Boyd, 1967.
2. Lee. R. B. Kung Bushmen Subsistence. In *Environment and Cultural Behavior*, p. 47, Ed., Vayda, A. P. New York: Natural History Press, 1969.
3. *Colliers Encyclopedia*, Vol. **5**, p. 191. Crowell-Collier, 1968.
4. Pike, A. H. *Soil Conservation Among the Matengo Tribe*. Tanganyika Notes and Records, No. 6, p. 79, 1938.
5. Allan, W. *The African Husbandman*, p. 199. London: Oliver and Boyd, 1967.
6. Uchendu, V. C. Anthropology and Agricultural Development in Sub-Saharan Africa. In *The Anthropology of Development in Sub-Saharan Africa*, p. 5. Monograph No. 10. The Society for Applied Anthropology, University Press of Kentucky, 1969.

7. Robson, J. R. K. Unpublished data.

8. Knutsson, K. E., Selinus, R. "Fasting in Ethiopia, an Anthropological and Nutritional Study." *Amer. J. Clin. Nutr.* **23**: 956, 1970.

9. Rappaport, R. A. *Pigs for the Ancestors.* Yale University Press, 1967.

10. Meshkat, A. "Improvement of Fish Consumption in Developing Countries Through Influence on Food Habits, with Special Reference to Africa," *Proceeding, 7th International Congress on Nutrition, Hamburg,* Vol. **4**, p. 1038. London: Pergamon Press, 1967.

11. van Veldhoven, M. "The Change of Food Habits and Their Causes During the Last Half Century in Curacao." *Proceeding, 7th International Congress on Nutrition, Hamburg,* Vol. **4**, p. 91. London: Pergamon Press, 1967.

12. Jelliffe, D. B. "Parallel Food Classifications in Developing and Industrialized Countries." *Amer. J. Clin. Nutr.* **20**: 279, 1967.

13. Edwards, C. H., McDonald, S., Mitchell, J. R., Jones, L., Mason, L., Kemp, A. M., Laing, D., Trigg, L. "Clay and Cornstarch Eating Women." *J. Amer. Diet. Ass.* **35**: 810, 1959.

14. Halsted, J. A. "Geophagia in Man: Its Nature and Nutritional Effects." *Amer. J. Clin. Nutr.* **21**: 1384, 1968.

15. Oberle, M. W. "Lead Poisoning: A Preventable Childhood Disease of the Slums." *Science* **166**: 991, 1969.

16. Gopalan, C. Observations on Some Epidemiological Factors and Biochemical Features of Protein Calorie Malnutrition. In *Protein Calorie Malnutrition,* p. 79, Ed., von Muralt, A. New York: Springer-Verlag, 1969.

17. Jelliffe, D. B. Observations on Protein Calorie Malnutrition in the Caribbean. In *Protein Calorie Malnutrition,* p. 63, Ed., von Muralt, A. New York: Springer-Verlag, 1969.

18. Gokulanathan, K. S., Verghese, K. P. "Socio-cultural Malnutrition." *J. Trop. Ped.* **15**: 118, 1969.

19. *Ceres.* The F. A. O. Magazine, **2**: 19, No. 5, 1969.

20. *Focus: Hope 68.* Food and Drug Survey, Hope Inc., Detroit 1968.

21. van Veen, A. G., Steinkraus, K. H. "Nutritive Value and Wholesomeness of Fermented Foods." *J. Ag. Food Chem.* **18**: 576, 1970.

22. Hollingsworth, D. F. "Effects of Some New Production and Processing Methods on Nutritive Value." *J. Amer. Diet. Ass.* **57**: 246, 1970.

23. Phillips, W. E. J. "Changes in Nitrate and Nitrite Contents of Fresh and Processed Spinach During Storage." *J. Ag. Food Chem.* **16**: 88, 1968.

24. Konlande, J. "Nutritive Value of Cooked Camas Bulbs." *Ecology of Food and Nutrition* **1**: 120, 1971.

25. Layrisse, M., Cook, J. D., Martinex, C., Roche, M., Kuhn, I. N., Walker, R. B., Finch, C. A. "Food Iron Absorption: A Comparison of Vegetable and Animal Foods." *Blood* **33**: 430, 1969.

26. Friedman, T. E., Witt, N. F., Neighbours, B. W., Weber, C. W. "Determination of Carbohydrate in Plant and Animal Foods." *J. Nutr.* **91**: 1 (Supplement 2), 1967.

27. Chow, B. F., Blackwell, R. Q., Blackwell, B. N., Hou, T. Y., Anilane, J. J. Sherwin, R. W. "Maternal Nutrition and Metabolism of the Offspring, Studies in Rats and Man." *Amer. J. Public Health* **58**: 668, 1968.

28. Craig, J. W. "Present Knowledge of Nutrition in Inborn Errors of Metabolism." *Nutr. Rev.* **26**: 161, 1968.

29. Malcolm, S. Research Reports No. 6 and 7, South Pacific Commission, Noumea New Caledonia, 1952.

30. Morley, D. C., McWilliam, K. M. "Measles in a Nigerian Community." *W. Afr. Med. J.* **10**: 246, 1961.

31. Gordon, J. E., Jansen, A. A. J., Ascoli, W. "Measles in Rural Guatemala." *J. Pediatrics* **66**: 779, 1965.

32. Robson, J. R. K., Jones, E. L. "Is the Child with Poor Crowth Achievement More Likely to Die of the Measles" *Clin. Pediat.* **10**: 270, 1971.

33. Gordon, J. E., Behar, M., Scrimshaw, N. S. "Acute Diarrhoeal Disease in Less Developed Countries." Bull. W. H. O. **31**: 15, 1964.

34. Jelliffe, E. F. P. "Low Birth Weight and Malaria Infection of the Placenta." Bull. W. H. O. **38**: 69, 1968.

35. Schneider, H. A. "Some Nutritional Parameters in the Ecology of Infectious Disease." *Proc. Nutr. Soc.* **26**: 73, 1967.

36. Brown, R. E., Katz, M. "Antigenic Stimulation in Undernourished Children." *E. Afr. Med. J.* **42**: 221, 1965.

37. Budiansky, E., da Silva, N. N. "Formacao de Anticorpus no Distrofia Plurocarencial Hidropigenica." *O Hospital (Rio de Janeiro)* **52**: 251, 1957.

38. O'Connor, P. A. "Nutritional Anemia, Role of Excessive Milk Intake." *Mich. Med.* **66**: 432, 1967.

39. "Hypocalcemia in New Born Infants Fed Cows Milk." *Nutr. Rev.* **26**: 299, 1968.

40. "Lactase Deficiency in Thailand." *Nutr. Rev.* **27**: 278, 1969.

41. Floch, M. H. "Whither Bovine Milk." *Amer. J. Clin. Nutr.* **22**: 214, 1969.

42. Gunther, M., Cheek, E., Matthews, R. H., Coombs, R. R. A. "Immune Responses in Infants to Cow's Milk Proteins Taken by Mouth." *Arch. Allerg.* **21**: 257, 1962.

43. Parish, W. E., Barrett, A. M., Coombs, R. R. A., Gunther, M., Camps, F. E. "Hypersensitivity to Milk and Sudden Death in Infancy." *The Lancet* **2**: 1106, 1960.

44. Dahl, L. K. "Salt in Processed Baby Foods." *Amer. J. Clin. Nutr.* **21**: 787, 1968.

45. Fomon, S. J., Thomas, L. N., Filer, L. J. "Acceptance of Unsalted Strained Foods by Normal Infants." *J. Pediat.* **76**: 243, 1970.

46. W. H. O. Expert Committee on Prematurity, W. H. O. Technical Report Series 27, 1950.

47. Davies, P. A. "Feeding the New Born Baby." *Proc. Nutr. Soc.* **28**: 66, 1969.

48. Drummond, J. C., Wilbraham, A. *The Englishmans Food*, p. 246, London: Jonathan Cape, 1964.

49. von Liebig, J. *Food for Infants: A Complete Substitute for that Provided by Nature.* 2nd. Ed. London: J. Walton, 1867.

50. Hytten, F. E. "Clinical and Chemical Studies in Human Lactation." *Brit. Med. J.* **1**: 249, 1954.

51. *Ibid*, p. 151.

52. Walker, A. R. P. "Nutritional, Biochemical and Other Studies on South African Populations." *S. Afr. Med. J.* **40**: 817, 1966.

53. Hytten, F. E. "Clinical and Biochemical Studies in Human Lactation." *Brit. Med. J.* **2**: 844, 1954.

54. Walker, A. R. P. "Nutritional and Biochemical Studies on South African Populations." *S. Afr. Med. J.* **40**: 817, 1966.

55. Committee on Nutrition. "Prepared Infant Formulas and Commercial Formula Services." American Academy of Pediatrics. *Pediatrics* **36**: 282, 1965.

56. Southgate, D. A. T., Widdowson, E. M., Smits, B. J., Cooke, W. T., Walker, C. H. M., Mathers, N. P. "Absorption and Excretion of Calcium and Fat by Young Infants." *The Lancet* **1**: 487, 1969.
57. Darrow, D. C., Cooke, R. E., Segar, W. E. "Water and Electrolyte Metabolism in Infants Fed Cows Milk Mixture During Heat Stress." *Pediatrics* **14**: 602, 1954.
58. Joint Committee, Maternal and Child Health and Nutrition. "Economy in Nutrition and Feeding of Infants." *Amer. J. Publ. Health* **56**: 1756, 1966.
59. Townsend, P. "Subsistence and Social Organization in a New Guinea Society." Ph. D. Thesis, The University of Michigan, 1969.
60. Quin, P. J. *Foods and Feeding Habits of the Pedi*, p. 257. Witwatersrand University Press, 1959.
61. Eggum, B. O. "The Protein Quality of Cassava Leaves." *Brit. J. Nutr.* **24**: 761, 1970.
62. Leichenger, H., Eisenberg, G., Carson, A. J. "Margarine and the Growth of Children." *J. Amer. Med. Assoc.* **136**: 338, 1948.
63. "The Green Revolution." *Nutr. Rev.* **27**: 133, 1969.
64. Mullick, M. A. "Back to Man." *Ceres* **3**: 63, No. 4, 1970.
65. Weeks, J. Personal Communication.
66. Pirie, N. W. *Food Resources Conventional and Novel*, p. 144. Baltimore: Penguin Books, 1969.

CHAPTER 3

Normal Nutrition

The physiology of nutrition

In the two previous chapters an account has been given of the manifestations of inadequate and improper nutrition. These may appear on the one hand as dramatic clinical diseases, or on the other, as disturbances of function that may be hard to discern. The remote and immediate reasons for improper nutrition have been discussed in the last chapter. The following discussion is concerned with normal nutrition and the disturbances in function which may occur when the nutrient intake is either inadequate, improperly balanced, or in excess.

The role of nutrients in the diet

Carbohydrates, fats, proteins, minerals, vitamins, and water are all necessary for proper body functions. These include the production of energy for body activities, the promotion of growth and the maintenance and repair of body tissues, the regulation of body processes, and the maintenance of a proper internal environment.

Energy can be produced from proteins, fats, or carbohydrates, but the body places such importance on the maintenance of energy production that it will divert and use any of the above as a source of energy, even though the body may be deprived of a nutrient which has an important role in other body functions.

The promotion of body growth is principally the responsibility of protein, vitamins, and minerals. The maintenance of proper body function is primarily the role of vitamins, minerals, and water.

In order to maintain health, the body requires a regular supply of nutrients in the correct amounts, of proper quality, and in the right proportions. In Chapter 2 it was shown that foods as sources of nutrients have a great variation, some food groups are good sources of proteins, others are good sources of calories or vitamins. It follows, therefore, that if the nutrient requirements of the body are to be met, it will be necessary to consume a variety of foods. These must be consumed in the right proportion to ensure that an excess, a deficiency, or imbalance of nutrients does not harm the body. These is the concept of a *balanced* diet.

Before nutrients can be utilized, they have to undergo physiological "processing". The first stage involves the breakdown of the food and the conversion of nutrients into a form which may be absorbed. This process is *digestion* which is facilitated by mastication and the muscular contractions of the intestine. *Absorption* is the process by which the food leaves the lumen of the intestine and enters the circulation of the blood. Having arrived in the blood stream the nutrients are transported through the circulation to the tissues where *metabolic* processes change the chemical nature of the nutrient. Any excess nutrients may be stored or broken down. These end products of metabolism are *excreted* from the body, either in the urine, the feces, the skin, or in respiration. These processes will be discussed in outline only, the reader who requires further detail is advised to refer to standard texts on physiology.

The gastro-intestinal tract

The gastro-intestinal tract starts at the mouth and ends at the anus (see Figure 10). It has specialized functions throughout its length which dictate its shape and anatomical form. From the mouth cavity, the pharynx leads to the esophagus. This passes through the thoracic cage and enters the stomach. The small intestine continues from the stomach, the first part of which is the duodenum. This leads into the jejunum which in turn becomes the ileum. The ileum leads into the colon which terminates in the rectum and the anal canal.

The stomach and the small and large intestines are found in the abdominal cavity. This also contains other viscera including the liver.

The gastro-intestinal tract has basically the same structure throughout its length but is modified in accordance with specific functions. It is a tube having four coats (see Figure 11). The first outer coat or serous coat consists of fibrous tissue in which there is some adipose tissue, with blood and lymph vessels. Within this there is a muscular coat consisting of two layers of smooth muscle tissue arranged in a longitudinal form in its outer layers and a circular form in its inner layers. Within the muscular coat there is a submucous coat consisting of dense fibrous tissue in which there are blood vessels, lymphatic vessels, and a nerve plexus which coordinates the motor and secretory activities of the mucosa. The internal mucous coat has specialized functions in different parts of its length. The cells in this coat lie on a loose fibrous tissue bed which contains capillaries and lymph vessels. The functions of the layers may be summarized as follows:

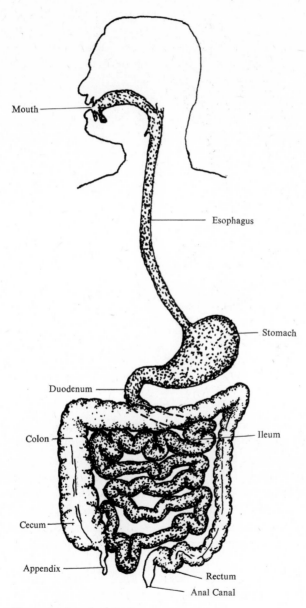

Figure 10   The gastro-intestinal tract

The serous coat carries nerves, blood vessels, and lymphatic vessels to and from the intestinal tract. The muscular coat controls the diameter of the tube and mixes and propels the contents. The submucous coat

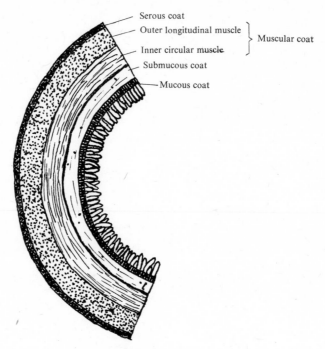

Figure 11   Transverse section of part of a typical section of gastro-intestinal tract showing the four coats

carries blood and lymph vessels and coordinates the motor and secretory activities of the mucosa. The mucous coat is responsible for secretion of substances that assist in the digestion and absorption of nutrients into the blood stream.

The stomach is the first specialized organ in the gastro-intestinal tract. It serves as a storage organ for food; it mixes the food mechanically. It is also concerned with the absorption of some nutrients and the adjustment of the osmotic pressure of the ingested fluids. It initiates the digestive process; gastric juice is secreted by glands situated in the gastric pits in the mucous coat of the stomach. Some cells produce mucus, others, the peptic or chief cells, produce enzymes. These include *pepsinogen*, which in the presence of hydrochloric acid starts the breakdown of protein, *rennin* which clots milk, and *lipase*, a weak fat splitting enzyme. The *parietal* cells secrete hydrochloric acid; this activates *pepsinogen* and renders the stomach contents more or less sterile. The stomach contents are held in the stomach by the pyloric sphincter; this relaxes from time to time and allows some of the stomach contents to pass into the duodenum. In the duodenum, the stomach contents meet digestive juices that have drained from the gall bladder and liver, via the hepatic and bile ducts, and also from the pancreas via the pancreatic duct. The digestive secretion contains enzymes that act on proteins, fats, and carbohydrates breaking the molecules into smaller units. The respective roles of the varions enzymes are discussed later in this chapter.

The bile salts help to produce a stable emulsion of fats and increases the surface area exposed to the fat splitting enzyme lipase, which it activates. The bile salts also form water soluble complexes with cholesterol and fat

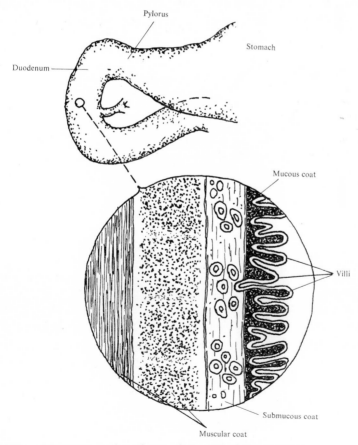

Figure 12   Transverse section of part of the wall of the duodenum

soluble vitamins that are normally insoluble in water. This greatly facilitates the absorption of these nutrients.

The mucous coat of the duodenum has fingerlike projections which add to the surface area of the intestine (see Figure 12). These processes are known as villi and they are covered by epithelial cells. In the submucosa there are specialized cells which produce an alkaline secretion; this protects the mucosa from the stomach acid.

The jejunum and ileum are the continuation of the remainder of the small intestine. Of this remainder the jejunum constitutes about two-fifths and the ileum three-fifths. In order to increase the surface area still more, the mucosa of this part of the small intestine is thrown up into folds (see Figure 13).

If the intestinal mucosal coat is examined microscopically it will be seen that, in addition to the villi, there are also pits which add to the area

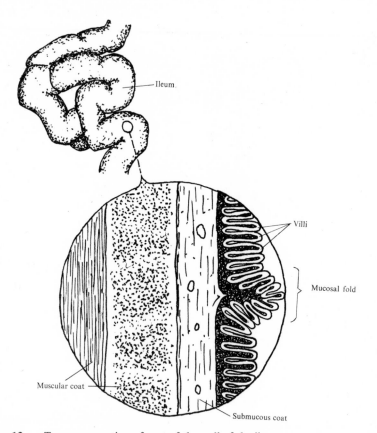

Figure 13   Transverse section of part of the wall of the ileum

of the intestine (see Figure 14). Some of the epithelial cells that line the villi produce mucus. Others secrete digestive enzymes. Formerly it was thought that these constituted a special digestive juice (the *succus entericus*) that acted in the lumen of the intestinal tract. It is currently believed that the further breakdown of nutrients in the intestinal contents is much more intimately associated with the surface of the epithelial cells. The net result of the action of the secretions of the small intestine is the reduction of the nutrients to small molecules of protein, fat, and carbohydrate that are able to pass readily through the mucous membrane of the small intestine.

In the ileum, *lymphoid* tissue in the submucous layer protects the intestinal mucosa from harmful bacteria ingested in the food (see Figure 15). In addition to the external secretions of mucus and the secretions of the intestinal mucosa, hormones are also secreted. This includes *enterogastrone, secretin, pancreozymin,* and *cholecystokinin.* These enter the blood stream

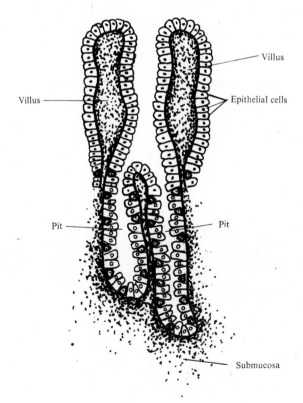

Figure 14   Section of the mucosa of the small intestine showing villi and pits

11*

and regulate the gastro-intestinal digestive secretions and the motility of the alimentary tract.

The small intestine terminates at the ileo-cecal valve at which point the large intestine commences.

The first part of this is called the cecum and from it the appendix forms a short diverticulum; the cecum becomes the ascending colon. In the region of the liver, the colon takes a right angled turn to become the transverse colon. In the region of the spleen it turns again to become the descending colon. As it crosses the floor of the pelvis, its tortuous appearance has led to it being termed the sigmoid colon. As it passes into the pelvis it becomes the pelvic colon; this opens into the rectum and then the anal canal. The large intestine is devoid of villi as digestion has now been completed.

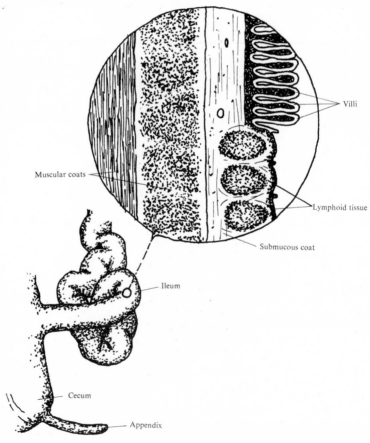

Figure 15   Transverse section of part of wall of ileum showing lymphoid tissue

The mucosal coat still serves an important function by absorbing water and salts, to conserve the body fluids, and dry the bowel excreta. Mucus secreting cells are more frequent and they provide a thick, alkaline fluid that lubricates and neutralizes the feces. Within the lumen of the intestinal tract some bacteria are able to synthesize certain vitamins that may be absorbed.

Gastro-intestinal absorption

One of the remarkable features of the small intestine is its enormous area for the absorption of nutrients. The inside, mucosal layer, is heaped up

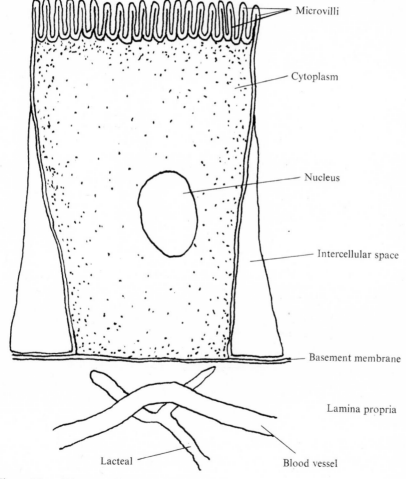

Figure 16   Diagram of intestinal epithelial cell

into folds which are covered by villi. Each villus is covered by epithelial cells; these bear several hundred bristles (*microvilli*) on their free or lumenal surface (see Figure 16). These microvilli, the villi, the crypts or pits between the villi, and the folds increase the effective surface area of the intestine to some 600 times that of the inside area of a simple tube of the same dimensions. The epithelial cell lies on a basement membrane which rests on a layer of connective tissue (the *lamina propria*) containing blood vessels and lymphatics. The process of absorption requires the movement of nutrients from the intestinal lumen through the epithelial cells into the lymphatics and blood vessels.

The process is extremely complicated because many of the nutrients are not soluble in the watery solutions of the cell. The passage through the cells is tortuous, and may depend on chemical transformation of the nutrients. The shift of nutrients from inside the lumen of the intestine to the cell, means that the concentration of nutrient molecules within the cell has to be adjusted by movement of water. The absorptive process is extremely

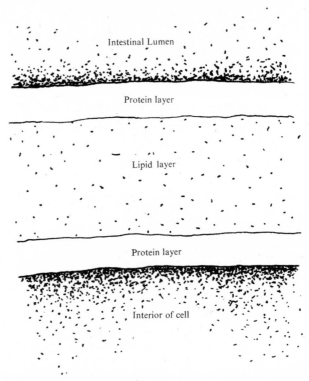

Intestinal Lumen

Protein layer

Lipid layer

Protein layer

Interior of cell

Figure 17   Diagram of the cell wall showing the three layered cell membrane

sophisticated and has to be maintained in perfect order if severe dysfunction is to be avoided.

The various mechanisms involved in absorption depend on the micro-anatomical and chemical features of the epithelial cell, the physical and electrical properties of the contents of the cell, and special transport systems capable of moving certain nutrients across the cell membrane.

The micro-anatomy and chemistry of the intestinal cell   The brush border, or microvilli, is covered by a polysaccharide coat (the *glycocalyx*) to which enzymes, secreted by the pancreas, adsorb. In association with this covering

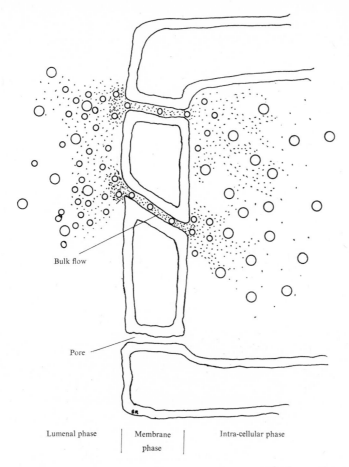

Bulk flow

Pore

| Lumenal phase | Membrane phase | Intra-cellular phase |

Figure 18   Osmotic pressure and *bulk flow*. The larger particles are unable to pass through the pores; they are more highly concentrated in the cell. The osmotic pressure causes water to flow through the pores from the lumen into the cell. The flow of water takes dissolved particles with it, a phenomenon known as *bulk flow*

there are the digestive enzymes believed formerly to be part of the *succus entericus*.

The cell wall is a three layered membrane, the inner and outer layers being composed of protein and the middle layer of fat (see Figure 17). While it is impervious to water and water soluble materials, it facilitates the passage of lipid materials into the cell.

The physical and electrical properties of the cell   The membrane of the intestinal cell is semipermeable which means that it allows the passage of

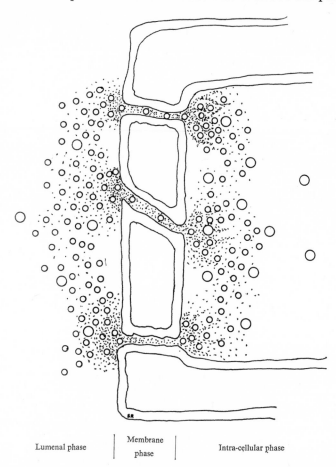

| Lumenal phase | Membrane phase | Intra-cellular phase |

Figure 19   Diffusion. Particles small enough to pass through the pores of the cell are more highly concentrated in the lumen. According to the laws of diffusion, they pass through the pores until the concentration of the particles in the cell, and the lumen, are equal. In the situation shown, particles too large to pass through the pores are more highly concentrated in the cell; the osmotic pressure causes water to flow into the cell

molecules of a certain size, but not larger. The presence of molecules in a greater concentration on one side of the membrane than the other, attracts the movement of water across the membrane, in an attempt to balance the concentration of the molecules on either side. This flow of water constitutes the osmotic pressure, one of the mechanisms governing the passage of water between the cells and the extra-cellular fluids. The water passes through pores in the cell membrane and carries with it dissolved particles of nutrients and other suspended particles small enough to pass through

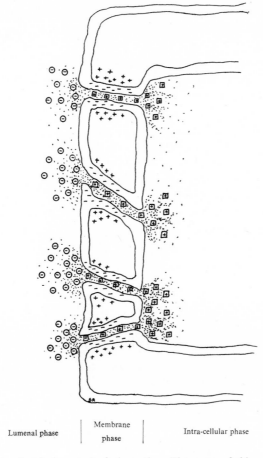

| Lumenal phase | Membrane phase | Intra-cellular phase |

Figure 20 The electrical control of absorption. The pores of this cell are negatively charged. The admission of positively charged particles and the exclusion of negatively charged particles increases the osmotic pressure of the cell. Water passes from the lumen into the cell

the pores. This phenomenon is known as *bulk flow* (see Figure 18). By the laws of diffusion, particles move from an area of high concentration to an area of low concentration. This mechanism is responsible for the movement of many nutrients from the lumen of the intestine to the cell. Substances small enough to pass through the pores may enter the cell either by diffusion, or by the bulk flow, or by both mechanisms (see Figure 19).

If the particles have an electric charge they will attract other particles of opposite charge, and take them through the membrane. Sometimes the pores have a negative electric charge which repels similarly charged ions. The electrical barrier may keep negatively charges particles in the lumen of the intestine and help to maintain osmotic pressures that hold water in the cell (see Figure 20).

Transport systems   The physical property of diffusion is random, haphazard, and wasteful of energy. The function of the cell is so planned that unorganized diffusion is discouraged. For example, catalysts and enzymes are frequently arranged in sequential order within the cell; this helps to ensure the product of one reaction is immediately dealt with by a succeeding mechanism. The diffusion of a nutrient in one particular direction, may be physiologically desirable. The energy liberated by this diffusion may be used to provide the energy for movement of a nutrient in the opposite direction. For example, the accumulation of sodium ions in a cell may be harmful; as the concentration of sodium in the cell rises above that in the extra-cellular fluid, it diffuses out. In doing so, the sodium links to a chemical transport system bringing other materials into the cell. There are other carrier systems in cells to facilitate the movement of nutrients against concentration gradients. Sodium, calcium, iron, glucose, galactose, amino acids, and vitamin B_{12} are absorbed in this way.

The ability of the cell to move sodium against the concentration gradients, as opposed to the downhill diffusion described above, is essential to the proper function of the body (see Figure 21). It allows sodium to move from the intestinal lumen into, and through the epithelial cell and then into the extra-cellular fluid. The movement of the positively charged sodium cations attracts negative anions (usually chloride anions) which are drawn from the lumen of the intestine as well. The effect of this *sodium pump* is to increase the molecular concentration in the extra-cellular fluid. This has the effect of drawing water out of the intestinal contents into the intra-cellular fluid. If this mechanism were not present the body would be dehydrated. At the same time, the fluid in the intestinal lumen would cause severe diarrhea. The sodium pump may be inactivated by toxins from the *cholera vibrio* which would explain the devastating and fatal diarrhea that is a feature of the disease.

The physical, chemical, and electrical properties of the cell and its contents, combined with passive diffusion and the active transport mechanisms, enable the intestinal contents to continue to give up nutrients. The normal function of the intestinal epithelium therefore permits fluid uptake by the body and adjustment of the pH of the intestinal contents to favor the digestive and absorptive processes. The epithelia also help to maintain a fluid balance between the tissues and the circulating blood, and a normal acid-base balance in the internal environment. Disturbed function of the epithelia has obvious serious consequences. It will be seen that the normal function of these cells depends on them receiving a proper supply of nutrients.

Nutrients from the intestinal cells pass either into the blood circulation or, in the case of most lipids, into the lymphatics. The small lymphatics unite and eventually form the *thoracic duct* which enters the venous circulation shortly before the large veins join the heart. The blood from the intestinal tract is collected in the *portal vein* and passes into the liver. Here the portal vein breaks up into branches which eventually surround the liver

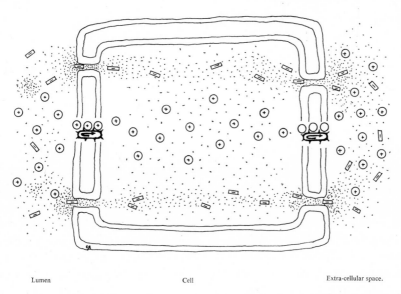

| Lumen | Cell | Extra-cellular space. |

Figure 21   The sodium pump. The "pump" takes sodium cations ⊕ across the membrane. Chloride anions ⊟ are attracted by the movement of the sodium and they pass through the pores. The increase in concentration of the particles creates an osmotic pressure and water is drawn out of the lumen into the extra-cellular space

lobule (see Figure 22). This brings the nutrients in close proximity to the liver cells which are very active in metabolism. The liver can synthesize and break down proteins; it can store energy in the form of glycogen, and other nutrients including protein, fat, and vitamins A, D and B_{12}. It can detoxify substances potentially harmful to the body. Liver cells are also concerned with the formation and destruction of red cells and the secretion of bile.

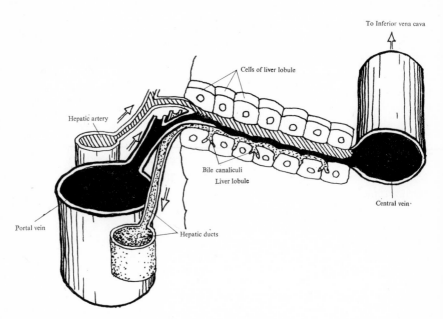

Figure 22   Diagram showing the blood supply to the liver

The liver is an extremely important organ; it receives a large branch from the aorta, the principle artery of the body. This brings a well oxygenated supply of blood to the cells and assures the efficient working of the liver. The products of metabolism are collected in the central vein within each liver lobule. The veins unite with one another and form the hepatic vein which drains into the vena cava and then into the heart. The circulation of the blood ensures that the nutrients drained from the intestinal tract are transported immediately to the main organ of metabolism; it also ensures that the products of liver metabolism are circulated to organs, tissues, and cells throughout the body without delay. It is now necessary to discuss the role of the cell and its normal function.

The cell

The cell is the lowest level of organization of living matter, and all plants and animals are made up of one or more cells. They are complex structures and they vary in size and shape depending on their function. Although cells are highly individual, for the present purpose a "typical" cell will be described.

The outer living boundary of the cell is called the cell or plasma membrane. It is a semipermeable membrane and controls the passage of materials in, and out, of the cell. The membrane is thought to be a lipoprotein structure with a double middle layer of lipid molecules and an outer single layer of protein molecules (see Figure 17). There is over still controversy the composition of the membrane. Some investigators have found that the layers on either side of the lipid core differ in chemical reactivity, and they suggest that there may be protein on one side and a carbohydrate layer on the other side of the lipid. The diversity in structure of the membranes of different cells is consistent with a known diversity in cell function. The selective permeability of the membrane is related to the constituents of the lipid core and the character of the nonlipid layers, as well as the metabolic condition and activity of the cell.

It is postulated also that the membrane structure includes pores or open spaces that allow the entrance of some materials into the cell. The size of the pores can be regulated to control what enters and leaves the cell. Nutrients must enter the cell, and end products must be removed, before reactions can occur in it. The constancy of the internal environment of the cell is dependent on the membrane, and of it does not function properly the cell will die.

There are several different ways for substances to enter the cell; the first is simple diffusion which has already been discussed. It involves the movement of molecules from a high concentration or electric potential to a lower one and it requires no energy expenditure. Small molecules such as water, oxygen, and carbon dioxide, that can easily pass through the membrane pores, enter and leave the cell in this way.

Facilitated diffusion is another process that allows substances to enter the cell and then proceed "downhill" along the concentration gradient. It requires a carrier to link with the solute and carry it across the membrane. In this way, the molecule to be transported joins with the carrier at one surface of the membrane, it diffuses through the membrane as a carrier-solute complex, and is finally released on the opposite side of the membrane (see Figure 23). Different molecules may compete for the same carrier.

As one molecule is attached to the carrier, perhaps by some facilitating mechanism, so others are prevented from being moved. This preferential treatment results in molecules being transported at different rates. The sugars are an example of this and their affinity to transport depends on their molecular configuration.

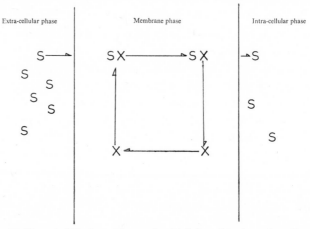

Figure 23   Facilitated diffusion. The carrier X links with the solute S and diffuses across the membrane, it releases the solute and diffuses back to the extra-cellular surface where it links with another molecule

Exchange diffusion also depends on a carrier. For each molecule transported across the membrane in one direction a similar molecule must be transported on the return trip of the carrier (see Figure 24). Exchange diffusion is involved in the exchange of ions and amino acids. In exchange diffusion the rate of diffusion is dependent on the number of carriers available and not on the concentration of the solute.

The method of active transport is similar to facilitated and exchange diffusion except it is energy-dependent. Complex enzyme systems on the surface, or in the membrane, are involved. First the solute links with an active carrier and crosses the membrane as a complex. At the inner surface of the membrane the solute molecule is released into the cell, and the carrier becomes inactive (see Figure 25). As the carrier passes back through the membrane it becomes active again by receiving a new charge of energy from the chemical adenosine tri-phosphate (see page 187).

Active transport may be compared to a pumping system; the energy for the pumping reactions comes from cellular metabolism. The mechanism of energy supply is described later in this chapter. In addition to sodium, glucose, amino acids, and salts enter the cell by active transport.

Active transport may work in several ways, depending on which direction the solute is moved. First, movement along the gradient may be accelerated. This occurs in the transport of glucose from a high concentration in the intestine, to a lower one in the plasma. The movement takes place at a much greater rate than is possible by simple diffusion alone. Secondly, movement with the gradient may be prevented. For example, sodium ions may be kept out of cells even when the extra-cellular sodium ion concentration exceeds

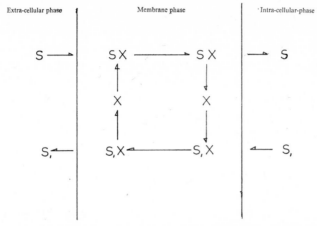

Figure 24   Exchange diffusion. Solute S is transported from the extra-cellular phase to the intra-cellular phase by carrier X. On its return journey it must transport a similar molecule S′ from the intracellular phase to the extra-cellular phase

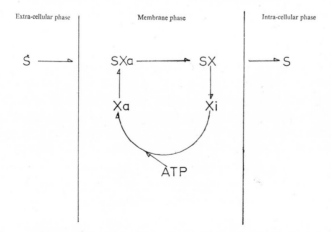

Figure 25   Active transport. The active carrier Xa transports solute S across the membrane. After release of the solute at the inner surface of the membrane the inactive carrier receives a new charge of energy from ATP

the intra-cellular concentration. The active transport system ensures the maintenance of a low concentration of sodium ions within the cells. The third possibility is movement of molecules against the gradient. This occurs when potassium ions are taken up by the cell even when the intra-cellular concentration exceeds the extracellular concentration. The cell actively maintains a high concentration of potassium ions.

The various reactions of active transport all help the cell maintain its electrical and concentration gradients in a favorable condition.

Phagocytosis is another process used by the cell to take in large molecules and other solid particles. First, a particle sticks to the membrane which then forms a cup around the particle and eventually separates it, as a watery bubble inside the cell (see Figure 26). *Pinocytosis* is similar to phagocytosis except water and dissolved particles are taken into the cells. *Endocytosis* is the term used to refer to the introduction of any foreign materials into the cell. The material is completely surrounded by a membrane and there-fore separated from the cytoplasm as a *vacuole* and is used to store food, water, or waste material.

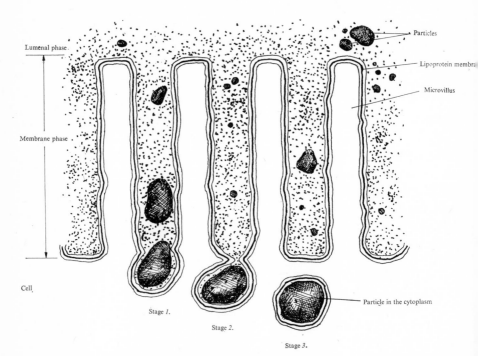

Figure 26   Phagocytosis and pinocytosis. The incorporation of solid and dissolved particles

The *cytoplasm* of the cell is the protoplasm outside the nucleus. It is a thick, viscous fluid and contains dissolved salts, proteins, carbohydrates, and fats. The dissolved salts contribute to cytoplasmic function by controlling the quantity of water in the cell by osmosis through the cell membrane. They also cause electrical currents to flow through the cytoplasm thereby promoting and regulating chemical reactions.

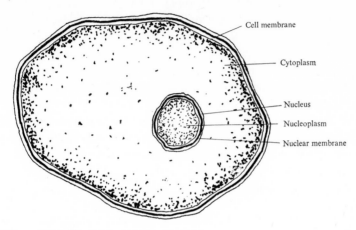

Figure 27   The cell

The cytoplasm contains *organelles*, and inclusions, which will be discussed individually. The production of new molecules for growth and the release of energy for cell functions, takes place within these structures, in the cytoplasm.

The *nucleus* is the largest and densest of the structures in the animal cell and it is basic to the life of the cell. It is composed of *nucleoplasm* and is similar in composition to cytoplasm (see Figure 27). There is a *nuclear membrane* separating the nucleus from the cytoplasm. The nuclear membrane is similar to the cell membrane but the pores are larger. This allows substances to pass more easily from the nucleoplasm to the cytoplasm, than from the exterior of the cell into the cytoplasm. The size of the pores in the nuclear membrane varies with cell type and function. The membrane is continuous with the *endoplasmic reticululum* discussed later.

The *nucleolus* is a round structure which looks dark when stained; it is found in the nucleoplasm. It has no membrane separating it from the nucleus. The nucleolus contains *ribonucleic acid* (*RNA*) and may be a storage place for RNA after it is made by the *desoxyribonucleic acid* (*DNA*) of the chromosomes (see Figure 28).

The nucleus has a controlling influence on the activity of the cell, consequently all metabolically active cells have a nucleus. The nucleus is the site of cell reproduction therefore cells without a nucleus cannot reproduce. (This is the reason why each red blood cell has to be replaced with a new cell.) Before cell division, a tangled network of structures called *chromatin* can be seen in the nucleus. This network is composed of individual threads of the chromosomes which carry *genes*. Each gene is composed of DNA a protein material carrying the hereditary information of the cell. Molecules af the nucleus of every cell are precisely the same as those of the parent cell, so genes are an inherited part of each nucleus. This ensures that the functions of the cells remain essentially the same from one generation to the next. The amount of DNA in each set of chromosomes is constant and is characteristic of the species.

The DNA molecules located on the chromosomes make the messenger RNA that transfers the hereditary information from the nucleus to the ribosomes. The ribosomes are minute structures containing RNA which regulates protein synthesis within the cell. In the ribosomes, RNA derived from the chromosome DNA serves as a template for protein synthesis (see Figure 29).

The *centrosome* is an organelle located near the center of the cell. It consists of two *centrioles*, each of which is an open cylinder surrounded by nine longitudinally arranged fibers of protein. The centrioles function in cell division.

The *lysosome* is a vacuole containing 12 or more powerful enzymes. The lysosome may fuse with a vacuole containing nutrient material. The enzymes in the lysosome break down the material which then becomes available to the cell. If the membrane of the lysosome is destroyed, or damaged, the freed enzymes will digest the cell. The membrane may be harmed by agents that disturb the cellular pH, the osmotic equilibrium, temperature, chemical stability, or the electrical charge of the membrane. *Ultraviolet* light and *ionizing* radiation are very damaging to the lysosome membrane and allow the enzymes to leak out into the cytoplasm, causing damage which usually leads to death of the cell.

The *endoplasmic reticulum* is a system of channels leading from the cell membrane to the nuclear membrane. They form a network throughout the cytoplasm (see Figure 30). The walls of the channels are continuous with, and have the same structure as, the plasma, or cell membrane. Since the endoplasmic reticulum is involved in the production of proteins, its complexity varies with the degree of protein synthesis that occurs within the cells.

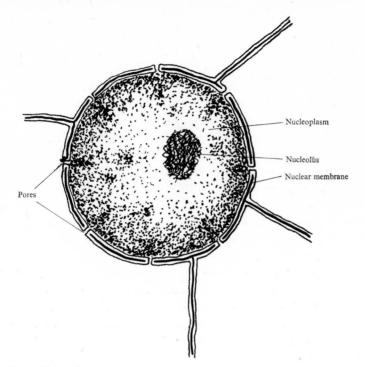

Figure 28   The nucleus

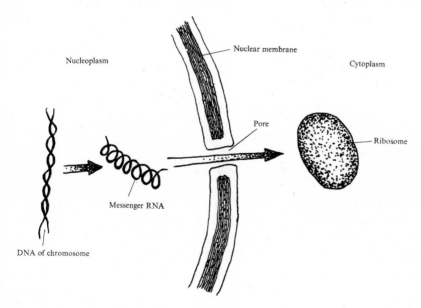

Figure 29   DNA and RNA and protein synthesis. The RNA derived from the chromosome DNA serves as a template for protein synthesis.

The endoplasmic reticulum provides a means of communication between the extra-cellular and intra-cellular environments. Materials flow slowly through the endoplasmic reticulum and are exchanged with the contents of the cytoplasm. Other organelles are dependent on the endoplasmic reticulum for supplying nutrients and removing waste products.

The *mitochondria* are granular, rod-shaped structures found in the cytoplasm thay have been called the "power houses" of the cell. Mitochondria are formed from two membranes which resemble the cell membrane in structure but they are arranged in the form of two sacs, one enclosing the other. The inner membrane is also folded to provide a greater surface area; it is probably involved in active transport and in the maintenance of osmotic pressures. The inner surface of the inner membrane is covered with small particles that have been called *electron transport particles* or *elementary* particles. These particles are believed to be the respiratory assemblies that carry out the metabolic activity of the mitochondria. The lumen of a mitochondrion is filled with a fluid matrix which contains proteins and lipids. The mitochondria contain many proteins with enzyme activity that promotes chemical reactions. The *Kreb's Cycle* enzymes and the *respiratory chain* enzymes are found in the mitochondria (see page 189). The enzymes are placed in the sequence of the chemical reactions in which they take part. This arrangement of enzymes produces the product of one reaction at a site where it can be used for the next step.

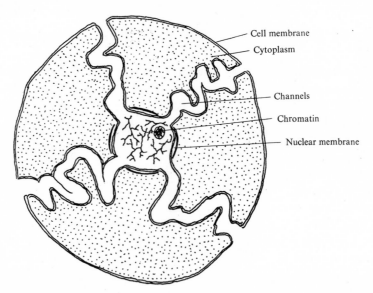

Cell membrane
Cytoplasm

Channels

Chromatin

Nuclear membrane

Figure 30   The endoplasmic reticulum

The main function of the mitochondria is to oxidize simple forms of proteins, fats, and carbohydrates, into carbon dioxide and water. During this process energy is released and becomes available for other cell functions. The mitochondria have the ability to actively transport and accumulate certain ions, and participate in the maintenance of the correct intra-cellular environment.

From this brief description of the structure of the cell an insight is gained into the processes that occur in the cell.

Cellular respiration is a process of simple diffusion and not an active process which requires energy. It involves the movement of dissolved oxygen to the inside of the cell and the utilization of the oxygen by the cell. The net diffusion of oxygen is in an inward direction because there is a higher concentration of oxygen in the fluids surrounding the cell than in the inside of the cell. Conversely, the concentration of carbon dioxide is higher inside the cell than out, so more carbon dioxide molecules diffuse to the outside.

Metabolism refers to chemical reactions that take place in the cell as it performs its functions. Metabolism is actually a series of reactions; these include *catabolism* and *anabolism*. Catabolic reactions disassemble larger molecules into smaller ones with the release of energy. Anabolic reactions assemble smaller molecules into larger ones and require energy supplied by the oxidation reactions taking place in the mitochondria. Metabolic reactions in the cell convert the potential energy of carbohydrate, protein and fat, into chemical energy. The conversion of nutrients into energy is the main function of the mitochondria.

The energy is stored in the chemical compound adenosine triphosphate (ATP). Every cell has a storehouse of ATP to provide the energy needed for physiological processes. These processes include muscular contraction, active transport, the development of membrane potentials, synthesis of chemical compounds and many other activities. Any energy not stored in ATP is transformed to heat energy. In this form, the energy cannot be used for work, and it is wasted.

The cell uses anabolic reactions to form needed compounds. Amino acids, the building blocks of proteins, cannot be made by the cell and they must be furnished from the surrounding fluids. Within the cells, the amino acids are built up into proteins; these are needed for most of the structural elements of the cells and enzyme formation. The types of proteins synthesized by the cell are a reflection of their prospective function.

Three types of fats are used by the cell. Neutral fat can be used for energy but if an excess of fats is available, the excess accumulates in the fat cells pending further use.

Cholesterol and phospholipids are more solid than neutral fat and can be used by the cell to form structures immiscible with the fluid of the cytoplasm. These lipid compounds are deposited in the cellular and nuclear membranes. Cholesterol is also used in the manufacture of other chemical compounds such as bile salts and some hormones.

Cellular excretion involves the transfer through the membrane of substances harmful to, or no longer needed by the cell. Urea, carbon dioxide, and some small molecules diffuse out. There may also be some active excretory process for large chemical compounds but the mechanism for this is unknown. Water and dissolved wastes may be released by reversing the process of pinocytosis and solids may leave by reverse phagocytosis.

This very brief review of the physiology of nutrition has outlined the fate of ingested food. The role of nutrients in the diet will now be discussed in detail. These are considered systematically but it should be remembered that nutrient relationships are extremely complex and it is virtually impossible to consider one nutrient in isolation. Wherever possible the function of each nutrient will be considered in relation to its normal function, and the abnormal function that may arise from deficiency or excess.

The role of carbohydrates in the diet

Carbohydrates provide most of the energy that is needed by man. The percentage of carbohydrates in the diet, however, depends on the economic status of the people. Since carbohydrates are the cheapest course of energy, they contribute as much as 90 per cent of the calories in poor countries and as little as 50 per cent in the prosperous countries.

Functions of carbohydrates

These are threefold, First they supply a cheap source of energy, second they add flavor, color, and variety to food, and third they are constituents of some vital body compounds such as nucleic acids, high energy compounds, flavins, and the matrix of connective tissue.

Photosynthesis

Chlorophyll is the green pigment of leaves and stems of plants; these use the energy of light to synthesize sugars from carbon dioxide in the air, and water from the soil. Part of the sugar is converted to cellulose which forms the structure of plants and gives them support; the rest is converted to starch which is stored in seeds, tubers and roots. The chemical reaction is:

$$6CO_2 + 6H_2O \xrightarrow[\text{chlorophyll}]{\text{sunlight}} C_6H_{12}O_6 + 6O_2$$

$$\text{glucose}$$

cellulose   starch

Chemistry

Carbohydrates are composed of carbon, hydrogen, and oxygen. The ratio of hydrogen to oxygen is 2 : 1; this is the same as in water and is the reason why the name *carbohydrates* is given to this class of compounds.

Classification   Carbohydrates are divided into three classes according to their relative complexity and the size of their molecules.

Monosaccharides   These are the simple sugars having the smallest molecules. They require no digestion and they are absorbed without undergoing further chemical change. Monosaccharides are classified according to the number of carbon atoms in their molecules; the trioses have three carbon atoms, the tetroses four, the pentoses five, the hexoses six, and the heptoses seven. The most important monosaccharides in the human diet are glucose, fructose, galactose, and mannose. They are all hexoses having the same formula, $C_6H_{12}O_6$, but they differ in the arrangement of the hydrogen atom and the hydroxyl group (OH) around the carbon chain (see Figure 31).

CHO	CHO	CHO	CH_2OH
HCOH	HCOH	HOCH	C=O
HOCH	HOCH	HOCH	HOCH
HCOH	HOCH	HCOH	HCOH
HCOH	HCOH	HCOH	HCOH
CH_2OH	CH_2OH	CH_2OH	CH_2OH
glucose	galactose	mannose	fructose

Figure 31   The configuration of hexoses

Of the pentoses, ribose, arabinose, and xylose are consumed by man, but these do not make a significant contribution to the diet.

Disaccharides   These are composed of two molecules of monosaccharides with elimination of one molecule of water.

$$2C_6H_{12}O_6 \xrightarrow{-H_2O} C_{12}H_{22}O_{11}$$

The disaccharides that are encountered in foods are sucrose (glucose + fructose), lactose (glucose + galactose), and maltose (glucose + glucose).

Polysaccharides   These include starch, cellulose, and glycogen; they are composed of several monosaccharides but unlike monosaccharides they do not have a sweet taste. Cellulose forms the structure and support of plants, whereas celluloses, starches, and glycogen, are storage forms of carbohydrate; the former is found in plants and the latter in animals. Cellulose, starches, and glycogen, are made up of many molecules of glucose linked together (*polymers*). Fifteen to twenty per cent of starch is in the form of a straight chain molecule made up of several hundred units of glucose and having a molecular weight of 4,000 to 150,000. This type of starch is called amylose. The rest is a branched polymer having a molecular weight of 500,000 and it is called amylopectin. The structure of glycogen is even more branched than amylopectin; each chain is made up of 10 to 20 glucose units instead of the 30 which are found in amylopectin. Cellulose is the most important structural carbohydrate; it has a molecular weight of 200,000 to 2,000,000.

Food sources of carbohydrates

With the exception of lactose in milk and glycogen in shellfish and liver, dietary carbohydrates are of plant origin. The percentage of carbohydrates in foods varies greatly and ranges from more than 99 per cent in sugar to 6 per cent in milk.

Monosaccharides   These seldom occur free in nature. Some glucose (dextrose) is found in a free form in grapes and honey but mainly it is combined in starch, glycogen, sucrose, lactose, and maltose. In industry, glucose is obtained by hydrolysis of starch. Fructose or levulose is found in a free form in honey and fruits and in a combined form in inulin and sucrose. Commercially fructose is obtained by the hydrolysis of inulin present in the Jerusalem artichoke. Galactose is not found in a free form but is a constituent of lactose. Mannose is found in nature chiefly as the polysaccharide mannosan which occurs in plants and certain seeds; from these mannose is prepared commercially. Some pentoses, such as ribose, arabinose, and xylose exist in fruits and root vegetables but they are not utilized by the body and are excreted in the feces and urine. Pentoses are found as complex polysaccharides called pentosans in certain gums from which the free pentoses may be obtained by hydrolysis. Although pentoses are constituents of important compounds such as nucleoproteins, high energy compounds, and flavins, they are not essential to the human diet because the body can synthesize them from glucose.

Disaccharides Sucrose is also known as saccharose. It occurs widely in plants; sugar beet, sugar cane, sorghum syrup, and certain palms and maples, are the most important sources. Lactose or milk sugar is found only in dairy products. Maltose or malt sugar is found in germinating cereal grains, usually barley. It is formed from the hydrolysis of starch by the action of the enzyme amylase. Raffinose is a trisaccharide made up of galactose, glucose, and fructose. It is found in molasses prepared from beet sugar, cotton seed, and manna the syrupy exudate of certain shrubs.

Polysaccharides *Starch* is stored in the form of granules in the plant cell. The size and shape of starch granules is peculiar to that species; this permits identification of each source. Cereal grains, potatoes, sweet potatoes, beans, and peas are the chief food sources of starch.

Glycogen. This is the form in which carbohydrate is stored in animals where it is mostly found in liver and muscle tissue. However, the total amount in storage is small and inadequate to meet daily human energy needs. The chief food sources of glycogen are liver and shellfish.

Cellulose. Although this carbohydrate is the most abundant, the body lacks the necessary enzyme (*cellobiase*) to break down the linkages of the cellulose molecule, so its component glucose units cannot be used. However, it contributes bulk to the diet which facilitates movement of the bowel contents.

Inulin. In its natural form, the fructose units of the molecule are un-available to the body. It is found in the leaves and tubers of Jerusalem artichokes, and in various other bulbs, tubers, and roots, such as those of the elecampane, dahlia, camas, chicory, dandelion, and burdock. Cooking and commercial preparation can liberate fructose from the inulin, therefore the nutritional value of the prepared food may be much greater than that indicated by the chemical analysis of the raw food.

Pectins. These are polymers of galacturonic acid, a derivative of galactose. They fill the inter-cellular spaces of plant tissues and, as a colloid, they are capable of absorbing large quantities of water. Commercial pectin is prepared from apples and citrus rind. Coagulation and the formulation of a gel can be brought about in the presence of acids and sugar. *Agar* is a polymer of galactose. It is used as a food by the Japanese but in other countries it is mainly used as a growth medium for micro-organisms, and as a stabilizer which maintains the colloid properties of gelling agents in food. *Gum Arabic* which is obtained from the bark of acacia trees is made up of the pentose sugar, arabinose. It is used as a thickener and emulsifier in food in industry.

The classification of carbohydrates, the main food sources from which they are derived and the end-products of their digestion are summarized in Table 17.

Table 17   Food sources and end-products of digestion of carbohydrates

Carbohydrate	Chief food sources	End-products of digestion
I—*Monosaccharides*		
a Hexoses		
Glucose	fruits, honey, corn syrup	glucose
Fructose	fruits, honey	fructose
Galactose	dairy products	galactose
Mannose	mannosan in certain plant seeds	mannose
b Pentoses		
Ribose, xylose	fruits and root vegetables	ribose, xylose
and arabinose		and arabinose
II—*Disaccharides*		
Sucrose	sugar beet, sugar cane	glucose + fructose
Lactose	dairy products	glucose + galactose
Maltose	malt products	glucose
III—*Trisaccharides*		
raffinose	molasses	glucose + fructose + galactose
IV—*Polysaccharides*		
Starch	seeds, tubers, roots	glucose
Glycogen	liver, sea foods	glucose
Inulin	Jerusalem artichoke	fructose
Pectin	fruits and vegetables	galacturonic acid
Pentosans	fruits and gums	pentoses

Digestion

The digestion of the polysaccharides starts in the mouth where the enzyme *ptyalin* of saliva breaks down starches and glycogen into intermediary breakdown products called *dextrins*. The optimum pH for ptyalin is neutral so that when the food meets the hydrochloric acid of the stomach its action is inhibited, and there is no further digestive breakdown of carbohydrates in the stomach. In the small intestine the food is mixed with the pancreatic juice; this contains a powerful digestive enzyme, amylase, which breaks the dextrins down further into the disaccharide maltose.

Maltose, together with other dietary disaccharides in the glycocalyx of the microvilli of the intestinal epithelial cells, is subjected to the enzymes maltase, lactase, and sucrase; these split the disaccharides into their constituent monosaccharides. The digestive process is summarized in Figure 32.

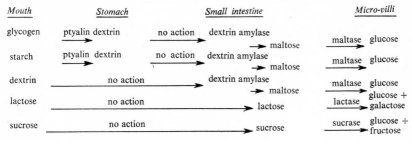

Figure 32   Summary of digestion by enzymes

Absorption

Monosaccharides cannot be broken down further, and they are absorbed by a mechanism that actively transports simple sugars from the mucosal cells to the blood capillaries which drain into the portal vein. The rate of absorption of galactose is faster than that of glucose, this in turn is faster than fructose.

Metabolism   The portal vein carries nutrients to the liver where glucose, fructose, and galactose enter the liver cells, and where phosphate is added to the monosaccharide molecules. This process requires the expenditure of energy which is provided by adenosine triphosphate (ATP). This compound yields chemical energy when it gives up its phosphate component. After phosphorylation, fructose and galactose are converted into glucose. This phase of metabolism may be summerized schematically as in Figure 33.

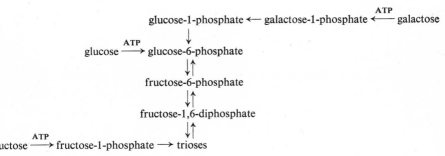

Figure 33   The metabolism of glucose

Other compounds such as amino acids, lactic acid, citric acid, and glycerol may also be converted to glucose in the liver. The formation of glucose from these non-carbohydrate compounds is called *gluconeogenesis*.

Glucose-6-phosphate is either broken down by catabolic processes torelease energy which is then available for tissue metabolism, or it is polymerized to form glycogen (a process known as *glycogenesis*), which is stored mainly in the liver and muscle.

Catabolism (or breakdown) of glucose or glycogen takes place in two stages: The first stage takes place in the cytoplasm of the cell where both products are broken down to pyruvic acid (see Figure 34). The second stage takes place in the mitochondrion where there is an accumulation of energy,

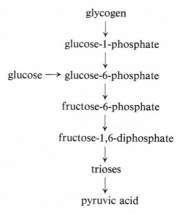

Figure 34   The catabolism of glucose and glycogen

in the form of ATP, from the breakdown of chemical compounds into carbon dioxide and water. Pyruvic acid, which has three carbon atoms, enters the mitochondrion and is converted into the 2 carbon atom compound, acetyl coenzyme A. This in turn combines with the four carbon atom compound, oxalo-acetic acid, to form citric acid, which has 6 carbon atoms.

$$\text{pyruvic acid} \xrightarrow[-2H]{-CO_2} \text{acetyl coenzyme A}$$
$$(3\,\text{C}) \qquad\qquad\qquad (2\,\text{C})$$

In subsequent reactions in the citric acid cycle (Kreb's Cycle) two molecules of CO_2 are lost, and oxalo-acetic acid is regenerated (see Figure 35). Four pairs of hydrogen atoms are also released. These are transported by coenzymes (NAD, NADP, FAD) and cytochromes and combine with oxygen with the production of energy and four molecules of water, two of which are used in the cycle. The overall reaction is:

$$C_6H_{12}O_6 + 6O_2 \rightarrow 6CO_2 + 6H_2O + 686000 \text{ calorie (or 38 ATP)}$$

Unlike other tissues, liver contains the enzyme glucose-6-phosphatase, which can convert glucose-6-phosphate to free glucose and discharge it in the bloodstream whenever needed. When excess carbohydrate is ingested the liver converts the extra glucose to glycogen, thus maintaining the level of glucose in the blood at 80 mg per 100 ml.

When the ingestion of carbohydrates exceeds the storage capacity of the liver and muscle, the excess is converted to fat and deposited in the adipose tissue.

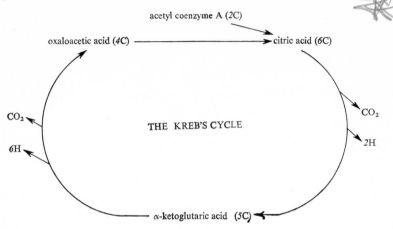

Figure 35   The Kreb's Cycle

Carbohydrates and Muscle

The body can use carbohydrate, fat, and protein as a source of energy, but both fat and protein require chemical modification before they can be used as a fuel. This conversion requires the expenditure of energy therefore they are less efficient as a source of energy than carbohydrates which can be oxidized without further chemical changes. Glycogen is also an important immediate source of energy in muscle but, as the amount available is sufficient for only short periods of activity it must be repleted from the blood glucose. The provision of energy from glycogen in muscle normally requires oxygen; when the blood circulation fails to provide sufficient amounts for immediate needs, the breakdown of glycogen can continue in the absence of circulating oxygen. This *anaerobic* process results in the breakdown of glycogen to lactic acid with the release of some energy. When oxygen again becomes available, some of the lactic acid enters the Kreb's Cycle and is broken down into carbon dioxide and water yielding more energy.

When the oxygen supply is severely depleted, as in prolonged exercise, the lactic acid accumulates in the tissue causing muscle fatigue. The continued breakdown of glycogen to lactic acid without oxygen incurs an *oxygen*

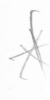

debt to the body which is "repaid" when the lactic acid is resynthesized to glycogen in the liver. There is no mechanism to convert lactic acid to glycogen in muscle. The sequence of these reactions is known as the Cori Cycle which is summarized in Figure 36.

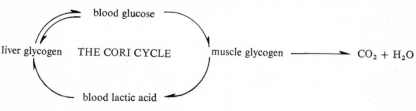

Figure 36   The Cori Cycle

Carbohydrates and the central nervous system

Glucose is essential for maintaining the functional integrity of the nervous system. Although some glycogen is present in nerve tissue, it appears to be bound up in its structure and is unavailable for metabolic use.

The proper function of the central nervous system is more dependent on the regular supply of glucose from blood than all the other tissues and organs of the body. If the blood glucose level is decreased, mental confusion takes place, a phenomenon which is utilized by some psychiatrists who give excessive doses of insulin (insulin shock treatment) in treating mental disease. Hypoglycemia (low blood glucose levels) in low birth weight babies can seriously impair brain function (see page 118).

Carbohydrates and the kidney

In the kidney, glucose escapes from the blood into the fluid filtrate (glomerular filtrate). It is however, almost completely reabsorbed back into the blood stream in the kidney tubule; sometimes the tubules become overloaded so that the glucose is incompletely reabsorbed. The resultant overspill of glucose into the urine is termed *glycosuria* and usually occurs when the blood glucose level exceeds 180 mg per 100 ml of blood.

Hormonal regulation of carbohydrate metabolism

A variety of hormones influence metabolism of carbohydrates, consequently they may cause elevation or reduction of blood glucose levels.

Insulin   This hormone is secreted into the blood by the β-cells of the Islets of Langerhans of the pancreas. Insulin lowers the blood glucose level by acting on the cell membrane to facilitate the entry of glucose into muscle and adipose tissue, and other highly specialized tissues in the mammary gland, anterior pituitary gland, peripheral nerves, spinal cord, white blood cells, and the lens of the eye.

Glucagon   This is secreted by β-cells of the Islets of Langerhans of the pancreas. It elevates blood glucose levels by stimulating the breakdown of liver glycogen to glucose.

Epinephrine   This hormone is also known as *adrenalin* and is secreted by the adrenal medulla. Its effect and mechanism of action are similar to those of glucagon in that it activates the enzyme phosphorylase, but it does so both in liver and muscle (see Figure 37). Epinephrine also influences carbohydrate metabolism indirectly, by stimulating the anterior pituitary to release *adrenocorticotrophic hormone (ACTH)*. *Norepinephrine* produces very slight changes in carbohydrate metabolism.

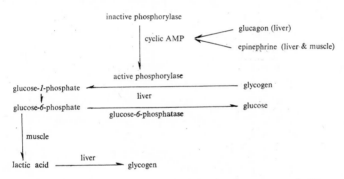

Figure 37   The role of glucagon and epinephrine in glycogen metabolism

ACTH (Adrenocorticotrophic hormone)   This hormone increases blood glucose levels. First by stimulating the release of glucocorticoids of the adrenal cortex; these hormones promote the production of glucose from protein (*gluconeogenesis*). Second, by inhibiting the phosphorylation of glucose to glucose-6-phosphate which is the first reaction in the catabolism of glucose.

Growth hormone   This is one of the hormones manufactured by the *anterior pituitary* gland. It increases blood glucose levels by reducing glucose uptake in tissues (the anti-insulin effect), presumably by inhibiting phosphorylation of glucose to glucose-6-phosphate. It also increases glucose output from the liver and it is suggested that it causes secretion of an unidentified blood glucose-elevating factor by the pancreas.

Thyroxine   This secretion of the thyroid gland enhances absorption of monosaccharides from the intestine and causes some degree of liver glycogen depletion, presumably through the liberation of epinephrine. It may also accelerate degradation of insulin.

The influence of various hormones on carbohydrate metabolism is shown in Figure 38.

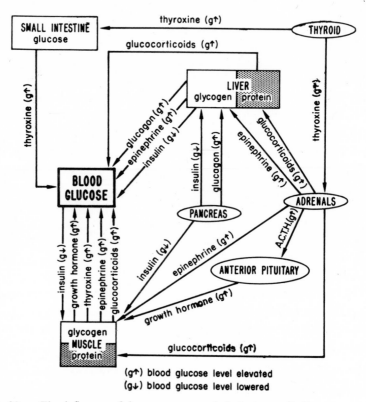

Figure 38   The influence of hormones on carbohydrate metabolism

Carbohydrates and atherosclerosis

This subject will be discussed later in this chapter.

Carbohydrates and tooth decay

The exact causation of tooth decay is still unknown. There is little doubt however, that microorganisms present in the mouth, and dietary carbohydrates, are important etiological factors. The carbohydrates in food may support the growth of certain acid-producing microorganisms that may cause some dissolution of tooth enamel and erosions of the tooth surface. The erosion appears to be more liable to occur where food adheres to the surface of the teeth. As it is impossible to eliminate carbohydrates from the diet, carbohydrate foods which tend to stick to tooth surfaces should be avoided; these include toffee, fudge, candies, and dried fruit.

Disturbances in carbohydrate metabolism

Diabetes   This disorder is due to a reduction in the production of insulin; consequently, less glucose enters the cells and accumulates in the blood stream. The elevation of blood sugar levels (*hyperglycemia*) may be so high that the kidney tubules become overloaded. Above a concentration of 180 mg per 100 ml of blood, the sugar will spill over into the urine. Treatment depends on carbohydrate restriction and the provision of insulin from some external source. It should be remembered however, that the diet should contain adequate calories and protein so that weight may be maintained.

Disturbance in fructose metabolism   Fructose contributes between one-sixth and one-third of the total carbohydrate intake of most diets. More than fifty per cent of the fructose in the body is metabolized by a specific fructose pathway. In some persons, one of the enzymes in this pathway is deficient, so that an abnormally high level of fructose accumulates in the blood. Eventually, this may result in fructose appearing in the urine, thereby giving the disease its name *fructosuria*.

In fructose intolerance, there is a deficiency of a liver enzyme so that fructose accumulates in the cells but, as it is not converted into glucose there is a hypoglycemia. Treatment involves the omission from the diet of fruit and cane sugar which are the main sources of fructose.

Galactosemia   This is caused by a deficiency of an enzyme which converts the galactose-1-phosphate to glucose-1-phosphate; consequently, the former accumulates in the blood, while the blood glucose level is lowered. The signs of this disease occur shortly after birth when milk, the principle source of galactose, is introduced to the child. Continued ingestion of milk sugar results in vomiting and diarrhea. This is followed by jaundice and liver enlargement, the formation of cataracts in the lens of the eye, and mental retardation; these latter conditions may be attributed to hypoglycemia. Treatment lies in the use of lactose-free formulae.

Glycogen deposition disease   These are group of diseases associated with the genetic absence of an enzyme involved in the breakdown or structural modification of stored glycogen. Glucose-6-phosphatase is probably the most commonly deficient. The absence of enzymes leads to an excessive accumulation of glycogen in the liver and other organs and tissues.

Disaccharidase deficiency   When one of the disaccharidases (maltase, lactase, and sucrase) is deficient, digestion of that particular disaccharide cannot take place. Therefore the osmotic pressure of the unabsorbed sugar retains water in the intestine producing diarrhea. This is further aggravated when unabsorbed sugar is broken down by bacteria in the colon into smaller molecules causing an additional increase in osmotic pressure. The bacteria produce organic acids and gas which lead to passage of watery and foamy stools. The diarrhea may be severe enough to cause dehydration. Other symptoms are vomiting, abdominal distention, and cramps. In lactase deficiency, lactose cannot be tolerated and in sucrase, maltase, and iso-maltase deficiency, sucrose, maltose, and isomaltose cannot be utilized. Treatment consists merely of excluding the offending disaccharides and substituting monosaccharides.

The role of fats in the diet

Fats and oils are widespread in nature, being found in food of animal and vegetable origin. In animals, energy is mainly stored in the form of fat.

In poor countries, where most of the land is used to produce carbo-hydrate-rich foods which provide cheap energy, only about 10 per cent of the daily calorie intake is derived from fats. In the highly industrialized countries this figure is in the region of 40–45 per cent of which two-thirds comes from animals and one-third from vegetable sources.

There is a wide variation in preferences for fat. In the Middle East many ethnic groups prefer mutton fat; in England, beef dripping and lard are the fats of choice, where as in many European countries olive oil is preferred. In the United States, butter, margarine, and corn oil are widely used.

Function in the diet

In addition to their chemical and biochemical properties, dietary fats im-part palatability to food by acting as a frying medium, as a seasoning for vegetables, or as a "spread". They also give a feeling of satiety as they delay the emptying of the stomach thereby postponing the onset of hunger sensations. They are also slowly digested. The biochemical functions in-clude the provision of a concentrated source of energy, each gram of fat providing 9 kilocalories compared with the 4 yielded by carbohydrate and protein. Fats supply the essential fatty acids that the body is unable to synthesize and they act as carriers of the fat soluble vitamins A, D, E, and K.

Function of fat in the body

Fats serve as a reservoir of potential chemical energy which is available in times of need. It is also a poor conductor of heat; in its subcutaneous locations it insulates the body and protects it from excessive heat loss. The depots of fat surrounding the vital organs such as the heart and the kidneys provide some protection from physical trauma. Chemically, fats are constituents of the cell membrane and are therefore concerned with the organization of cell function and its permeability to various nutrients.

Chemistry

Fats are composed also of carbon, hydrogen, and oxygen but the proportions of carbon and hydrogen to oxygen are higher in fats than carbohydrates. Fats are esters of fatty acids and alcohol. The alcohol moiety of all food fats is glycerol, a 3 carbon compound to which fatty acids attach (CH_2OH—$CHOH$—CH_2OH). All the fatty acids found in nature have an even number of carbon atoms, a methyl group (—CH_3) at one end, and a carboxyl group (—$COOH$) at the other end; the basic chemical formula for fatty acids is $CH_3(CH_2)n$ $COOH$, where n represents an even number. Fatty acids are either saturated or unsaturated with hydrogen atoms; the unsaturated fatty acids lack one or more pairs of hydrogen atoms. A double bond is formed between the carbon atoms at each point where a pair of hydrogen atoms are absent (see Figure 39).

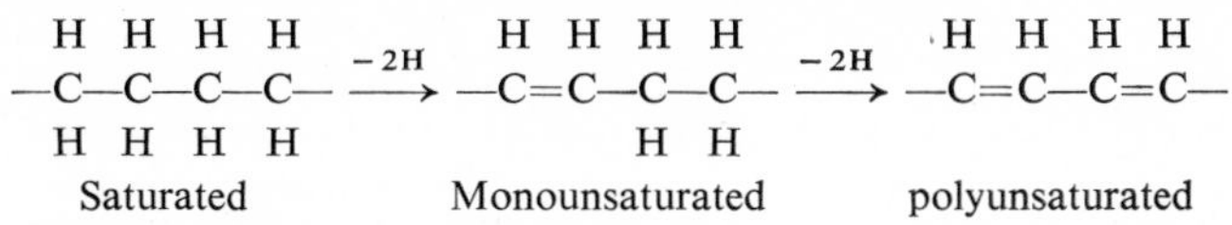

Figure 39   Fatty acids

The most important saturated fatty acids are butyric acid (C_4) found in butter, and palmitic (C_{16}) and stearic (C_{18}) acids found in most vegetable and animal fats. There are several important unsaturated fatty acids. Oleic acid has 18 carbon atoms and one double bond; it is found in most vegetable and animal fats. Linoleic acid (C_{18}, two double bonds) is found in animal and vegetable fats; linolenic acid (C_{18} and three double bonds) is found in vegetable fats and egg yolk. Arachidonic acid (C_{20} and four double bonds) is found in animal tissues.

If only one fatty acid is attached to glycerol, it is called a monoglyceride; if two are attached it is referred to as a diglyceride. If three fatty acids are attached the molecule is called a triglyceride. The three fatty acids in

13*

a triglyceride are seldom the same, so their composition as described by the different fatty acids, could be oleo-dipalmitin or stearo-palmito-olein.

The chemical formulae for the various glycerides are shown in Figure 40.

CH_2OH CH_2OH CH_2OFA_1 CH_2OFA_1

$CHO\text{—}FA_1$ $CHOFA_1$ $CHOFA_2$ $CHOFA_1$

CH_2OH CH_2OFA_2 CH_2OFA_3 CH_2OFA_1

monoglyceride   diglyceride   mixed triglyceride   simple triglyceride

In each case FA_1 FA_2 etc. represents a different fatty acid.

Figure 40   Glycerides

Classification

The term lipid includes true fats and also fat-like substances which are related physically or chemically.

Several types of lipids are of importance in nutrition.

Neutral fats (or *true* fats) are esters of one molecule of glycerol and three molecules of fatty acid. These are the triglycerides described above and they constitute 98 to 99 per cent of food and body fats.

Derived fats are the monoglycerides and diglycerides described above.

Phospholipids are organic esters of fatty acids but they also include phosphoric acid and a nitrogeneous base which could be choline (in lecithins) or ethanolamine or the amino acid serine (in cephalins).

Glycolipids (*cerebrosides*) are present in nervous tissue and contain a carbohydrate (galactose or glucose) in combination with a long chain fatty acid and sphingosine.

Lipoproteins are composed of lipids bound to protein and are found in mammalian plasma.

Sterols, such as cholesterol, are also considered as lipids because they have the same solubility properties as other members of this group. Sterols contain the phenanthrene ring (see Figure 41). Cholesterol is an essential

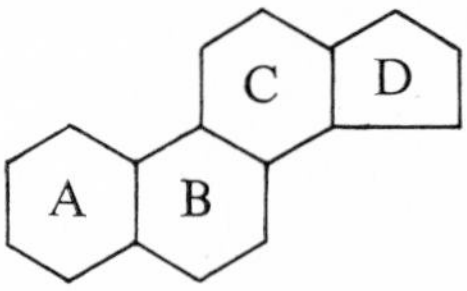

Perhydrocyclopentanophenanthrene

Figure 41   The phenanthrene ring

constituent of many cells, including nerve and glandular tissues. It is found in high concentrations in the liver where it is stored, and in blood where it is transported.

Properties of fats

Pure fats are odorless, tasteless, and generally colorless. The color of natural fats and oils is due to the presence of pigments dissolved in the fat.

Fats are insoluble in water but they are readily dissolved in organic solvents, such as benzene, ether, chloroform, and boiling alcohol. When oil is shaken up in water it forms a transitory emulsion which can be made more permanent by the addition of emulsifying agents such as soaps, bile salts, monoglycerides, and diglycerides. The emulsifying agents act by lowering the surface tension of the water phase; in addition, they are adsorbed on the surface of minute oil droplets. This coating prevents them coalescing. It will be seen later that emulsification is important in the digestion and absorption of fats.

The specific gravity of fats is lower than that of water; this is the reason why cream rises to the surface of milk.

Each fat has a specific melting point. Low molecular weight fats and unsaturated fatty acids have a lower melting point than high molecular weight fats and saturated fatty acids. Thus, glycerides containing unsaturated fatty acids are liquid at room temperature and are called oils, while those containing saturated fatty acids are solid at room temperature and are called fats. For example, while tristearin (C_{18}, saturated) melts at 70°C, tripalmitin (C_{16}, saturated) melts at 66°C, and triolein (C_{18}, unsaturated) melts at −5°C.

Hydrogen can be introduced into the molecules of vegetable oils; this converts them into solid fats, such as margarines and shortenings. This process of hydrogenation eliminates double bonds and changes unsaturated fatty acids into saturated fatty acids.

When a fat containing unsaturated fatty acids comes in contact with air and moisture it becomes rancid, a chemical change caused by the production of peroxides of fatty acids. This takes time, but the process is accelerated by light and heat. Rancid fats are unpalatable and seem to be slightly toxic for some individuals, and destructive to other nutrients in food such as vitamin A. To prevent fat spoilage, food has to be preserved by antioxidants; these are compounds which retard the rate of development of rancidity and they include phenols and hydroquinones. Vegetable oils are more resistant to rancidity than are animal fats because the former contain some natural antioxidants such as vitamin E.

Food sources of fats

Some foods are almost entirely made of fat, these include butter, margarine, shortenings, and cooking oils. These are called *visible* fats and constitute about 45 per cent of dietary fats in highly developed countries.

Foods such as cream, cheese, meat, poultry, fish, nuts, and chocolate contain 20 to 70 per cent fat, while whole grain cereals contain 2 to 9 per cent and seeds 4 to 17 per cent. Fats in these foods are called *invisible* or *hidden*.

Over 98 per cent of lipids that are present in diets are triglycerides. About 31 per cent of the fatty acids present in dietary fats are palmitic and stearic acids, about 40 per cent is the monounsaturated fatty acid oleic acid, and about 12 per cent are the polyunsaturated fatty acids mainly linoleic acid.

Fats of animal origin are butter, suet, tallow, lard, and fish oil, the latter being derived from the liver which stores fat instead of glycogen. Oils can be extracted from many plant sources; these include olives, corn, soyabean, peanuts, cottonseed, rape seeds, sesame seeds, sunflower seeds, poppy seeds, coconuts, oil palm nuts, and pecan nuts.

Digestion and absorption

When the ingested fat reaches the stomach, proteolytic enzymes free fat which may be chemically bound to protein. The mixture is churned up by contractions of the stomach so that the fats form a coarse emulsion. The emulsion is discharged in small amounts into the duodenum where it is mixed with bile and the pancreatic juices. The bile assists in the further emulsification of the fat, it helps to maintain the emulsion and it accelerates the action of pancreatic lipase. The pancreatic lipase acts on the triglycerides (see Figure 42); in complete hydrolysis the triglyceride molecule is broken down into fatty acids and glycerol. Many molecules are not completely hydrolyzed however, so that the molecule may only be reduced to a diglyceride or monoglyceride. Between 50 and 70 per cent of the fatty acids of the ingested triglycerides are hydrolyzed prior to absorption; as digestion proceeds the action of the pancreatic lipase causes the formation of a finer emulsion of triglycerides and diglycerides which are then subjected to further hydrolysis. Formerly, it was believed that very minute oil droplets consisting of triglycerides and diglycerides might be absorbed directly into the intestinal epithelial cell, a process known as *pinocytosis*. Biochemical evidence however, suggests that this is not so, but that absorption of lipids into cells is achieved in two other ways. In the first method, the fatty acids and monoglycerides liberated by the hydrolysis of the emulsified fat are incorporated

directly into the membrane of the intestinal epithelial cell. In the second
method, the fatty acids and monoglycerides combine with bile salts to
form a minute complex (*micelle*) that facilitates absorption of the fatty
acids and monoglycerides (see Figure 43). When the complex is in opposition with the cell membrane, the fatty acids and monoglycerides may
detach and enter the cell leaving the bile salts free to form other micelles;
alternatively, the micelle itself may enter the cell. Whichever method of
absorption is employed, it is independent of enzymes and does not require
the expenditure of energy.

Within the intestinal mucosal cell, triglycerides are resynthesized from
glycerol, monoglycerides, diglycerides, and fatty acids. This helps to maintain a positive concentration gradient which will attract these nutrients
from the lumen of the intestine into the epithelial cell. It should be noted
that the glycerol derived from fats is inactive and cannot combine with

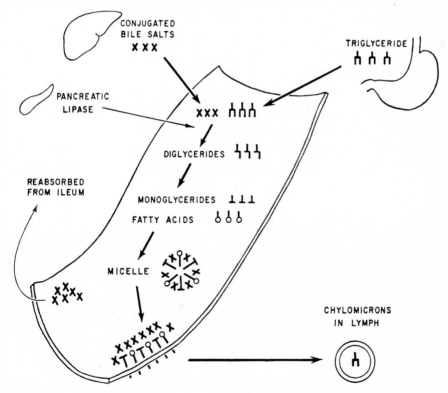

Figure 42   Schematic summary of fat digestion. (Reproduced with the permission of
the Federation of the American Society of Experimental Biology. From Federation Proceedings, **26**, page 1421, 1967)

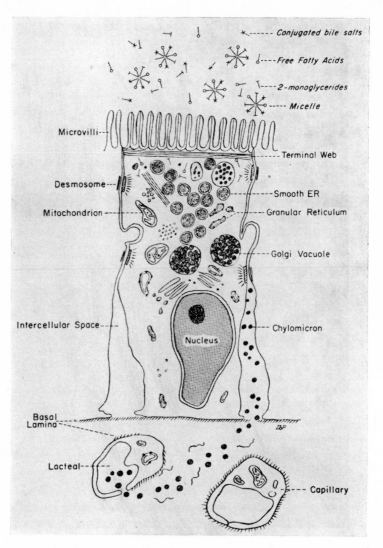

Figure 43   The absorption of lipids. This diagram of a cell of the intestinal mucosa shows the formation of a micelle which facilitates absorption of monoglycerides and fatty acids. Within the cell, triglycerides are resynthesized, coated with lipoprotein, and extruded into the intercellular space as *chylomicrons*. From here, the chylomicrons enter the lacteals. (Reproduced from an original figure by J. F. Trier in Federation Proceedings, **26**: 1392, 1967, by permission of the Federation of American Societies for Experimental Biology)

fatty acids; however, glycerol which has been derived from the metabolism of glucose is in an active form (see Figure 44). The resynthesis of fatty acids to triglycerides in the epithelial cell therefore uses glycerol derived from glucose metabolism. The triglyceride molecules are then coated with lipoprotein and transported as a droplet of microscopic size termed a chylomicron (see Figure 43). Chylomicrons are extruded from the cell by a process of reverse pinocytosis into the intercellular space, and from there, they move through the basement membrane into the lacteals of the mesentery which eventually drain into the thoracic duct. Fatty acids with a chain length of less than 10 carbon atoms are transported directly into the blood capillaries of the basement membrane and eventually drain into the portal vein; all the longer chain fatty acids are absorbed into the lymph system.

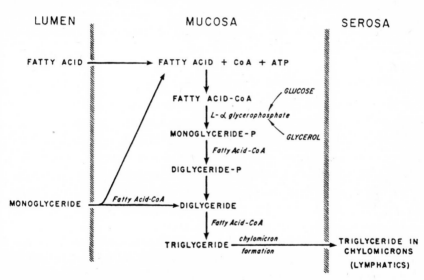

Figure 44   The resynthesis of lipids in the intestinal mucosa. (Reproduced from an original figure by K. J. Isselbacher in Federation Proceedings **26**: 1421, 1967, by permission of the Federation of American Societies for Experimental Biology)

Factors affecting fat absorption

Chain length   The absorption of saturated fatty acids depends on the length of their carbon chain. The longer the chain length the more difficult it is for absorption to take place.

Degree of saturation   Saturated fatty acids are less well absorbed than unsaturated fatty acids.

Bile   The presence of bile salts facilitates the formation of micelles and therefore enhances absorption.

Protein   Increasing the intake of protein stimulates the secretion of pancreatic enzymes; these facilitate the absorption of fat.

Calcium   A high intake of calcium inhibits the absorption of fats because the calcium and the fatty acids form insoluble soaps which are excreted in the feces.

Steatorrhea

This is a condition in which more than 10 per cent of the ingested fat appears in the stools. The etiology of this condition has been discussed on page 70. Steatorrhea can often be treated without reducing the total amount of fat in the diet. This is accomplished by substituting the more readily absorbed triglycerides of medium chain length (MCT) in place of some of the long chain triglycerides normally present in the diet.

Transportation and deposition of fat

The chylomicrons which have been transported through the lymph system reach the blood stream via the thoracic duct. From here they may be taken up by the liver, the fat depots, or other tissues throughout the body. In the liver, the fat is combined with protein and in the form of a lipoprotein it is readily soluble in plasma and can be transported to other tissues. Lipoproteins can be separated by ultracentrifuging into high and low density groups; the former containing more protein and less fat than the latter. Lipoproteins are taken up by the tissues either as a source of energy or, when the intake of energy exceeds the expenditure, for storage in fat depots. When fat is needed it is liberated from the depots and becomes bound to plasma albumin and is carried to those cells which require energy.

 ### Metabolism of fats

Catabolism   Before fats can be oxidized they must be broken down, the first step is into fatty acids and glycerol which follow different paths during subsequent oxidation. The glycerol is oxidized in a similar fashion to that of carbohydrates, finally entering the Kreb's (citric acid) Cycle. The degradation of fatty acids proceeds by a series of reactions in which fragments containing 2 carbon atoms are removed from the fatty acid molecule. This removal is carried out in successive steps; it starts at the carboxyl end of the chain and continues until the molecule is completely broken up. Each fragment forms a molecule of acetyl coenzyme A. Thus for a 16 carbon atom fatty acid such as palmitic acid, this reaction must take place seven times in order to produce 8 molecules of acetyl coenzyme A.

Acetyl coenzyme A may either combine with oxaloacetic acid in the Kreb's Cycle and be completely oxidized to carbon dioxide and water, or it may be resynthesized into fatty acids, *ketone bodies*, or cholesterol.

Anabolism   The basic mechanism for building up fatty acids consists of the combination of molecules of acetyl coenzyme A in a head-to-tail linkup.

Animals can use acetyl coenzyme A derived from any source and build up fatty acids by adding 2 carbon molecules at a time. In this way palmitic acid (C_{16}) can gain 2 carbon atoms and be converted to stearic acid; similarly it can lose 2 carbon atoms and be converted to myristic acid (C_{14}). Mammals can also dehydrogenate saturated fatty acids to the corresponding unsaturated fatty acids. For example, stearic acid becomes oleic acid by losing two hydrogen atoms (see Figure 45). The fatty acids thus formed may be incorporated into phospholipids or triglycerides.

$$\text{myristic acid} \underset{-2C}{\overset{+2C}{\rightleftarrows}} \text{palmitic acid} \underset{-2C}{\overset{+2C}{\rightleftarrows}} \text{stearic acid}$$
$$\downarrow -2H$$
$$\text{oleic acid}$$

Figure 45   Anabolism, and dehydrogenation, of fatty acids

Essential fatty acids

The body is incapable of synthesizing certain unsaturated polyunsaturated fatty acids (linoleic, linolenic, arachidonic) which are necessary for growth and the well-being of man, especially in infancy. Such fatty acids are termed *essential fatty acids*. However, the only real essential fatty acid is linoleic acid because the body can convert it into linolenic and arachidonic acid (see Figure 46).

$$\text{linoleic} \xrightarrow{-2H} \text{linolenic} \xrightarrow[+2C]{-2H} \text{arachidonic}$$
$$(C_{18}, 2 \text{ double bonds}) \quad (C_{18}, 3 \text{ double bonds}) \quad (C_{20}, 4 \text{ double bonds})$$

Figure 46   Synthesis of essential fatty acids

Animals kept on diets deficient in essential fatty acids have poor growth and they develop skin lesions. Feeding of linoleic acid is completely effective in restoring growth and curing the skin lesions of deficient animals.

A diet providing 1 per cent of its calories from linoleic acid meets the human requirement for the essential fatty acids.

Ketosis

When carbohydrate is not available for the production of energy, fat is metabolized instead. This state of affairs occurs in starvation when the intake of carbohydrate is low, or in diabetes when insulin deficiency does not allow glucose to be used. The fatty acid oxidation results in an excess of acetyl coenzyme A which cannot be handled by the Kreb's Cycle so there is a condensation of 2 molecules of acetyl coenzyme A; this results in the formation of acetoacetic acid. A large portion of the acetoacetic acid is reduced in the liver to hydroxybutyric acid; a minor part is converted to acetone by the removal of carbon dioxide from the molecule (see Figure 47). These three substances, acetoacetic acid, beta-hydroxybutyric acid, and acetone, are termed ketone bodies.

$$2 \text{ acetyl coenzyme A} \longrightarrow \text{acetoacetic acid} \xrightarrow{+2H} \text{beta-hydroxy-butyric acid}$$
$$\downarrow -CO_2$$
$$\text{acetone}$$

Figure 47   Ketone bodies

The peripheral tissues, especially muscle, have an efficient mechanism for the oxidation of ketone bodies. Under the above conditions when the rate of production of ketone bodies exceeds the rate of oxidation there is an increase in the concentration of ketones in the blood (*ketonemia*) which may spill over into the urine (*ketonuria*). This condition characterized by a high concentration of ketone bodies in the tissues and tissue fluids is called *ketosis*.

Since acetoacetic acid and beta-hydroxybutyric acid are moderately strong acids, they exist in urine as anions. Cations are excreted by the kidney in order to maintain the electron neutrality of urine. There is therefore a loss of sodium ions from the body; as the plasma and other body fluids become depleted of cations, acidosis develops. In order to maintain adequate dilution of the salts of acetoacetic and beta-hydroxybutyric acids which are excreted in the urine, large quantities of water are also excreted causing dehydration.

Hormonal regulation of fat metabolism

A number of hormones coordinate various phases of lipid metabolism. Insulin stimulates the formation of lipids from glucose in adipose tissue and inhibits the liberation of free fatty acids into the blood stream. Epinephrine and norepinephrine activate tissue lipase thereby promoting the hydrolysis of lipids in adipose tissue. They also cause a rise in plasma-free fatty acid levels, although the presence of adrenocortical and thyroid hormones are required also.

ACTH promotes the release of fatty acids from adipose tissue. Thyroid hormone lowers plasma cholesterol, phospholipids, and lipoprotein levels. This could be caused by the hormone altering the biosynthetic and catabolic rates of cholesterol; the catabolic effect however, predominates over the synthetic.

Cholesterol

The type of fat with which ingested cholesterol is associated, undoubtedly affects cholesterol levels in blood. For example, cholesterol dissolved in butter, or cholesterol dissolved in eggs, causes a greater increase in blood cholesterol levels than the same quantity of cholesterol dissolved in vegetable oil. Ingestion of animal fats, which have a high content of saturated fatty acids, increases the level of blood cholesterol. Conversely, consumption of a higher proportion of vegetable oil and fish oil which are rich in polyunsaturated fatty acids lowers blood cholesterol levels.

Vegetable oils are hydrogenated during the processing of margarine and shortenings; this process makes the fats more saturated. For some reasons which are as yet unknown, consumption of such fats results in an elevation of blood cholesterol levels. However, restricting the quantity of cholesterol-containing foods, such as eggs, does not lower blood cholesterol levels because the body synthesizes about 2 grams of cholesterol per day. This quantity is greater than that supplied by a normal diet (0.5 to 1 gram per day) and is used for several physiological functions including the synthesis of sex hormones, the transport of lipids, as a constituent of skin, and as a covering of nerve fibers.

Nutrition and coronary heart disease

Between 1955 and 1960 a possible relationship between diet patterns and coronary heart disease was suggested. Epidemiological studies indicated that mortality from coronary heart disease and blood cholesterol levels were low in populations consuming a diet which contained little fat from animal sources. Conversely, populations consuming large amounts of animal fat had high cholesterol levels and a high mortality from coronary heart disease.[1,2] It had already been shown that serum cholesterol levels could be lowered by replacing the saturated fat of animals with unsaturated vegetable fats. This phenomenon explains the low cholesterol levels in populations consuming a diet which is predominantly vegetable in origin. Misinterpretation of scientific data, and improper reporting of facts, have led the public to believe that there is a direct cause and effect relationship between the intake of animal fat, high cholesterol levels, and mortality from coronary heart disease. However, there is no scientific evidence that high cholesterol levels are caused entirely by high intakes of animal fat nor is there evidence that the high cholesterol levels are responsible for atherosclerosis. The role of the diet in coronary artery disease is much more complex and consideration must be given to dietary components other than fat.

Protein   Diets incorporating animal fats usually contain animal protein. The effect of protein intake on serum lipid levels should therefore be assessed. Serum cholesterol levels can be lowered by reducing the amount of animal protein in the diet and it is well known that serum lipid levels are low in protein calorie malnutrition.

Epidemiological studies have shown that populations increasing their protein intake also increase their chance of coronary artery disease. Japanese immigrants to the United States and Sephardic and African Jews immigrating to Israel experienced increased lipid levels and coronary artery disease in their new environment. While the transition to the more sophisticated society is associated with increased intakes of animal fat, protein, and refined carbohydrate, sophisticated living also brings a more sedentary life, a greater exposure to stress, a greater chance of living to an age when degenerative diseases are important, and a more prolonged exposure to the effects of smoking and alcohol. All of these factors may be important in the etiology of coronary heart disease.

Carbohydrates   Any carbohydrate ingested in excess of requirements is converted into fat. The increase in fat may be responsible for the high blood triglyceride level which appears to add to the risks of coronary heart disease. It has also been observed that in certain circumstances (perhaps abnormal) high cholesterol and high triglyceride levels can be lowered by carbohydrate restriction. Epidemiological studies of the Masai and Sambura tribes of East Africa have revealed that they have a high fat and a low sugar intake and little coronary artery disease. The population of the Island of St. Helena has a low fat and a high carbohydrate intake and the mortality experience from coronary heart disease is high. In both of these populations the respective roles of stress and exercise cannot be measured, but the possibility that dietary carbohydrates may be important in the development of coronary artery disease cannot be ignored. The chemical characteristics of the sugar appears to be important for it has been noted that high triglyceride and cholesterol levels in persons consuming sucrose can be lowered by substituting starch for the sugar.

Lipidemia

The interplay between dietary carbohydrate and fats and the lipid levels in the blood has led to much study of the blood levels of cholesterol and triglycerides. The biochemical findings have been classified on this basis,[3]

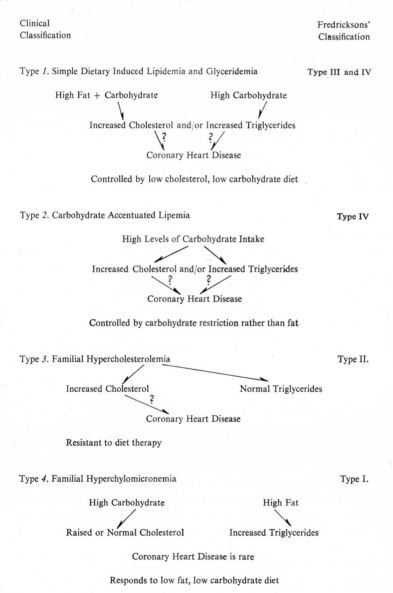

Clinical
Classification

Fredricksons'
Classification

Type *1*. Simple Dietary Induced Lipidemia and Glyceridemia   Type III and IV

High Fat + Carbohydrate   High Carbohydrate

Increased Cholesterol and/or Increased Triglycerides

?   ?

Coronary Heart Disease

Controlled by low cholesterol, low carbohydrate diet

Type *2*. Carbohydrate Accentuated Lipemia   **Type IV**

High Levels of Carbohydrate Intake

Increased Cholesterol and/or Increased Triglycerides

?   ?

Coronary Heart Disease

Controlled by carbohydrate restriction rather than fat

Type *3*. Familial Hypercholesterolemia   Type II.

Increased Cholesterol   Normal Triglycerides

?

Coronary Heart Disease

Resistant to diet therapy

Type *4*. Familial Hyperchylomicronemia   Type I.

High Carbohydrate   High Fat

Raised or Normal Cholesterol   Increased Triglycerides

Coronary Heart Disease is rare

Responds to low fat, low carbohydrate diet

Figure 48   The etiology of lipidemia

but for the nutrition worker it may be less confusing if the biochemical findings are related to epidemiological and dietary knowledge; these are summarized in Figure 48.

Simple dietary induced lipidemia and glyceridemia   This occurs in individuals with no apparent metabolic abnormality. A high fat and carbohydrate intake may lead to elevated blood cholesterol and triglyceride levels, and is associated with a high mortality experience from coronary heart disease. This type of lipidemia may be expected to respond to dietary restriction of cholesterol, animal products, animal fat, and carbohydrate. It should be remembered however, that the body is capable of manufacturing cholesterol itself and is not dependent on outside sources of this nutrient. The biochemical observations in this type of lipidemia correspond to Fredrickson's Type III and IV.

Carbohydrate accentuated lipidemia   This usually occurs in persons with a genetically transmitted metabolic abnormality but it may also occur in normal persons consuming large quantities of carbohydrate. It corresponds to Fredrickson's Type IV lipidemia. It is characterized by elevated cholesterol and triglyceride levels which either alone, or in combination, have been associated with coronary heart disease. The cholesterol and triglyceride levels are improved by restricting carbohydrate but the lowering of the lipids to normal levels does not seem possible.

Familial hypercholesterolemia   This is an inherited disease in which the patient has elevated blood cholesterol levels and normal triglyceride levels; it corresponds to Fredrickson's Type II lipidemia. Familial hypercholesterolemia is associated with a high mortality rate from coronary heart disease. It is resistant to diet therapy including the marked restriction of dietary cholesterol and saturated fats and the adoption of a low unsaturated fat diet.

Hyperchylomicronemia   This is a rare familial condition in which the body is unable to clear the blood of the chylomicrons that transport fat from the lacteals of the intestine. It does not necessarily carry the risk of coronary heart disease and it corresponds to the Fredrickson's Type I lipidemia.

In addition to the dietary influences on cholesterol levels, it is possible that there is also a genetic control; for men belonging to Blood Group A have higher mean cholesterol levels than men in Blood Groups 0 or B.[4]

The genesis of atherosclerosis

In rabbits, the development of atherosclerosis can be accelerated by providing a diet in which the fat is predominantly saturated and conversely the process can be inhibited by providing unsaturated fats. It has been assumed that human atherosclerosis is similarly affected by diet but there is no scientific evidence that this is so.

Atherosclerosis is a degenerative condition of the arteries. In the earliest stages, there is a fatty streaking or spotting of the wall of the vessel caused by the formation of new connective tissue which contains cells distended with fat and cholesterol. A fibrous plaque next develops between the internal and middle coats of the artery; at first these are small and discrete but they are elevated and may reduce the diameter of the vessel. Large plaques seriously interfere with the flow of blood and eventually they may block the lumen of the vessel completely. The consistency of the plaque is normal at first, but it undergoes softening and its surface may break down so that an ulcer is formed. When the ulcer is invaded by fibrous repair tissue it causes distortion of the lumen of the vessel. Calcification, hemorrhage, and clot may restrict or block the circulation. The obstruction of blood flow through the coronary arteries may be due to an atherosclerotic process alone or it may be combined with thrombus formation.

The mechanism of formation of atheroma is not understood but several theories have been advanced.

The lipid infiltration theory   The plasma lipid mixture normally permeates the inner portions of the arterial wall by simple diffusion and there is no deposition of lipid. Where tissues are damaged however, cholesterol is liable to accumulate. It is suggested that vessels may be subject to damage by temporary elevations of blood pressure such as occurs during times of stress. If the serum lipid levels are elevated at that time, then damage and the development of atheromata are more likely. This theory encourages the concept of lowering cholesterol levels in the blood by replacing saturated fats with unsaturated fats in the diet.

Deficiency of essential fatty acids   Experimental animals that have been deprived of essential fatty acids have capillaries whose walls are more permeable than normal. It is believed that this increased permeability allows large molecules, such as lipoprotein-bound cholesterol, to diffuse through arterial walls where they may establish an atheromatous plaque as described above. This theory is supported by the observation that the process of atherosclerosis in animals can be retarded (but not completely controlled) by including large amounts of linoleic acid in the diet.

Hemostasis   This theory postulates that atherosclerosis starts with blood platelets adhering to damaged endothelial cells of the arterial wall. If there is not immediate healing, the platelets aggregate and a clot forms; in time, the clot this will be invaded by fibrous tissue and may be incorporated in the wall of the vessel and overgrown by its endothelial lining.

Prostaglandins   Essential fatty acids are the precursors of *prostaglandins* which may form a link between the dietary fat and atherosclerosis. Prostaglandins synthesized in the tissues are released to the extra-cellular fluid and then to the blood. One of their functions is to inhibit the aggregation of platelets. It has been suggested that the prostaglandins permeate or coat the walls of the blood vessels and act as a protective mechanism against platelet aggregation. Prostaglandins also counteract hypertension for they are antagonistic to *catecholamines*. These latter substances induce high blood pressure and stimulate the mobilization of adipose tissue; they are released under conditions of emotional stress and by tobacco smoking. Normally, any release of catecholamines would be counteracted by the prostaglandins but if these are deficient there is no antagonism; in addition, the vessel wall would not be protected. Under the stimulus of catecholamines there would be lipolysis of fat and perhaps episodes of hypertension that could damage the cell wall. All these conditions would favor the development of atherosclerosis. There is still much to be learned of prostaglandins but they may provide an explanation for several phenomena which formerly appeared to be unrelated.[5]

It should not be overlooked that water is an essential nutrient. Recent studies have indicated a relationship between cardiovascular disease and the chemical quality of the drinking water. Populations living in England and Wales supplied by "hard" water (which contains more calcium) had a lower mortality experience than other populations served by "soft" water.[6] Further studies are required to assess the various influences of diet, stress, smoking, and other environmental conditions before any single cause and effect relationship can be established. It is still too early to incriminate any nutrient, including water, in the causation of atherosclerosis and coronary heart disease.

The role of proteins in the diet

Proteins are complex organic compounds containing nitrogen. They are found in all animal and plant cells where they constitute the vital part of protoplasm. The average protein content of the dry matter of the adult body is about 50 per cent but the distribution within the tissues varies; for example, muscle contains about 30 per cent, bone and cartilage 20 per cent, and skin 10 per cent.

Proteins play a significant role in the vital processes of all living organisms from the smallest virus to the largest mammals including man. As structural elements, or as biological catalysts, proteins participate in all body functions. They can also be used to provide energy, or thay may be converted into glucose or fat as required.

Unlike plants and bacteria, animals are unable to utilize the element nitrogen. In order to maintain proper body function protein of good quality has to be supplied in the diet in sufficient quantities throughout life.

In the highly industrialized countries, protein provides about 14 per cent of the daily calorie intake, but in less developed countries where cereals and starchy roots are the primary staples, protein may only account for 7 or 8 per cent of the calories in the diet. At such low levels of intake and where protein is also of poor quality, protein calorie malnutrition is inevitably prevalent.

Function of protein

Maintenance and growth   Proteins supply essential amino acids for growth of new tissue, and the repair of old and damaged tissue. Protein is involved in the synthesis of enzymes, hemoglobin, antibodies, and hormones such as insulin, thyroxin, parathyroid hormone, epinephrine, and pituitary hormones.

Production of energy   When dietary protein is in excess of that needed for maintenance and growth, or when diet does not contain sufficient carbohydrates and fat to meet calorie needs, proteins are burnt as body fuel.

Maintenance of water balance   Proteins are unable to penetrate capillary membranes so that they exert an osmotic pressure; this influences the exchange of water between the tissue fluids and the surrounding body fluids.

Regulation of acid-base balance   Proteins have amino ($-NH_2$) and carboxyl ($-COOH$) groups which can react with, and neutralize, acids or bases. They play an important role in ensuring a constant body pH.

Chemistry

Proteins are composed of carbon, hydrogen, and oxygen, but in addition they contain nitrogen; most proteins also contain sulphur, and several include phosphorus, iron, or iodine in their molecules. Proteins are made up of amino acids of which there are 20 (Table 18). Each amino acid consists of an amino acid group, a carboxyl group, and a radical (R) attached to the

14*

same carbon atom. Amino acids can be linked together through the carboxyl group of one and the amino group of another; this type of linkage is termed a *peptide* linkage. Several amino acids therefore form a *peptide*; groups of peptides form larger molecules called *polypeptides* and the linking of several polypeptides constitutes *a protein*.

Table 18   Amino acids

Essential	Non-essential
valine	glycine
leucine	alanine
isoleucine	serine
methionine	tyrosine
threonine	cysteine
phenylalanine	cystine
lysine	aspartic acid
tryptophan	glutamic acid
histidine*	arginine
	proline
	hydroxyproline

* Histidine is essential for infants only.

The general formula for amino acids is

$$R—\overset{\displaystyle H}{\underset{\displaystyle NH_2}{C}}—COOH.$$

Amino acids differ only in the character of the radical. Some amino acids have a *straight* chain, in others the radical is *branched* or in a *ring form* (see Table 19). Cystine with the radical $R = HS—CH_2$, cysteine which consists of 2 molecules of cystine, and methionine $(R = CH_3—S—CH_2CH_2)$ contain sulfur. Aspartic acid $(R = COOH—CH_2)$ and glutamic acid $(R = COOH—CH_2—CH_2)$ have 2 COOH groups and hence are known as diacidic amino acids. Arginine $(R = {}_2HN—C—NH—CH_2CH_2CH_2)$, lysine $(R = {}_2HN—CH_2CH_2CH_2CH_2)$, and histidine have 2 NH$_2$ groups and are therefore known as dibasic amino acids.

All amino acids except glycine have at least one asymmetric carbon atom. When the COOH is placed on top of the formula, NH$_2$ is written to the left of the carbon atom for L-amino acids, and to the right for D-amino acids. The naturally occurring amino acids in animal and plant proteins are of the L-form.

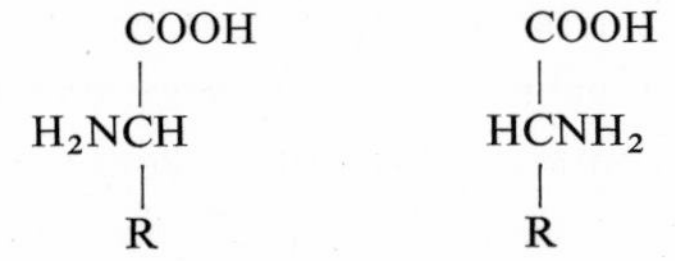

$$
\begin{array}{cc}
\text{COOH} & \text{COOH} \\
| & | \\
\text{H}_2\text{NCH} & \text{HCNH}_2 \\
| & | \\
\text{R} & \text{R} \\
\text{L-amino acid} & \text{D-amino acid}
\end{array}
$$

Table 19   Amino acid linkages

Straight chain amino acids.

glycine R = H

alanine R = CH_3

serine R = CH_2OH

threonine R = CH_3CHOH.

Branched chain amino acids

valine R = CH_3—$\overset{\overset{\displaystyle CH_3}{|}}{CH}$

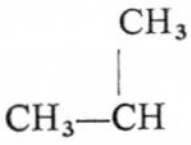

leucine R = CH_3—$\overset{\overset{\displaystyle CH_3}{|}}{CH}$—$CH_2$

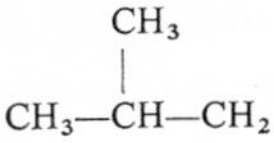

isoleucine R = CH_3—CH_2—$\overset{\overset{\displaystyle CH_3}{|}}{CH}$

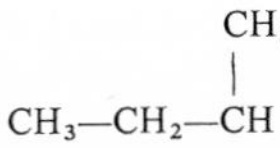

Amino acids with *ring form* radicles.

phenylalanine R = —CH_2

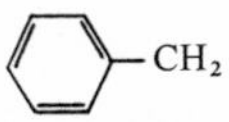

tyrosine R = HO——CH_2

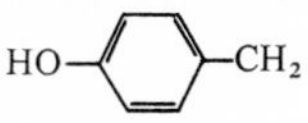

tryptophan R =

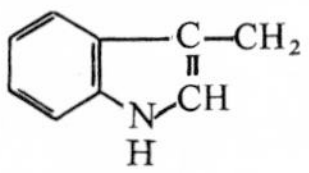

histidine R =

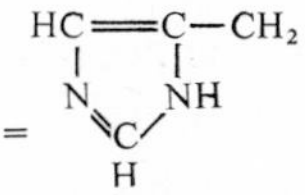

proline R =

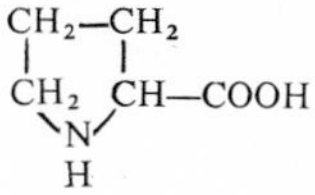

hydroxyproline R =

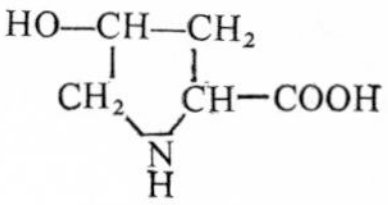

Amino acids are soluble in water. Since they have both COOH and NH_2 groups they can react with either bases or acids.

The percentage of nitrogen in different proteins varies; for example, milk contains 15.7 per cent, some nuts may contain up to 19 per cent. To convert nitrogen content into protein content, it is assumed that all proteins contain 16 per cent nitrogen and hence the nitrogen value is multiplied by the factor $6.25 \left(\dfrac{100}{16} = 6.25 \right)$. The discrepancy between the assumed nitrogen content and the actual content causes inaccuracies in the evaluation of the nutrient content of diets (see page 385).

Essential and non-essential amino acids

Essential amino acids are those which must be supplied by the food. Of the 9 amino acids listed in Table 18 which are essential to man, 8 of them cannot be synthesized. The ninth is histidine which cannot be synthesized rapidly enough for growth and maintenance in infants. Other amino acids may be essential for other species.

Non-essential amino acids are those which can be synthesized in the body in adequate amounts. This is achieved by combining an NH_2 group of one amino acid with the carbon skeleton residue of the intermediary products of carbohydrate and fat metabolism. The body has no difficulty in synthesizing amino acids whose carbon skeleton chains are straight. During the course of evolution it has lost the ability to form either the branched chains, which would be required to synthesize leucine, iso-leucine, and valine, and the cyclic chains, which are required to synthesize tryptophan and phenylalanine. Therefore, the main difference between essential and non-essential amino acids is the inability of the body to manufacture a carbon skeleton of the right configuration.

It should be noted that essential amino acids are not more important for growth and metabolism than the non-essential amino acids. The terms imply only the necessity for a supply of essential amino acids from the diet. For efficient protein synthesis, both essential and non-essential amino acids must be available simultaneously, and in sufficient quantities, to meet the needs of the body.

Classification of proteins

Proteins which yield only amino acids on hydrolysis are called simple proteins. Table 20 shows some of the sources of simple proteins. Simple proteins are differentiated from each other by their solubility in water, salt solutions, alcohol, dilute acids and bases, and by their physical response to heat.

Proteins may conjugate with several substances in various sites (see Table 21); the chemical group which joins up with the protein (in addition to the amino acids) is known as the *prosthetic* group.

Table 20   Sources of protein

Protein	Source
Albumins and globulins	Blood serum, eggs
Histones and protamines	Cell nuclei
Scleroproteins	Keratin in nails, collagen in skin and bone, elastin in ligaments
Glutelins	Wheat
Prolamines	Zein in maize
Oryzinin	Rice

Table 21   Protein conjugation

Prosthetic Group	Product	Site
Nucleic acid	Nucleoproteins	Chromosomes
Fats	Lipoproteins	Serum
Carbohydrates	Glycoproteins	Intestinal mucous membrane
Phosphoric acid	Phosphoproteins	Milk casein
Porphyrins	Hemoprotein	Hemoglobin
Riboflavin derivatives	Flavoproteins	Enzymes
Iron	Metalloproteins	Ferritin in cells
Zinc	Metalloproteins	Carbonic anhydrase enzyme

Food sources of proteins

The dietary protein intake is derived from animal and plant sources. However, proteins are not stored in large quantities in either animals or plants; even protein-rich foods have relatively low concentrations of protein. There is also a wide variation in the protein content among species in both the animal and vegetable kingdom (see Table 22).

Protein quality

The quality of protein depends on a number of factors:

Amino acid composition   Various proteins differ in their amino acid content. A good quality protein or a *complete* protein such as meat, eggs, or milk supplies sufficient quantities of all the essential amino acids to meet body needs for maintenance and growth. A poor quality protein, or an *incomplete* protein such as zein of corn which lacks tryptophan and lysine, can support neither maintenance nor growth. A protein such as gliadin of wheat, which provides enough lysine for maintenance but not growth, is called *partially complete*.

Table 22   Protein content of foods

Food	Content (%)
Meat	14–30
Poultry	9–30
Fish	9–26
Egg	12
Milk	3.5
Vegetables	1–5
Legumes	1–23
Fruits	0.5–3.0

Balance of amino acids   A balanced protein such as that of egg and milk contains amino acids in the right proportions. Other food proteins may be imbalanced with respect to one or more amino acids, e.g. zein of maize. is imbalanced by leucine and isoleucine.

Amino acid imbalance is brought about by a change in the proportion of amino acids in the diet. The imbalance inhibits growth but it can be overcome by supplementation with those essential amino acids which are present in the least quantity in the diet. Such amino acids are termed *limiting amino acids* (*L.A.A.*).

Amino acid antagonism refers to a pattern of amino acids in the diet in which the excess quantity of one amino acid causes retardation of growth; thus excess leucine depresses the utilization of isoleucine and valine, and excess lysine depresses the utilization of arginine.

Amino acid antagonism or imbalance, may actually increase the requirement for an individual amino acid. Consequently if some amino acids are present in excess, the remainder may be inadequate although they may be present in quantities that would be considered adequate when the amino acids are in balanced proportions.

Amino acid availability   The rates at which amino acids are liberated from different proteins vary widely and they depend on the nature of the linkages within the protein molecule. These linkages, which determine the digestibility of various proteins, may be affected by the manner of food preparation. Heat, for example, uncoils the folded proteins and exposes a larger surface area to the digestive enzymes. Excessive, or prolonged heat, may encourage the formation of additional linkages; this is especially liable to occur when protein is heated in the presence of carbohydrates and is the reason why toasting bread, reduces the availability of lysine.

Proteins of animal origin are usually of a better quality than plant proteins which may lack one or more of the essential amino acids. The deficiency in protein quality is not confined to plant proteins. Gelatin, a protein of animal origin, lacks tryptophan and contains only small amounts of tyrosine and cysteine.

Lysine and threonine levels in cereals are generally low, in addition, maize is also deficient in tryptophan. Legumes are good sources of lysine and threonine but they are deficient in methionine and tryptophan. Green leafy vegetables are well balanced with respect to all the essential amino acids with the exception of methionine. Despite these shortcomings, it is possible to devise meals containing good quality protein by combining proteins from several sources. These supplement the amino acid content of each other and consequently assist in making the amino acid mixture of the meal as a whole complete. Such mixtures of proteins are a feature of most traditional diets. In the Middle East, for example, wheat bread which lacks lysine is frequently eaten with cheese which has a high lysine content.

Effective supplementation only occurs, however, when the deficient and supplementary proteins are ingested simultaneously or within a short interval of time. For this reason the complementary proteins of maize and beans are better utilized when ingested together.

It can be seen that it is not absolutely essential to consume expensive animal proteins to support growth nor is there any reason why vegetarians should suffer from protein deficiency.

The biological value of deficient protein foods may also be improved by supplementing the missing or limiting amino acid with pure, synthetic amino acids, for example, lysine may be added to cereals and methionine to legumes.

Evaluation of protein quality

A number of biological and chemical methods are available for determining protein quality. Most techniques are based on growth response, nitrogen balance, or amino acid concentrations. The most popular methods will be described in brief.

Estimation of Biological Value (B. V.) This is determined from the proportion of absorbed nitrogen retained in the body.

$$\text{B. V.} = \frac{\text{body nitrogen}}{\text{absorbed nitrogen}} = \frac{I - (U + F)}{I - F} \times 100,$$

where I = nitrogen intake, U = urinary nitrogen, F = fecal nitrogen. The biological value is an index of the percentage of absorbed nitrogen retained for growth and maintenance, but it does not take into consideration incomplete absorption. The biological values of various food items are given in Table 23.

Table 23 Biological value of food

Food item	Biological value
Egg	100
Milk	93
Rice	86
Fish	75
Beef	75
Maize	72
Cottonseed flour	60
Groundnut flour	56
Wheat gluten	44

Digestibility This represents the proportion of food nitrogen absorbed. It is calculated as follows:

$$\text{Coefficient of Digestibility} = \frac{\text{absorbed } N \times 100}{N \text{ intake}} = \frac{I - F}{I} \times 100$$

Net Protein Utilization (NPU) The NPU is the proportion of food nitrogen retained in the body. It is the product of the biological value and digestibility and is calculated from the equation

$$\text{NPU} = \frac{B - B_0}{I}$$

where B = body nitrogen (measured at the end of the test period on animals fed the test diet), B_0 = body nitrogen at zero time (measured on a control group of animals at the beginning of the test period). Since the efficiency of protein utilization decreases when the caloric intake is low or when the protein intake is high, the NPU must be measured under standard conditions. It is unfortunate that these standards can seldom be achieved under normal situations of food intake. Table 24 shows the NPU of various foodstuffs.

Table 24 Chemical Score and Net Protein Utilization of selected proteins

Food	Score	Limiting amino acid	NPU
Egg	100	—	100
Milk (cow's)	60	S*	75
Casein	60	S	72
Pork	80	S	84
Fish	75	Tryptophan	83
Rice	75	Lysine	57
Corn meal (maize)	45	Tryptophan	55
Millet	60	Lysine	56
White flour	50	Lysine	52
Peanut flour	70	S	48
Soy flour	70	S	56
Sesame seed	50	Lysine	56
Sunflower seed	70	Lysine	65
Navy bean	42	S	47
Peas	60	S	44
Potato	70	S	71
Sweet potato	75	S	72
Spinach	90	S	—
Cassava	40	S	—

* S = Sulphur-containing amino acids (methionine and cystine)

Source. *Health Aspects of Food and Nutrition*. W. H. O. 1969

Protein Efficiency Ratio (PER)   The PER is the weight gain of growing animals divided by the weight of the protein they consume.

$$PER = \frac{\text{weight increment (gram)}}{\text{protein consumed (gram)}}$$

The shortcomings of this method are twofold; first the PER varies with the food intake, and second it is limited to growing animals.

Nitrogen Balance   Nitrogen balance is the apparent nitrogen retention by the body and is calculated:

$$\text{Nitrogen Balance} = I - (F + U)$$

where I = nitrogen intake, F = fecal nitrogen, and U = urinary nitrogen. When the nitrogen intake equals nitrogen excretion, the individual is in nitrogen equilibrium, indicating that the protein intake is sufficient to support maintenance but not growth. When the intake exceeds excretion, the individual is in positive nitrogen balance, indicating that the intake is able to support growth. Finally, if the intake is less than excretion, the individual is in negative nitrogen balance, and is losing some tissue proteins.

Protein repletion method In this method the influence of protein on the rate of regaining body weight is measured and is determined from increases in the amount of protein in the liver, or increases in plasma protein levels in previously depleted animals.

Chemical Score (C. S.) The chemical score is the percentage of the limiting amino acid in a food protein compared with the amount of the same amino acid in a standard protein.

$$\text{C. S.} = \frac{\text{per cent limiting amino acid} \times 100}{\text{per cent same amino acid in standard protein}}$$

Although the chemical determination of protein quality is a valuable means of assessment of protein quality, the availability of the amino acids cannot be estimated; consequently, the chemical scores are often higher than indicated by biological evaluation. Furthermore, chemical assessment cannot take into account the effects of one or more amino acids on others present in the food so that evaluation of protein quality on chemical criteria has serious limitations. The chemical score may serve a useful role in identifying poor quality protein (see Table 24); it does not necessarily give a proper indication of the true quality of good protein for some of the amino acids may not be available for absorption and utilization by the body.

The utilization of protein depends on the caloric intake, so evaluation of protein should take this into account. A theoretical unit *NDpCal%* is being increasingly used to evaluate not only protein in a food or a diet but also the protein requirements of individuals and groups (see page 396).

Net Dietary protein Calories per cent (NDpCal%) The first step in the determination of NDpCal% is to relate the quantity of the protein in the food (or diet) to the total calories in the food (or diet). The protein calories per cent is estimated from the following:

$$\text{Protein Cal\%} = \frac{\text{No. of calories contributed by protein in the food} \times 100}{\text{total No. of calories in the food (or diet)}}$$

$$= \frac{\text{protein in grams} \times 4 \times 100}{\text{total calorific value of food (or diet)}}$$

If, for example, a given quantity of food contains 40 grams of protein and the total calorie value of the food is 1600 calories then,

$$\text{Protein Cal\%} = \frac{40 \times 4 \times 100}{1600} = 10.0$$

The next step is to evaluate the quality of the protein. This is done by comparing the value of protein in the food with a theoretical "perfect" or "ideal" protein. For this purpose, the amount of limiting amino acid

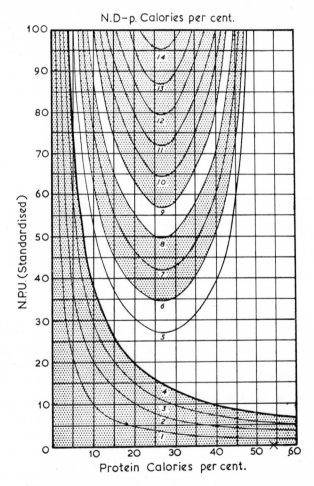

Figure 49   Nomograph for the prediction of the protein value of diets. The parabolas are lines of equal NDpCal %. (Reproduced from *Health Aspects of Food and Nutrition*, original figure by Miller D. S. and Payne PR in *Journal of Nutrition* **74**: 413, 1961)

present in the protein is compared with the amount of the same L. A. A. which would be present in the "ideal" protein. From a practical point of view it is only necessary to consider one or two L. A. A.s in most diet patterns. For mixed diets the quality of the protein is usually limited by the sulphur-containing amino acids, methionine, and cysteine; in diets based on a wheat staple it is lysine, and for maize diets it is tryptophan. The perfect protein which would have a score of 100 would contain 0.27 g of sulphur amino acids, 0.27 g of lysine, and 0.09 g of tryptophane per gram of nitrogen.

If the amount of sulphur amino acid in the above food is part of a mixed diet, the total sulphur amino content of the food is determined from food composition tables; in this example the tables showed that the food contains 0.21 g of sulphur amino acids per gram of nitrogen. The score of the food protein is now obtained by comparisons with the "perfect" protein, the results being expressed as a percentage.

$$\text{Protein Score} = \frac{\text{amount of Limiting Amino Acid in food} \times 100}{\text{amount of Limiting Amino Acid in "perfect" protein}}$$

$$= \frac{0.21 \times 100}{0.27}$$

$$= 78$$

The values of the Protein Calories and the Protein Score can now be used to determine the Net Dietary protein Calories Per cent (NDpCal%) directly from a nomograph (see Fig. 49). In this example the Protein Calorie Per cent of 10 and a Protein Score of 78 has an NDpCal% of 7.2. This technique can also be used to evaluate food mixtures (see page 392). Although this evaluation is theoretical there is a close relationship between the calculated values for NDpCal% and those observed in experimental conditions (see Table 25). This unit has undoubted important significance, because alone, neither the protein quantity in a diet nor its quality reflect the true value of proteins to the body.

Digestion

Since proteins are macromolecules under normal conditions, they can neither be absorbed across the intestinal barrier nor can they be utilized by the body even when introduced parenterally. Even peptides containing only a few amino acids are usually eliminated in the urine. Thus, for dietary proteins to be utilized by the body they must be first broken by proteolytic enzymes to amino acids. Digestive enzymes attack specific linkages in the

Table 25 Comparison of observed and calculated values for protein quality

Origin	Staples	Additional effective sources of protein	Total no. of components	NPUop (%)	Observed values Protein calories (% total calories)	NDpCal(%)	Score e	Calculated values d Protein calories (% total calories)	NDpCal(%)
Gambia	Cassava	Pulses	4	45	2.8	1.3	53	2.1	1.1
Papua	Sago	Fish	3	75	3.5	2.6 ± 0.2	74	4.1	3.0
Jamaica	Sugar	Cornmeal	3	66	4.9	3.2 ± 0.1	45	4.3	2.0
Gambia	Cassava	Fish	5	65	6.1	4.0 ± 0.3	64	8.9	5.3
E. Pakistan	Rice	Pulses, milk	14	59	9.2	5.4 ± 0.2	69	9.3	5.9
Jamaica	Maize	Fish	4	60	10.0	6.0 ± 0.2	58	14.0	6.8
Britain	Wheat	Cheese	6	73	9.4	6.9 ± 0.3	76	10.7	7.1
Nigeria	Sorghum	Pulses, fish	12	58	12.5	7.3 ± 0.4	72	12.5	7.7
Gambia	Maize	Pulses, fish	6	57	13.9	7.9	68	14.2	8.0
Persia	Wheat	Meat, eggs, milk	11	55	15.0	8.3 ± 0.3	76	13.0	8.3
Nigeria	Sorghum	Milk fish	13	63	14.0	8.8 ± 0.3	76	15.1	9.0
Turkey	Wheat	Meat, pulses	11	59	15.7	9.2 ± 0.2	71	15.3	8.7
Britain	Wheat	Milk	5	44	29.0	12.8 ± 0.2	80	29.0	11.8

Source: *Health Aspects of Food and Nutrition*. W. H. O. 1969.

peptide chain as shown in Table 26. Gastric pepsin breaks the protein molecule in an acidic medium to shorter polypeptides, known as *proteoses* and *peptones*. In the alkaline medium of the small intestine trypsin and chymo-

Table 26   Action of proteolytic enzymes

Enzyme	Source	Major action
Pepsin	Stomach	splits peptide bonds in which phenylalanine or tyrosine provide NH_2
Trypsin	Pancreas	splits peptide bonds in which arginine or lysine provide COOH
Chymotrypsin	Pancreas	splits peptide bonds in which tyrosine, phenylalanine or tryptophan provide COOH
Carboxypeptidase	Pancreas	splits peptide bonds of terminal amino acid with free COOH
Aminopeptidase	Small intestine	splits peptide bonds of terminal amino acid with free NH_2
Dipeptidase	Small intestine	splits peptide bonds adjacent to both NH_2 and COOH

trypsin from pancreatic juice break down proteoses and peptones to shorter *peptides*. Carboxypeptidase of pancreatic juice splits the peptide bonds of the terminal amino acids which have a free COOH radical, and aminopeptidase of the small intestine splits peptide bonds with a free NH_2 radical. Finally, dipeptidase of the small intestine breaks the dipeptides into 2 amino acids (see Figure 50). About 92 per cent of ingested protein material can be digested, the actual amount being dependent on the method of preparation of the food.

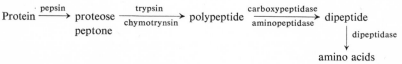

Figure 50   The digestion of protein

Fecal nitrogen consists partly of undigested or unabsorbed food nitrogen. The remainder is endogenous nitrogen, consisting of residues of digestive enzymes, bacteria, and desquamated epithelial cells, of the gastrointestinal tract.

Absorption

Amino acids are mostly absorbed from the duodenum and the upper jejunum. As the concentration of amino acids is much higher in the plasma than in the intestinal contents, an active transport mechanism is required to move the amino acids into the bloodstream. They are carried by the portal blood to the liver and from there they enter the general circulation from which they are rapidly removed by the tissues.

Some insignificant quantities of short chain peptides are also absorbed occasionally. In early infancy it is believed that whole protein molecules are able to penetrate the intestinal mucosa. In some cases this leads to immunologic sensitization and the development of milk allergy (see page 117).

Protein metabolism

The fate of amino acids in each tissue varies according to immediate needs. They may be used to synthesize tissue proteins, enzymes, hormones, hemoglobin, antibodies, or be converted into non-essential amino acids, urea, glucose, fat, pharmacologically active amines, or they may be oxidized to carbon dioxide and water with production of energy.

Biosynthesis of protein   For protein synthesis to take place, all the essential amino acids needed for its structure along with many non-essential amino acids must be present simultaneously and in adequate amounts. A biosynthetic process may be delayed for up to 4 or even 6 hours if an essential amino acid is missing but if the delay is further prolonged the amino acids will be metabolized.

The genetic information necessary for protein synthesis is coded in the chemical structure of deoxyribonucleic acid (DNA). The DNA molecule is very large and consists of two intertwining chains of polymers forming a long helical molecule. DNA is composed of units called *nucleotides*, each of which consists of a *purine* base (adenine or guanine) or *pyrimidine* base (thymine or cytosine) attached to a phosphorylated pentose. Since proteins may contain up to 20 different amino acids and there are only 4 bases in DNA, each triplet of nucleotides comprises a code for each amino acid. The specificity of nucleotides for amino acids determines the genetic code.

Although DNA is found in the nucleus, protein synthesis occurs in ribosomes in the cytoplasm. The genetic message or code is brought to ribosomes by a special kind of ribonucleic acid (RNA) known as messenger RNA (mRNA). Ribonucleic acid, which is similar to DNA, is made up of a series of nucleotides but it differs from DNA in that it consists of one chain not two, its pentose is ribose instead of deoxyribose, and it contains the pyrimidine uracil instead of thymine.

Amino acids are attached to another type of RNA known as soluble RNA (sRNA) or transfer RNA (tRNA) and are conveyed to the ribosomes. For each amino acid there is a specific tRNA.

On the ribosomes, amino acids are linked together by peptide bonds and form protein. Amino acids are linked together through the carboxyl groups of one amino acid and the amino group of another with release of one molecule of water (see Figure 51).

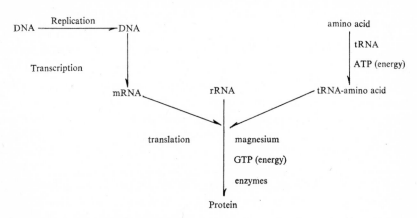

Figure 51   The linkage of amino acids by the peptide bond

Once synthesis is completed, the protein is stripped off the ribosomes and released into the soluble portion of the cell. Thus, there are three kinds of RNA involved in protein synthesis; *messenger* RNA, *transfer* RNA, and the *structural* RNA of ribosomes (rRNA). The main features of protein synthesis are summarized in Figure 52.

DNA ——Replication——► DNA   amino acid

                                                                                           tRNA

            Transcription   ATP (energy)

                              mRNA   rRNA   ◄ tRNA-amino acid

                      translation   magnesium

                                         GTP (energy)

                                         enzymes

                              Protein

Figure 52   Summary of protein synthesis

Biosynthesis of non-essential amino acids   The non-essential amino acids can be synthesized in the body by the process of transamination. The amino group of one amino acid is transferred to an alpha-keto acid leading to the formation of another amino acid. If, for instance, the meal is rich in glutamic acid and poor in alanine, the body can synthesize the latter by transferring the amino group of glutamic acid to pyruvic acid (see Figure 53).

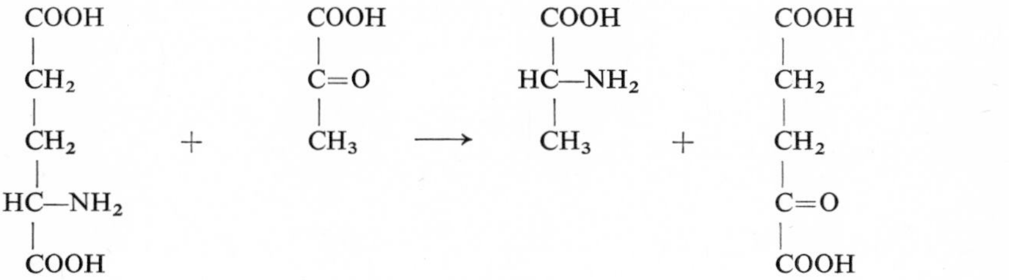

$$
\begin{array}{ccccccc}
COOH & & COOH & & COOH & & COOH \\
| & & | & & | & & | \\
CH_2 & & C{=}O & & HC{-}NH_2 & & CH_2 \\
| & & | & & | & & | \\
CH_2 & + & CH_3 & \longrightarrow & CH_3 & + & CH_2 \\
| & & & & & & | \\
HC{-}NH_2 & & & & & & C{=}O \\
| & & & & & & | \\
COOH & & & & & & COOH
\end{array}
$$

Glutamic Acid	+	pyruvic acid	→ alanine	+	alpha-keto-glutaric acid

Figure 53   Transamination

Urea formation If an excessive amount of protein, or an incomplete protein is ingested, the amino acids which comprise the protein are neither utilized by the body for protein synthesis nor can they be stored in the body. Therefore their amino group is removed by L-amino acid oxidases. This process which usually takes place in the liver and kidney is known as deamination (see Figure 54). During the process of deamination, ammonia is formed; if this was to be allowed to accumulate in excess of the normal 0.1–0.2 mg per 100 ml of blood, it would cause toxic effects. To avoid this, man and other mammals detoxify the ammonia by converting it to urea; in reptiles and birds, detoxification is achieved by conversion of the ammonia to uric acid.

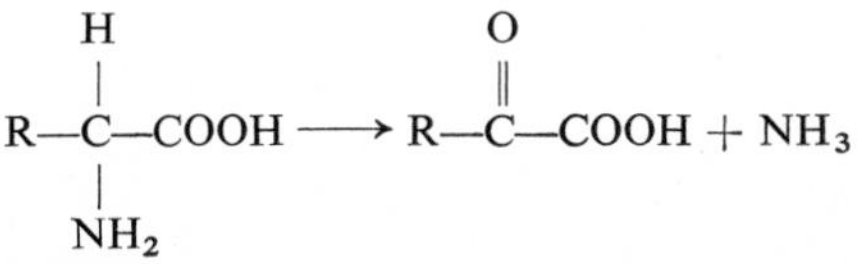

$$
\begin{array}{cc}
H & O \\
| & \| \\
R{-}C{-}COOH \longrightarrow & R{-}C{-}COOH + NH_3 \\
| & \\
NH_2 &
\end{array}
$$

Figure 54   Deamination

Formation of urea is by a cyclic mechanism which is summarized in Figure 55.

Energy production During starvation, or when the caloric intake is insufficient to meet the energy needs of the body, the alpha-keto acid (the non-nitrogenous fraction or the carbon-skeleton) formed by the removal of amino groups, is either directly oxidized for energy production or it is converted first to glucose or fat, and then oxidized. It finally enters the Kreb's Cycle for energy production. In general, amino acids which become

15*

pyruvic acid make glucose (glucogenic), while those which become acetyl coenzyme A or acetoacetic acid make fats (ketogenic). For instance, alanine is glucogenic while leucine is ketogenic.

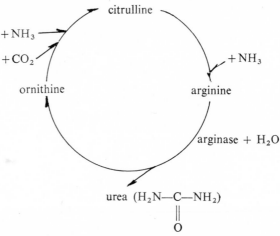

Figure 55   The urea cycle

Formation of active amines   Specific enzymes are able to split off the carbon dioxide group from amino acids; this process converts pharmacologically inert amino acids into highly active amines. Histidine, for example, can be decarboxylated to histamine which is a powerful vasodilator; aspartic acid when decarboxylated to beta-alanine becomes part of the vitamin pantothenic acid. The reaction is as follows:

$$R—CH_2—CH—COOH \rightarrow R—CH_2—CH_2NH_2 + CO_2$$
$$\quad\quad\quad | $$
$$\quad\quad NH_2$$

Protein metabolism is summarized in Figure 56.

Hormonal regulation of protein metabolism

Anabolic hormones   Insulin, growth hormone, and testosterone are anabolic hormones which promote synthesis. Insulin stimulates the entrance of amino acids into cells and promotes amino acid incorporation into muscle protein. Growth hormone causes growth of almost all tissues and an increase in cell size and promotes the penetration of amino acids into the cells.

Catabolic hormones   Adrenal corticoids and thyroxine are catabolic hormones which influence the transfer of muscle proteins through the plasma amino acid pool into the liver. Where they may be broken down and even-

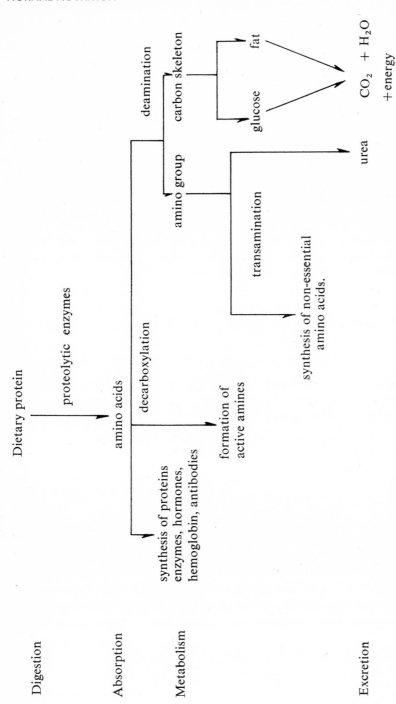

Figure 56   A summary of protein metabolism

tually eliminated from the body. Thyroxine increases nitrogen excretion by increasing the basal metabolic rate, while adrenal corticoids are involved in the deamination of amino acids resulting in nitrogen loss and the formation of glucose (gluconeogenesis).

Disorders of amino acid metabolism

Phenylketonuria Because of a hereditary lack of the enzyme phenylalanine hydroxylase, the normal oxidation of phenylalanine to tyrosine in the liver cannot take place. There is a consequent accumulation of phenylalanine in the serum and excessive amounts of some of the metabolites of phenylalanine are excreted in the urine.

Alcaptonuria In the absence of the enzyme homogentisic acid oxidase, homogentisic acid which is produced during the metabolism of phenylalanine and tyrosine, cannot be further broken down, either in the liver or the kidney. As a result, there is an accumulation of homogentisic acid in the blood which spills over into the urine. Cartilage and other connective tissues become pigmented and the patient is susceptible to arthritis in later years. Severe restriction of phenylalanine and tyrosine intake in the diet is not practical except for brief periods so treatment is largely symptomatic.

Albinism Because of insufficient amounts of the enzyme tyrosinase, melanocytes fail to produce normal quantities of melanin in the skin, hair and eyes. Tyrosine does not accumulate in serum because it can be oxidized or converted into epinephrine or thyroxine (see Figure 57).

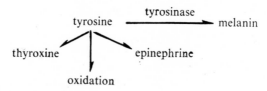

Figure 57   Tyrosine metabolism

Maple syrup urine disease In this condition, the oxidative decarboxylation of branched chain amino acids (leucine, isoleucine, and valine) is blocked therefore both the amino acids and their associated alpha-keto acids accumulate in the blood and are excreted in large quantities in urine (see Figure 58). The disease, which may be fatal, becomes apparent in the very young infant; survivors are inevitably mentally retarded. A diet containing small amounts of branched chain amino acids prevents the serious complications of the disease.

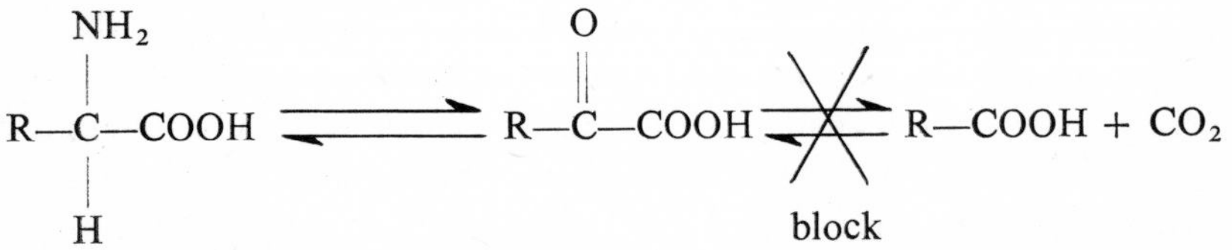

$$
\underset{\text{H}}{\overset{\text{NH}_2}{\underset{|}{\overset{|}{R-C-COOH}}}} \rightleftharpoons \underset{}{\overset{\text{O}}{\overset{\|}{R-C-COOH}}} \overset{}{\underset{\text{block}}{\cancel{\rightleftharpoons}}} R-COOH + CO_2
$$

Figure 58   The inborn error in metabolism in Maple syrup urine disease

Histidinemia   Due to a lack of the enzyme histidase, histidine cannot be metabolized. There is an accumulation of histidine in the serum and excretion of excessive amounts of this amino acid and certain of its imidazole metabolites in urine. Patients are mentally retarded and have speech difficulties. Restriction of the dietary level of histidine may be beneficial.

Other inherited diseases   Several other disorders related to the metabolism of amino acids have been reported. These include prolinemia, hydroxyprolinemia, cystathionuria, homocystinuria, and deficiency of urea cycle enzymes. In all these disorders the subjects are mentally retarded.

Adaptation of protein metabolism to low protein intakes

The range of protein intake is wide and therefore the metabolic machine must be flexible enough to compensate for differences in this range.

The immediate adaptation to a reduced protein intake is a fall in urinary nitrogen excretion; this is achieved by a decrease in activity of the urea cycle enzymes in the liver. At the same time, a more efficient use is made of amino acids; for example, muscle reduces its demands for amino acids and the body makes better use of the amino acids freed by the breakdown of tissue protein. These mechanisms help to ensure that loss and wastage of nitrogenous material is minimized. The control of these changes may depend on an increase in activity of cortisone and growth hormones which promote protein synthesis in the liver, or a decrease in insulin activity which normally promotes the entry of amino acids in the muscle. This hypothesis is supported by the observation that growth hormone levels are raised and insulin secretion is frequently deficient in protein calorie malnutrition.[8]

Protein requirement

The requirement of the body for protein is discussed in detail in Chapter 4.

Role of calories in the diet

The living cell is not an engine which depends on heat for energy, although heat is generated as a by-product of cell function. Chemical energy is the fuel used by the cell and it is derived from the oxidation of foodstuffs (carbohydrates, fats, and proteins). This energy is either directly or indirectly provided by plants utilizing solar energy to synthesize our food. The types of work performed by cells are:

Chemical	biosynthesis
Mechanical	muscle contraction
Transport and concentration . .	absorption, secretion, excretion
Electrical	conductance of nerve impulses
Photochemical	luminescence
Osmotic	secretion of hypertonic urine

The cell is not 100 per cent efficient in carrying out this work and some energy appears as heat. Since this heat is continuously lost to the environment, there is a daily requirement for food energy to maintain the caloric balance and perform work. If the requirement is not met, man will burn up his own tissues in an effort to supply the energy needed for vital body functions.

The complete oxidation of 1 mole of glucose yields 686 000 calories:

$$C_6H_{12}O_6 + 6O_2 \rightarrow 6CO_2 + 6H_2O + 686000 \text{ calories}$$

If this amount of energy was to be released as a single burst of heat energy the cellular organization would be disrupted by the oxidation of only a few moles of glucose.

The energy in food exists as chemical energy in unstable "high energy" compounds, the most important being adenosine triphosphate (ATP). The molecule of this compound has three phosphate bonds; when these bonds are broken, energy is released. Most of the energy is in the form of chemical energy, but some escapes as heat. The breakdown of one bond of the molecule of ATP liberates the energy equivalent of 8000 calories per mole and leaves adenosine diphosphate (ADP). The breaking of a second bond liberates additional energy, equivalent to 6500 calories per mole, and leaves adenosine monophosphate (AMP). The breakdown of adenosine monophosphate to adenosine and phosphoric acid, liberates the energy equivalent of 2200 calories (see Figure 59).

Since ATP is the unit of energy, it is called the *energy currency* of body cells.

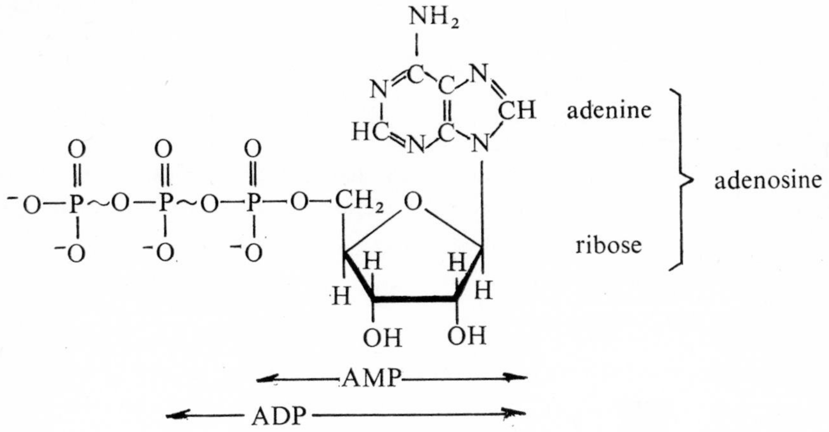

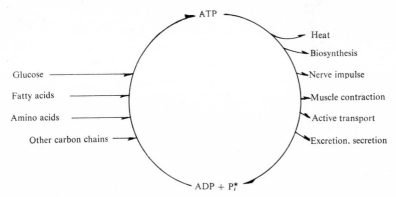

Adenosine triphosphate (ATP)

Figure 59   Breakdown and formation of ATP

The molecules of AMP, ADP, and ATP, can be resynthesized but in order to achieve this end, energy has to be supplied. This is obtained from the oxidation of glucose, fatty acids, amino acids, and other carbon chains in the Kreb's Cycle. The concept of work performance and the provision

ATP

Glucose

Fatty acids

Amino acids

Other carbon chains

Heat

Biosynthesis

Nerve impulse

Muscle contraction

Active transport

Excretion, secretion

$ADP + P_i^*$

* P_i is inorganic phosphate, i. e. phosphate that is not bound to an inorganic compound.

Figure 60   Work performance and the provision of energy

of energy to achieve this end is shown in Figure 60. If a fatty acid molecule is oxidized the reaction would be:

$$\text{Fatty acid} + O_2 \rightarrow CO_2 + H_2O + \text{Energy} \qquad \text{(Reaction 1)}$$

The energy may be used to form ATP by binding phosphate:

$$\text{Energy} + \text{ADP} + P_i \rightarrow \text{ATP} \qquad \text{(Reaction 2)}$$

The ATP may be used to synthesize protein from amino acids:

$$\text{ATP} + \text{amino acids} \rightarrow \text{Protein} + \text{ADP} \qquad \text{(Reaction 3)}$$

Reaction 1 is *exergonic* which means that energy is released, an event which occurs in catabolic reactions. Reaction 3 is *endergonic* which means that energy is required for anabolism.

ATP formation

The generation of high energy phosphates (phosphorylation) can be achieved in two ways; first from substrate level phosphorylation and secondly from oxidative phosphorylation.

Substrate level phosphorylation The substrate is first attached to a phosphate group and then it is utilized to produce ATP. The following reactions may occur in glycolysis and the Kreb's Cycle:

Glycolysis

1,3 diphosphoglyceric acid + ADP→3 phosphoglyceric acid + ATP
(contains 2 phosphate groups)   (one phosphate group)

phosphoenolpyruvic acid + ADP →pyruvic acid + ATP
(one phosphate group)   (no phosphate group)

Kreb's Cycle

a) succinyl coenzyme A + GDP (guanosine diphosphate) → succinic acid
                                                       + GTP + CoA

b) GTP + ADP → GDP + ATP

Oxidative phosphorylation In this process, various carriers or coenzymes (which include those containing the vitamins niacin and riboflavin) transfer hydrogen atoms or electrons from the substrate to oxygen with the formation of water. This takes place in the mitochondrion of the cell (see page 180). In passing over the carriers the energy levels diminish progressively; by the time water has been formed, all the energy has been drained from the hydrogen atoms. This energy is trapped in the ATP molecules. For each mole of hydrogen passing over the carriers, 3 moles of ATP are formed.

Energy storage

When an excessive amount of ATP is available to the cell such as occurs following glycolysis, most of the ATP which has been produced is stored in muscle tissue in the form of creatine phosphate. In the resting state muscle has 4 to 6 times as much creatine phosphate as ATP. Creatine phosphate cannot serve as an immediate source of energy for muscle contraction because it is unable to react with the proteins of the muscle fibril; therefore, it only serves as a store of energy. During contraction the muscle requires the almost instantaneous delivery of ATP; in muscular activity creatine phosphate yields ATP. During rest the creatine phosphate reserves are built up again. These events can be summarized in the following reactions:

creatine phosphate + ADP $\rightleftharpoons$ creatine + ATP + 1500 calories

ATP → ADP + P_i + phosphate + 8000 calories

The net result is:

creatine phosphate → creatine + phosphate + 9500 calories

$$\text{creatine phosphate} \overset{\text{creatine}}{\underset{}{\rightleftharpoons}} \begin{array}{l} \text{ADP during contraction} \\ \text{ATP during relaxation} \end{array}$$

Food sources of calories

The only nutrients that provide calories are carbohydrates, fats, and proteins. Vitamins, minerals, water, and fiber do not yield energy.

Various foods differ greatly in their energy content. The higher the proportion of fat in the diet and the lower its water content, the greater the caloric value. Some food items such as oil and sugar yield nothing but calories. Cheese, cream, nuts, cakes, pies, potato chips, olives, and avocado are energy-rich foods, while green leafy vegetables and fresh fruits have low fuel value.

Several factors such as cost, custom, and availability influence the choice of energy sources in the diet. In Southeast Asia most of the energy is supplied by the carbohydrate in rice, however, the Eskimos derive most of their calories from protein and fat.

Determination of food energy

The amount of energy locked up by the bonds which cement a molecule together can be determined by burning the food in a bomb calorimeter.

The instrument consists of an insulated water jacket containing a known
quantity of water (see Figure 61). An accurately weighed sample of food
is placed in the chamber containing pure oxygen and ignited electrically.
The temperature change of the water is an index of the amount of heat
released by oxidation of food. By dividing the amount of heat released by
the quantity of food sample, the caloric value in kilocalories per gram can

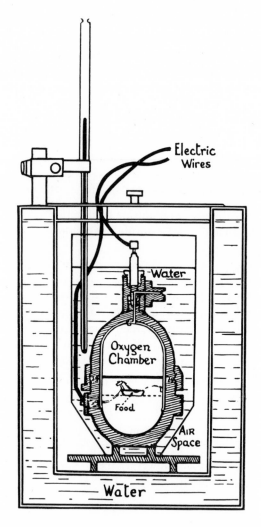

Figure 61   The Bomb Calorimeter (Reproduced from *Textbook of Physiology and
Biochemistry* 7th Edition 1968 by Bell, Davidson and Scarborough, with the permission
of E. & S. Livingsrone)

be calculated. The quantity of heat produced per gram of carbohydrates, fats, and proteins is 4.1, 9.45, and 5.65 kilocalories (C), respectively.

The heat produced is the result of oxidation of carbon to carbon dioxide, hydrogen to water, and nitrogen to nitrous oxide.

Fats have the greatest caloric value because their molecules contain large quantities of carbon and hydrogen relative to the amount of oxygen. Therefore, considerable oxygen is required from an external source to combine with carbon and hydrogen; this results in the release of much energy. Carbohydrates contain enough oxygen in their molecule to combine with their own hydrogen atoms so that external oxygen is only required for the carbon atoms. When proteins are oxidized completely, they are intermediate between fats and carbohydrates in their caloric value.

Kilocalorie or Calorie (C)   The calorie is the unit of energy and it is defined as the quantity of heat which is required to raise the temperature of 1000 g (1 litre) of water from 15°C to 16°C.

The calorific value of food burned in a bomb calorimeter differs from the calorific value of food burned in the body. There are two reasons for this; first, the food in the calorimeter oxidizes the food into its final products, carbon dioxide and water. In the body however, protein is not completely burned and oxidation stops when ammonia and urea are formed. The calorific value of one gram of this residue is 1.25 Cals which have to be deducted from the value of 5.65 Cals per gram of protein obtained by direct calorimetry. The calorific value of protein to the body is therefore only 4.4 Cals per gram. The second reason relates to the inability of the body to digest and absorb some of the nutrients in food. It is estimated that only 98 per cent of carbohydrates, 95 per cent of fats, and 92 per cent of protein are utilized. The small unused portions of these nutrients cannot therefore contribute to body energy. The following calculation shows show the physiological fuel values of nutrients are reached.

	Carbohydrates	Fats	Proteins
Bomb calorimeter value	4.10	9.45	5.65
Values of urinary end products	0	0	1.25
			4.40
Percent digestibility	98.00	95.00	92.00
Physiological fuel value	4.00	9.00	4.00

If the quantity of each nutrient in the food mixture is known, the energy value of that food can be obtained by multiplying these quantities by the physiologic fuel values and summing the calorific value of each component nutrient. For example: a sample of 100 grams of white bread containing 11 grams of protein, 2 grams of fat, and 78 grams of available carbohydrate would have its caloric value calculated as follows:

$$
\begin{aligned}
\text{Calories from protein} &= 11 \times 4 = 44 \\
\text{Calories from fat} &= 2 \times 9 = 18 \\
\text{Calories from carbohydrate} &= 78 \times 4 = 312 \\
\text{Total caloric value of bread} & = 374 \text{ per 100 grams}
\end{aligned}
$$

Utilization of dietary energy

Although dietary energy can be converted into the chemical energy of ATP this conversion is not very efficient. The oxidation of 1 mole of glucose releases 686,000 calories but only 38 ATP molecules are formed from the same amount of glucose. Each mole of ATP yields 8000 calories so the total

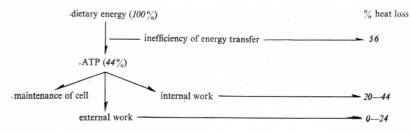

Figure 62   Utilization of food energy

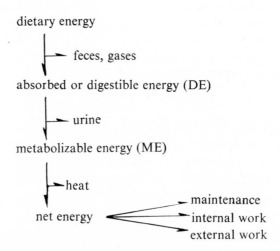

Figure 63   The derivation of net energy from dietary energy

yield of calories will be $38 \times 8000 = 304,000$. The efficiency of conversion is therefore $\dfrac{304,000}{686,000} \times 100 = 44\%$. The remaining 56 per cent of this reaction is emitted as heat. Figure 62 summarizes the utilization of food energy.

Some energy is lost in the feces if the food is not digested and there is a loss of 1 to 3 per cent of the total energy intake in the urine. In addition there are some insignificant losses via gases. The net energy available consists of the total energy minus heat energy and losses of energy in excreta; the net energy is employed for the various body functions (see Figure 63). Since there are physiological differences in the ability of animal species to digest and utilize foods, the amount of energy wasted varies.

Specific Dynamic Action (SDA)

After the ingestion of food there is an immediate rise in heat production above the basal level. The extra heat produced by the organism above the basal heat production, as a result of food ingestion, is known as the Specific Dynamic Action (SDA). Its magnitude varies with the type of nutrient; for example, when proteins are ingested there is a 30 per cent increase in heat, with carbohydrates 6 per cent, and with fats 4 per cent. The SDA of a mixture of nutrients is less than the sum of the SDA of individual constituents and is taken as 10 per cent of the fuel value of food. This heat is usually wasted except in cold weather when it helps to maintain body temperature.

The cause of SDA is unknown; it is not due to digestive or absorptive processes because it manifests itself even after an intravenous injection of amino acids. The SDA means, in practice, that the net energy is reduced; for example, food which yields 110 calories has only 100 of these available. In calculating calorie requirement, provision has to be made to meet this energy loss.

Respiratory quotient (R. Q.)

In the process of oxidation, carbohydrates, fats, and proteins react with oxygen and produce carbon dioxide. The ratio of the volume of carbon dioxide produced, to the volume of oxygen consumed, is called the Respiratory Quotient (R. Q.) and its magnitude depends on the proportion of carbon and oxygen in these nutrients.

$$R. Q. = \frac{\text{volume } CO_2 \text{ produced}}{\text{volume } O_2 \text{ consumed}}$$

The R. Q. of carbohydrates The complete oxidation of glucose, as a representative of carbohydrates, is as follows:

$$C_6H_{12}O_6 + 6O_2 \rightarrow 6CO_2 + 6H_2O$$

$$R.\,Q = \frac{6}{6} = 1$$

The R. Q. of Fats The oxidation of tristearin, as representative of fats, is as follows:

$$2C_{57}H_{110}O_6 + 163O_2 \rightarrow 114CO_2 + 110H_2O$$

$$R.\,Q. = \frac{114}{163} = 0.7$$

The R. Q. of protein Unlike carbohydrates and fats, proteins are not completely oxidized in the body; the final and most important breakdown product of protein is urea, which is excreted in the urine. As the excretion of urea is directly related to the nitrogen intake, urinary nitrogen can be used for calculating protein metabolism. Each gram of urinary nitrogen represents the metabolism of 6.25 grams of protein, the combustion of 5.94 litres of oxygen, and the production of 4.76 litres of carbon dioxide with the liberation of 26.51 Calories.

$$R.\,Q. = \frac{4.76}{5.94} = 0.8$$

R. Q. Greater than Unity Carbohydrates have more oxygen in proportion to carbon than do fats. During conversion of carbohydrates to fats, some of the oxygen of carbohydrates become available for oxidation, therefore there is less requirement for atmospheric oxygen. This means that carbon dioxide production exceeds oxygen consumption and the R. Q. would become theoretically greater than one. For instance, conversion of glucose to palmitic acid gives an R Q. of eight.

$$4C_6H_{12}O_6 + O_2 \rightarrow C_{16}H_{32}O_2 + 8CO_2 + 8H_2O$$

$$R.\,Q. = \frac{8}{1} = 8$$

Normally the R. Q. does not exceed one. The extent to which the R. Q. approaches one, reflects the degree to which oxidation of carbohydrates predominates in the food mixture. From the knowledge of urinary nitrogen, oxygen consumption, and carbon dioxide production, one can calculate the quantity of each nutrient metabolized and the heat produced by the body.

Calculation of heat production in the body

The amount of heat produced in the body can be determined by either direct or indirect calorimetry.

Direct calorimetry   This method is similar in principle to the bomb calorimeter. The subject is placed in a sealed insulated chamber (see Figure 64). The heat generated by the subject is removed from the chamber by water circulated through coils. Water which is present in the exhaled air is absorbed in sulfuric acid. The amount of heat loss is computed from the rise in water temperature as recorded by the thermometers and rate of flow of water. In addition, the quantity of heat utilized for vaporization of water is calculated by measuring the moisture content of the air leaving the chamber.

Although this method is accurate, it is costly and requires an elaborate instrument; for these reasons, its use is limited to specialized research.

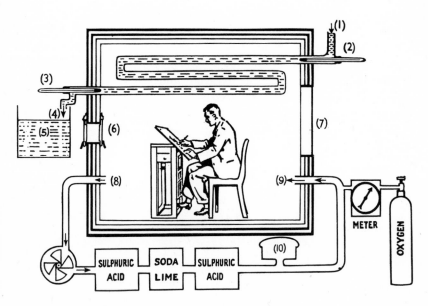

Figure 64   Diagram of the Atwater-Benedict respiration calorimeter. Water flows from (1) to (4), and its temperature is measured at the inlet and the outlet. Air leaves at (8), water is removed from it by sulfuric acid, CO is removed by soda lime, and O_2 is added at a measured rate; the gas mixture re-enters the chamber at (9). (2), inlet thermometer; (3), outlet thermometer; (6), porthole; (7), window; (9), air inlet; (10), air cushion. (Reproduced from *Textbook of Physiology and Biochemistry*, 7th Edition, 1968, by Bell, Davidson and Scarborough, with the permission of E. & S. Livingstone.)

The following is an example of how the heat production is calculated:

Volume of water absorbed in sulfuric acid = 2000 litres
Average rise in temperature   = 0.5°C
Amount of water vapor produced   = 1000 g
Heat of vaporization of water at 20°C   = 0.59 Cals
Heat production = 2000 × 0.5 + 1000 × 0.59 = 1590 Cals

Indirect calorimetry   In contrast to direct calorimetry which is a physical method, indirect calorimetry is a chemical method based on the measurement of the quantity of oxygen consumed, carbon dioxide produced, the output of urinary nitrogen, and a calculation of the R. Q.

There are two types of apparatus which can be employed involving a closed or open circuit system.

Closed circuit system (Benedict-Roth Respiration Apparatus)   The subject inhales pure oxygen through a mouthpiece or face mask; the carbon dioxide which is produced is absorbed by soda lime. By measuring the volumes of oxygen consumed and carbon dioxide produced, the R. Q. and the amount of heat produced may be calculated. This test takes 6 to 8 minutes.

The following is an example of the calculation to determine the heat produced by a subject over one hour.

Reduction in the weight of the oxygen cylinder = 1.15 g
Weight of carbon dioxide produced = 1.35 g
Duration of test = 6 minutes
Volume occupied by a gram molecular weight of any gas = 22.4 litres
Gram molecular weight of carbon dioxide = 44
Gram molecular weight of oxygen = 32

The volume of CO_2 = $1.35 \times \dfrac{22.4}{44}$ = 0.688 litre

The volume of O_2 = $1.15 \times \dfrac{22.4}{32}$ = 0.805 litre

The R. Q. = $\dfrac{0.688}{0.805}$ = 0.85

The caloric value for an R. Q. of 0.85 is 4.862 per litre of O_2
The heat produced in 6 minutes = 0.805 × 4.862 = 3.914 Cals
The heat produced over one hour will therefore be 3.914 × 10 = 39.14 Cals

The contribution of protein oxidation can be calculated from urinary nitrogen, however, 95 per cent of the heat produced by the body is derived from the combustion of carbohydrates and fat. The error incurred by ignoring the contribution of heat from protein sources is so small as to be negligible. When the test is carried out on subjects at rest, the R. Q. is assumed to be 0.83 which represents the R. Q. derived from a food mixture of carbohydrates, fats, and protein. If this is assumed, the carbon dioxide production is ignored and the heat production is calculated from oxygen consumption alone. If the data from the above example are used and the calorific value of one litre of oxygen at an R. Q. of 0.83 is 4.838, the heat produced in 6 minutes would be: $0.805 \times 4.838 = 3.895$ Cals. Over one hour this would be 38.95 Cals a figure very close to that calculated from both oxygen consumption and carbon dioxide production.

Open circuit system   In this method the subject breathes atmospheric air, the expired air being collected in a bag (*Douglas Bag*) or a mechanical measuring device (*Tissot Spirometer*). The measurement of the volume of the expired air and the composition of the air which has been collected permits an estimation of the volume of oxygen consumed and the volume of carbon dioxide produced. From this, the R. Q. and the amount of heat generated may be calculated. The following is an example of a calculation of heat production when 200 litres of air have been collected in a Tissot Spirometer over a period of one hour, and where the expired air contains 4.43 per cent of carbon dioxide and 15.44 per cent of oxygen.

If the concentration of CO_2 in atmospheric air is 0.03 per cent, the percentage of CO_2 produced will be $4.53 - 0.03 = 4.50$.

If the concentration of oxygen in atmospheric air is 20.94, then the percentage of oxygen consumed will be $20.94 - 15.44 = 5.50$.

The volume of CO_2 will therefore be $4.50 \times 200 = 9$ litres and the volume of oxygen will be $5.50 \times 200 = 11$ litres.

The R. Q. $= \dfrac{9}{11} = 0.82$

The caloric value per litre of O_2 at an R. Q. of 0.82 = 4.825.

The hourly heat production will therefore be $11 \times 4.825 = 53$ Cals

Basal metabolism

Basal metabolism is the quantity of energy required for maintenance and conduction of continuous and fundamental cellular, tissue, and organ activities, such as muscle tone, peristalsis, circulation, respiration, digestion, absorption, metabolism, secretions, excretion, and body temperature; it represents about 50 per cent of the total daily energy expenditure.

To measure basal metabolism, the subject must be lying down comfortably, awake and relaxed. The test is taken 12 to 15 hours after the last meal. In practice, basal metabolism is determined over 10 to 15 minutes and expressed as Cals per hour per square meter of body surface.

16*

The Basal Metabolic Rate (BMR) is influenced by many factors:

Size: The BMR increases with surface area because heat is lost from the skin. The surface area can be predicted from height (H) and weight (W) using the following formula:

$$\text{surface area (square meter)} = 0.202 \times W^{0.425(kg)} \times H^{0.725(m)}$$

Age: The BMR increases for some months after birth and then decreases with age.

Sex: In females the BMR is 6 to 10 per cent less than males; this is because they are generally less active. In addition, their muscular development is less but they have more subcutaneous fat which prevents heat loss and has little metabolic activity.

Body composition: The BMR increases as lean body mass increases, or as fat decreases.

Muscular training: The development of muscle in athletic training or other strenuous work activity leads to an increase in the BMR.

Climate: The BMR of people living in tropical climates is less than those in colder climates where more heat is needed to maintain body temperature.

Sleep: During sleep the BMR decreases by about 10 per cent.

Pathological conditions: In hyperthyroidism the BMR increases 50 to 75 per cent and in hypothyroidism it decreases by 40 per cent. Determination of the BMR is therefore of great value in the diagnosis of these conditions.

State of nutrition: The BMR of undernourished individuals is less than that of normal individuals.

Stress: Stresses such as pain, fear, and worry increase the BMR.

Fever: For each 1°C increase in body temperature, the BMR increases by 13 per cent.

Drugs: Certain drugs such as epinephrine, thyroxine, caffeine, and nicotine (smoking) increases the BMR, while sedatives lower it slightly.

Calorie requirement

To prevent loss, or wasting of body tissues, the daily diet must provide at least as much energy as is expended every day. The daily expenditure constitutes BMR, SDA, and external work. Calorie requirements should reflect a food intake which enables an active and productive life with no handicap through lack or excess of food.

Since a number of factors influence calorie requirements, recommendations are based on "Reference Man and Woman" and then adjustments are made to meet the variables.

The factors affecting calorie requirements are discussed in detail in Chapter 4. For the present time it should be noted that physical activity, body size and body composition, climate, age, and physiological status such as pregnancy and lactation, determine the body requirements for energy sources.

Energy imbalance

Energy balance depends on the food intake and the energy output which is a sum of internal and external work and the energy needed for maintenance and growth. Normally, several mechanisms in the body such as appetite, satiety, and external work maintain the energy balance. According to the first law of thermodynamics, energy can neither be created nor destroyed. Therefore, as long as the balance between calorie intake and energy expenditure is maintained, there will be no gain or loss in body weight. However, when the energy expenditure exceeds the intake, calories are derived from the body stores to meet the deficit and as a result the individual loses weight. On the other hand, if the intake exceeds output, the energy is stored as body fat and the person gains weight. The body has no mechanism for excreting excess fat (as it does for excess water or minerals), so that the fat is retained and there is a consequent gain in weight. The clinical condition of positive energy balance known as obesity, and calorie deficiency have been described in Chapter 1.

Role of vitamins in the diet

Definition

Vitamins and their precursors (provitamins) are organic compounds, distinct from the energy-yielding nutrients, carbohydrates, fats, and proteins. They occur in natural foods and are found in the body in very small concentrations, but they are essential for normal growth and maintenance of life. The dietary lack of a vitamin, or its poor absorption, causes vitamin deficiency disease. Vitamins differ from hormones in that they cannot be synthesized by animals and therefore they must be provided by the diet. A compound may be a vitamin for one animal species but not for others; for example, ascorbic acid is a vitamin for man alone. On the other hand, myo-inositol and para-aminobenzoic acid are vitamins for certain micro-organisms and animals but apparently not for man.

Vitamins are compounds which differ greatly from each other in chemical properties, structure, physiological action, and natural distribution.

Classification

Vitamins are divided into two classes according to their solubility in fat or water: fat-soluble vitamins which includes vitamins A, D, E, and K, and the water-soluble vitamins which comprise C and those of the B group (thiamine, riboflavin, niacin, pyridoxine, biotin, folic acid, pantothenic acid, cyanocobalamin). Choline and myo-inositol are sometimes also considered as vitamins.

Fat-soluble vitamins differ from water-soluble vitamins in several respects: First, their absorption follows the same path as fats, therefore any condition which affects fat absorption similarly affects these vitamins. For instance, in steatorrhea the absorption of fats and consequently the absorption of these vitamins is reduced.

Fat-soluble vitamins unlike water-soluble vitamins are not excreted in the urine.

Since they can be stored in the body (chiefly in liver), deficiency manifestations take longer to appear compared with water-soluble vitamins which are not stored in the body to any appreciable degree.

The ability to store, and the inability to excrete, fat-soluble vitamins means that toxicity can develop if large doses are ingested.

Some of the fat-soluble vitamins can be formed in the body from the inactive precursors of provitamins. Another property of some importance is that the activity of fat-soluble vitamins is not confined to a single compound; a group of chemically related substances can produce similar effects.

Function

Vitamins neither furnish energy nor provide building units for the organism. The exact biochemical role of many vitamins is still not known but in those vitamins whose mode of action is known, they catalyze metabolic reactions through the action of enzyme systems, or coenzyme systems which facilitate the action of enzymes.

Deficiency

Vitamin deficiency may be of either primary (dietary) or secondary (conditioned) origin. Primary deficiency results from inadequate ingestion of vitamins, and is easily alleviated by improving the diet or by providing vitamin supplements. To prevent primary vitamin deficiency, minimum daily requirements have been defined (see Chapter 4). Secondary deficiency results from an increased need or organic disease. For example, extra vitamins are required during pregnancy, lactation and growth, and under conditions of stress such as body injury or alcoholism. Organic defects may inhibit or prevent the absorption of vitamins from a diet which may contain sufficient quantities of vitamin. In obstructive jaundice, for example, bile salts cannot reach the intestine; they are, however, essential for the absorption of vitamin K. As a consequence vitamin K deficiency is a common complication of liver and biliary disease. Similarly, a lack of the gastric intrinsic factor causes pernicious anemia because vitamin B_{12} cannot be absorbed unless this factor is secreted by the stomach. Therapy will be ineffective unless the vitamins are given by injection or administered simultaneously with the missing factors. In the above examples, these would be bile salts and intrinsic factor. Deficiency symptoms may arise in several ways. The vitamin deficiency may mean that intermediate metabolites are unused, their accumulation in the body may disturb function. Alternatively, the metabolic process may not be carried out by the usual pathway and abnormal metabolites may be formed.

Hypervitaminosis Many populations have adopted the habit of consuming large quantities of vitamins. Any excess ingestion can bring no benefit to the body as they have no substrate on which to work. The fat-soluble vitamins on the other hand may have toxic effects (see page 24) when consumed in large amounts because they accumulate in the body. Normally the routine supplementation of a balanced and varied diet with vitamins is unjustified. In certain circumstances it may be advised for disadvantaged children and pregnant and lactating women.

Sources

Vitamins are found in both animal and plant tissues. The fat-soluble vitamins occur mostly in fatty foods such as egg yolk, liver, butter, seed germs, and nuts. Water-soluble vitamins on the other hand are found in milk, meat, whole grain cereals, fruits, vegetables, and legumes.

Several vitamins such as vitamin K and vitamins of the B group can be synthesized by intestinal micro-organisms and they can at least partially fulfill the requirements of the host. For this reason adult humans do not require an exogenous source of vitamin K and ruminants have no need for an external source of the B vitamins.

Vitamins can be destroyed by a number of chemical and physical agents such as acids, alkalis, heat, ultraviolet irradiation, oxidation, and light. Food processing, food preparation, and storage can also adversely affect the vitamin content of foods. Different vitamins vary greatly in their susceptibility to these agents and processes. Water-soluble vitamins are particularly subject to loss because they can be leached out of foods into the cooking water; in many cooking procedures this water is discarded, therefore the vitamin loss may be considerable.

Unknown vitamins

The chemical structure of all the vitamins which we know today are identified and all of them, with the exception of B_{12}, have been chemically synthesized. The question arises as to whether all the vitamins have been discovered. There is, however, much evidence to support the presence of agents which have metabolic effects and which are termed "unidentified factors". It seems probably that other vitamins which are engaged in physiological processes may still be waiting discovery.

Vitamin A

Chemistry

Vitamin A is a colorless compound found in nature as vitamin A_1, the most predominant form, and vitamin A_2 which is found only in the liver and other tissues of certain fresh water fishes. The biological activity of vitamin A_2 is about 40 per cent of vitamin A. Vitamin A occurs in nature in three chemical forms; alcohol (retinol), aldehyde (retinal), and acid (retinoic acid). The International Unit (I. U.) is no longer used and vitamin A is expressed as retinol; one I. U. of vitamin A being the equivalent of 0.3 μg of retinol. Vitamin A is found only in foods of animal origin. In plants it is present in the form of inactive precursors (provitamins) known as carotenoids which are yellow or red hydrocarbons. The most important carotenoids are beta, alpha, and gamma carotene and cryptoxanthin. One I. U. of vitamin is equivalent to 0.6 μg of beta carotene. Beta carotene contains two beta ionone rings while vitamin A and other carotenoids contain only one such ring. Therefore, two molecules of vitamin are formed by splitting one molecule of beta carotene (see Figure 65), but only one molecule of vitamin is formed by splitting the other three carotenoids. If the vitamin A activity of beta carotene is 100, then the relative activity of alpha carotene would be 53 while that of gamma carotene and cryptoxanthin would be

27 and 57, respectively. Carotenoids impart a yellow color to human fat and constitute as much as 12 per cent of the vitamin A stores of the body.

Vitamin A and carotenoids are stable to heat and to food processing but they are destroyed by oxidation or exposure to ultraviolet light.

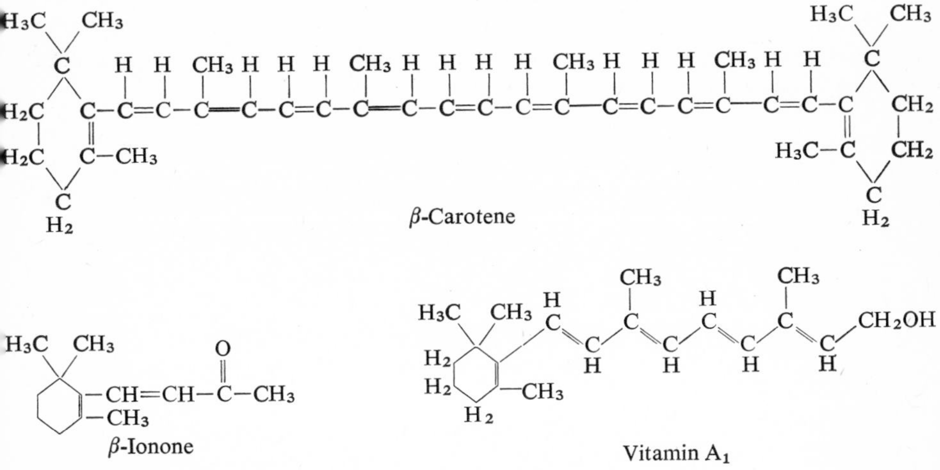

β-Carotene

β-Ionone

Vitamin A₁

Figure 65   The structure of vitamin A and its precursor.

Absorption

Vitamin A and its carotene precursors are mostly absorbed from the duodenum and jejunum. Dietary vitamin A is mainly in the form of esters which are hydrolyzed to retinol and fatty acid. This is achieved partly by pancreatic lipase in the intraluminal phase of digestion and partly by hydrolases situated on the outer surface of the brush border of intestinal epithelial cells. Retinol is then transferred inside the brush border cells, where it is re-esterified with a fatty acid (usually palmitic acid). These retinyl esters are incorporated into the lymph chylomicrons and transported in the intestinal lymphatics to the thoracic duct where they enter the bloodstream.

Since vitamin A is a fat-soluble vitamin, faulty absorption of fat will cause a reduction in absorption of vitamin A. This occurs in chronic diarrhea, sprue, or biliary and pancreatic dysfunction.

Biosynthesis of vitamin A from carotenes

The biosynthesis of vitamin A from beta carotene takes place mainly in the intestinal mucosa. The reaction takes place in two steps: First, beta carotene is cleaved into two parts by a dioxygenase reaction (see Figure 65) requiring molecular oxygen to form two molecules of retinal. Next, the retinal is reduced to retinol. The newly formed retinol is esterified with a fatty acid, and enters the lymphatic system. The human intestine is also capable of absorbing a small amount of unchanged dietary beta carotene directly into the lymph.

Thyroid hormone seems to be necessary for converting carotene to vitamin A, for despite there being an adequacy of vitamin A in the diet, night blindness frequently occurs in hypothyroidism.

Transport

Retinol is transported in human plasma bound to a specific protein, retinol-binding protein (RBP). The normal concentration of RBP in plasma is 3–4 mg per 100 ml and that of vitamin A is 30–50 µg per 100 ml. In the plasma, RBP circulates as a complex with another larger protein. The formation of this RBP-prealbumin complex preevnts filtration by the renal glomerulus of the relatively small RBP molecule and hence loss of RBP in urine.

RBP contains an unusually high level of aromatic amino acids which may be related to its ability to bind retinol. This has practical implications because the quality of the dietary protein might affect the biosynthesis of RBP and so modify retinol transport.

The release of retinol from the RBP complex may occur by an interaction with membrane lipids.

Storage and utilization

After entering the vascular compartment, the majority of the newly formed retinyl esters are taken up by the liver where they are stored and constitute about 95 per cent of total body vitamin A. The human liver stores are adequate to last for up to a year or even longer when the diet is completely deficient in vitamin A. The stored ester is hydrolyzed by a liver enzyme and released as free retinol to travel in the bloodstream to tissues where it is utilized. Protein is essential for removal of vitamin A from the liver and its utilization by the body is proportional to the protein intake when vitamin A intakes are low. This explains why vitamin A deficiency disease is so commonly a feature of populations experiencing protein calorie malnutrition.

Functions

These are many, several of them are important, that of maintaining normal growth being particularly vital.

It also has an important function in vision. The retina of the eye contains two kinds of light receptors. The first are known as rods; they contain rhodopsin (visual purple) and they are concerned with vision in dim light. The second are the cones; these contain iodopsin and they are concerned with vision in bright light and with color vision. Both pigments are photosensitive and are bleached upon exposure to light. This process causes a nervous excitation which is transmitted via the optic nerve to the brain where a visual sensation results.

Rhodopsin dissociates into retinene (11-cis retinal), a derivative of vitamin A, and a protein (opsin). In the presence of light, the retinene (retinal) is then reduced to retinol by the enzyme alcohol dehydrogenase. During visual activity, retinol diffuses out of the retina into the bloodstream and the pigment epithelium. The retina subsequently re-absorbs the retinol, which is resynthesized to retinal. In the dark, retinene and opsin recombine to form rhodopsin. Retinoic acid has no function in vision.

The photochemistry of vision is shown in Figure 66.

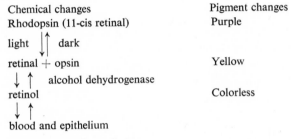

Figure 66   The photochemistry of vision

Vitamin A may be an integral structural component of cellular and intracellular membranes controlling their permeability and stability. It maintains mucous secreting epithelia and it influences mucopolysaccharide biosynthesis. It plays a role in the construction of normal bone by controlling the activity of the osteoblasts and osteoclasts of epithelial cartilage. It exerts an indirect influence on glycogen biosynthesis, by facilitating the synthesis of corticosterone from cholesterol in the adrenal cortex. It stimulates the synthesis of RNA and is thus associated with the nuclear mechanism of protein synthesis.

Deficiency

Vitamin A deficiency is a major public health problem in many developing countries and one of the most important causes of preventable blindness in infants and children. Among the most important etiological factors concerned in vitamin A malnutrition are inadequate intake of vitamin A by mothers during pregnancy and lactation, poor vitamin A content of supplementary foods after weaning, and kwashiorkor. This last disease is associated with vitamin A deficiency because of the reduced plasma protein which is needed to transport vitamin A. Vitamin A deficiency may also arise from faulty absorption caused by infections or sprue. It may be a consequence of cirrhosis of the liver which interferes with storage or it may arise because of interference with the conversion of carotenes to vitamin A such as occurs in hypothyroidism and in diabetes mellitus.

Deficiency symptoms appear after the tissue stores are depleted and the serum concentration is reduced from a normal value of 30–50 μg per 100 ml to less than 10 μg per 100 ml.

The clinical manifestations of night blindness, xeropthalmia, and keratomalacia have already been described.

There are other manifestations of the disease which include *keratinization* of hair follicles and atrophy of *sebaceous glands*. This results in the formation of dry, firm papules with protruding cornified plugs; a condition known as *follicular hyperkeratosis*.

Bone malformation may occur possibly because osteoclasts, which normally reabsorb bone, are reduced in activity while the osteoblasts, which form bone, continue with no curtailment of activity.

Growth retardation and deranged tooth formation may also occur and there may be lowered resistance to infection.

Treatment and prevention

Although vitamin A deficiency can be relieved by dietary means, large doses of vitamin bring about a rapid response. The vitamin therapy should be supported by a high protein diet and antibiotics. As a preventive measure it is useful to administer a single dose of an oil-soluble preparation of vitamin A to undernourished children. This quantity helps them to sustain a minimal level of serum vitamin A for as long as six months.

The mechanism of the toxic effects of vitamin A is not known but it could be due to the vitamin A (retinol or retinoic acid) causing a weakening of the lysosomal membrane and subsequent release of lysosomal enzymes into the circulation. The clinical state of hypervitaminosis A has already been described in Chapter 1.

When large amounts of carotene-containing foods are ingested, the concentration of plasma carotenoids increases, causing a yellow coloration of the skin, but, unlike jaundice, neither the conjunctivae nor the urine are colored. This condition is harmless and reversible.

Sources

Vitamin A is only found in animals, while carotenes are present in both plant and animal tissues. The richest sources of vitamin A are milk, cheese, butter, egg yolk, and some fish liver oils. The most important sources of carotenes (provitamins) are green vegetables such as spinach, parsley, kale, and broccoli. There is a direct relationship between the vitamin activity and the chlorophyll content of vegetables as shown by the degree of greenness. Yellow vegetables and fruits such as carrots, tomatoes, apricots, corn, squash, pumpkin, and sweet potatoes are also rich in carotenoids.

Requirement

Children under one year require 0.5 mg of retinol per day, increasing to 1.5 mg at adolescence. There is an additional requirement of 0.3 mg per day during pregnancy and 1 mg per day during lactation.

Vitamin D

Chemistry

There are at least 10 substances in nature which possess vitamin D activity. Chemically they are all sterols but there are differences in their side chains. Only two of them have biological activity: the first, vitamin D_2 (ergocalci-

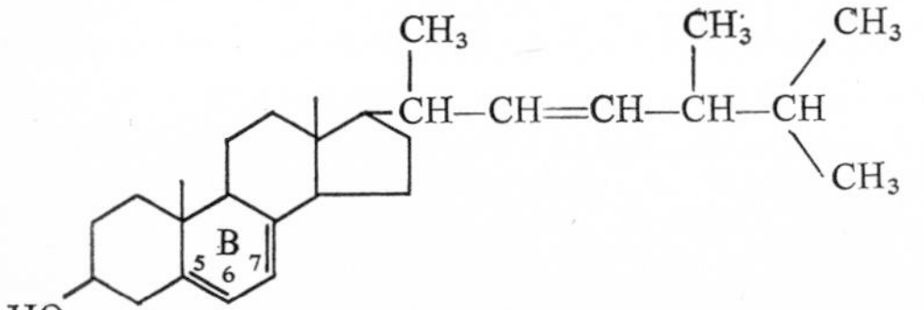

Ergosterol

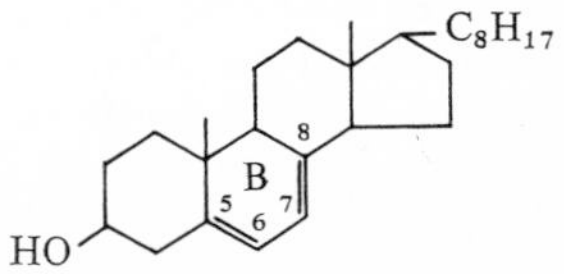

7-Dehydrocholesterol

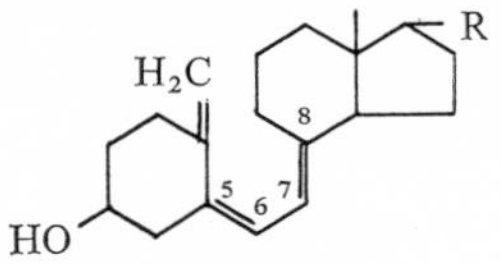

Vitamin D

$R = C_8H_{17}$ in vitamin D_3.
$R = C_9H_{17}$ in vitamin D_2.

Figure 67   Vitamin D and vitamin D provitamins

ferol), is formed by ultraviolet irradiation of ergosterol in plants; the second, vitamin D_3 (cholecalciferol), is formed by irradiation of 7-dehydrocholesterol in animals. D_2 and D_3 have equal biological activity in man. Irradiation opens up one of the rings of the sterol nucleus, thereby converting the inactive provitamins (ergosterol and 7-dehydrocholesterol) to active vitamins (D_2 and D_3) (see Figure 67).

Vitamin D is a white colorless heat-stable crystal.

Absorption and metabolism

Ergosterol is poorly absorbed but 7-dehydrocholesterol and vitamins D_2 and D_3 are readily absorbed from the small intestine. Since they are fat-soluble, their absorption will be inhibited if there is interference with fat absorption such as occurs when there is a deficiency of bile salts. The amount which can be stored in the body is limited; the major storage site being the liver, but the skin, brain, spleen, bone, and lung also contain significant amounts of the vitamin. Excretion takes place via the bile but most of it is reabsorbed. There is no urinary excretion and the metabolites of vitamin D are still unidentified.

Functions

Vitamin D, or its metabolic product 25-hydroxycholecalciferol, promotes calcium absorption across the intestine by inducing synthesis of a *calcium binding protein (CaBP)*.

Administration of vitamin D increases the activity of several enzymes in the brush border of the small intestine, namely, alkaline phosphatase, leucine aminopeptidase, and calcium-dependent adenosine triphosphatase.

Vitamin D seems to have a direct effect on bone, regulating the blood calcium level by mobilizing calcium from bone.

Phosphate exists in serum in both organic and inorganic forms but in the bone it occurs primarily in the inorganic form in a complex with calcium. Vitamin D retains phosphorus in the body by converting the organic into the inorganic form. Vitamin D may also promote absorption of phosphate from the intestine and its reabsorption by kidney tubules.

It is involved in the oxidation of citric acid, which is a major constituent of bone. The rate at which calcium can go into solution, and the regulation of calcium ion concentration varies with the tissue levels of citric acid; citric acid is subject to regulation by vitamin D. In rickets both the skeletal and serum citric acid concentrations decrease.

Deficiency of vitamin D

Rickets and children, and osteomalacia in adults, are caused by vitamin D deficiency. The clinical picture of these conditions is described in Chapter 1.

Vitamin D deficiency can be treated by giving vitamin D daily for 1–3 months or by giving a massive single dose of vitamin D intramuscularly, which lasts for 3 months.

Hypervitaminosis D

It is now being recognized that vitamin D overnutrition may be of public health importance (see page 24).

The regular use of large doses of vitamin D over a prolonged period of time will produce toxic symptoms which include anorexia, nausea, vomiting, thirst, constipation, fever, abdominal pain, pallor, fatigue, diarrhea, renal failure, calcification of soft tissues, and bone demineralization. Calcium and phosphorus serum levels increase and appear in the urine in high concentrations. If the vitamin D intake is reduced to normal levels, the symptoms will disappear.

Sources

Ergosterol is widely distributed in plants but it is of no nutritional value to man since is cannot be absorbed from the intestinal tract. The main animal sources of vitamin D are fish liver oil, butter, milk, and egg yolk. Humans can also synthesize this vitamin in skin exposed to ultraviolet light.

The vitamin D content of milk can be increased by either irradiating the cow or its milk, or by feeding the cow irradiated yeast or vitamin D concentrates.

Requirements

If the skin is adequately exposed to sunlight no exogenous source of vitamin D seems to be required by adults. However, it is recommended that all age groups should receive 400 I. U. of vitamin D per day. Each I. U. of vitamin D equals 0.025 µg of vitamin D_3.

Vitamin E

Chemistry

Four naturally occurring forms of vitamin E are found; these are alpha, beta, gamma, and delta tocopherols which differ slightly in chemical structure (see Figure 68). The biological activity of tocopherols in decreasing order are alpha, beta, gamma, and delta. Their antioxidant potency is in the reverse order so that alpha tocopherol has the highest biological activity and the lowest antioxidant activity. Because of their phenolic hydroxyl group, they can form esters, which are more stable than the free form.

Vitamin E is a yellow viscous oil, although stable to heat it is readily broken down when exposed to the air; this results in the loss of its biological activity.

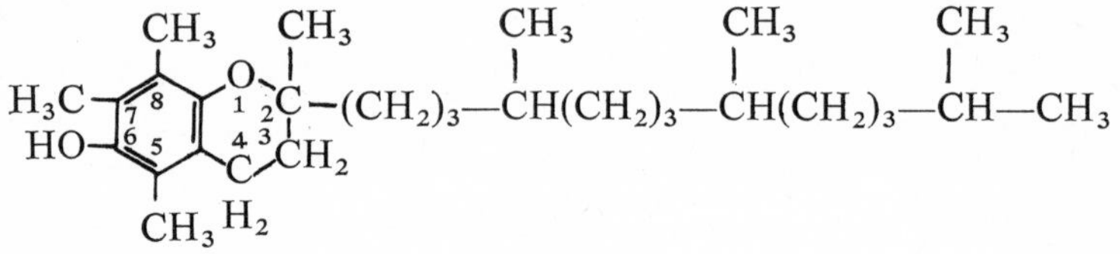

α-Tocopherol

Figure 68   Vitamin E

Absorption and metabolism

Vitamin E is readily absorbed both in its free and ester forms from the small intestine but bile is necessary for its absorption. It is transported in the blood stream chiefly in the alpha lipoprotein fraction of serum where its concentration is 1 mg per 100 ml. It is present in all the tissues, particularly in adipose tissue. Humans do not excrete significant amounts of vitamin E in the urine.

Functions

The biological activity of vitamin E is due to its antioxidant property. By being oxidized itself, it lowers the amount of oxygen available to oxidize other oxygen-susceptible compounds such as unsaturated fatty acids, vitamin C, and vitamin A. Vitamin E therefore maintains the structural integrity of membranes of organelles and cells. In the case of red blood cells, it protects them against hemolysis.

Vitamin E may have a role as a regulator of heme synthesis, probably by controlling the synthesis of enzymes.

It may also play a role in cellular respiration by being involved in the electron transport chain.

Deficiency of Vitamin E

Vitamin E deficiency is rarely seen in man. In the newborn it is characterized by macrocytic anemia, generalized edema, reticulocytosis, cell fragmentation, and thrombocytosis. Low birth weight babies are particularly susceptible to this syndrome at about 6–10 weeks of age. Vitamin E probably prevents these dysfunctions by helping to inhibit peroxidation of the lipids of the red cell membrane.

Selenium can replace vitamin E as a therapeutic agent in some of the vitamin E deficiency diseases.

Sources

Vitamin E is widely distributed in nature. Vegetable oils, particularly wheat germ oil, are the richest sources of vitamin E. They contain different forms of tocopherol. Other sources include egg, milk, butter, liver, legumes, and green leafy vegetables.

Requirement

The vitamin E requirement has a direct relationship with the intake of poly-unsaturated fatty acids. The daily requirement of infants is 5 mg, children 10–15 mg, male adults 20–30 mg, and female adults 20–25 mg. During pregnancy and lactation, the requirement increases to 30 mg per day.

Vitamin K

Chemistry

Two naturally occurring vitamins have been identified: vitamin K_1 (phyllo-quinone) which is found only in plants, and vitamin K_2 (farnoquinone)

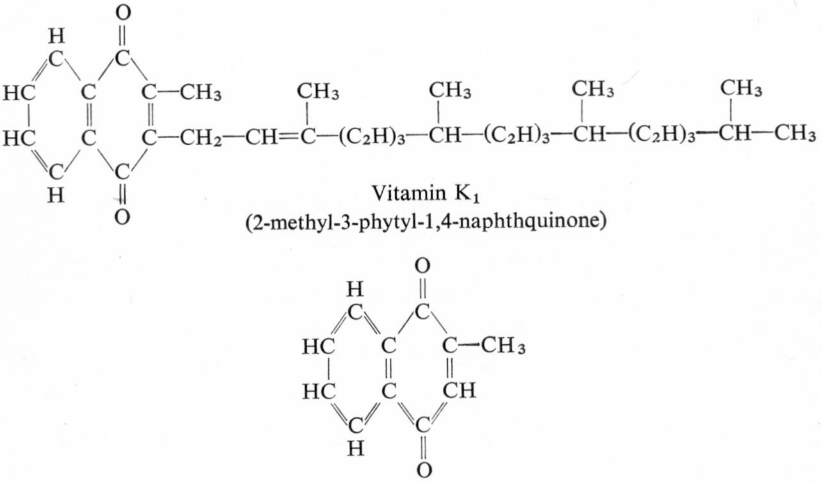

Vitamin K_1
(2-methyl-3-phytyl-1,4-naphthquinone)

Menadione
(2-methyl-1,4,-naphthoquinone)

Figure 69   Vitamin K

which is synthesized by intestinal micro-organisms. They differ in the length of the side chain which is attached to the quinone nucleus. A number of synthetic K vitamins have been prepared, the most potent of which is K_3 (menadione). In contrast to the naturally occurring vitamins which are fat-soluble, the synthetic forms of vitamin K are water-soluble, a property related to them having no long side chains (see Figure 69). The fat-soluble forms can be administered orally or intramuscularly, but the water-soluble analogues are given intravenously. All forms of vitamin K are yellow compounds which are stable to heat but they are readily destroyed by light, alkalis, and alcohol.

Absorption and metabolism

Vitamin K is absorbed mainly from the jejunum where it enters the lacteals and passes into the blood circulation via the thoracic duct. Bile salts are required for its absorption. It is primarily stored in the liver. Vitamin K_2 is the most active form of the vitamin in mammalian metabolism. Other forms of dietary origin are first converted to menadione and then to vitamin K_2. This is done partly in the liver and partly in other tissues. Vitamin K is not excreted in urine and most of the fecal vitamin K is of bacterial origin synthesized in the intestine.

Functions

Vitamin K facilitates blood *coagulation* by influencing the hepatic synthesis of *prothrombin* and *proconvertin*.

$$\text{prothrombinogen} \xrightarrow{\text{vitamin K}} \text{prothrombin} \xrightarrow[\substack{\text{proconvertin,}\\\text{Ca, other}\\\text{factors}}]{\text{thromboplastin}} \text{thrombin} \xrightarrow{\text{fibrinogen}} \text{fibrin}$$

It may also facilitate electron transport and oxidative phosphorylation reactions in the tissues.

Deficiency in vitamin K

Because vitamin K can be synthesized by the intestinal flora, deficiency rarely results from dietary inadequacy in adults. Newborn infants who do not have an intestinal flora capable of synthesizing vitamin K and who have inadequate body stores, do not receive sufficient vitamin K in milk and they may develop vitamin K deficiency, a condition which is known as "hemorrhagic disease of the newborn". It can be prevented by the routine prophylactic administration of synthetic vitamin K to mothers prior to delivery, or to the newborn infants. In adults, deficiency may be caused by faulty intestinal absorption. There may also be a conditioned deficiency caused by liver disease; the damaged liver cells being unable to utilize vitamin K for the manufacture of prothrombin. Antibiotics may inhibit the growth of intestinal flora and reduce synthesis of the vitamin.

Dicumarol is a derivative of a sweet smelling substance in clover; it resembles vitamin K and can replace it at its site of action in the liver or displace it from an enzyme system and so induce an effective vitamin K deficiency state.

Sources

Vitamin K_1 is found only in plant tissues, mainly in green leafy vegetables. Vitamin K_2 is synthesized by intestinal micro-organisms.

Requirement

Because vitamin K is widely distributed in nature and can be synthesized by intestinal flora, there is no known dietary requirement for vitamin K under normal physiological conditions. Infants, however, whose intestinal flora may not have developed sufficiently to supply enough vitamin K, may benefit from a single dose of the vitamin after birth.

Vitamin C

Chemistry

Vitamin C (ascorbic acid) is a white crystalline compound, having an empirical formula, $C_6H_8O_6$, and a configuration similar to that of carbohydrates; it is a relatively strong acid. The naturally occurring vitamin is

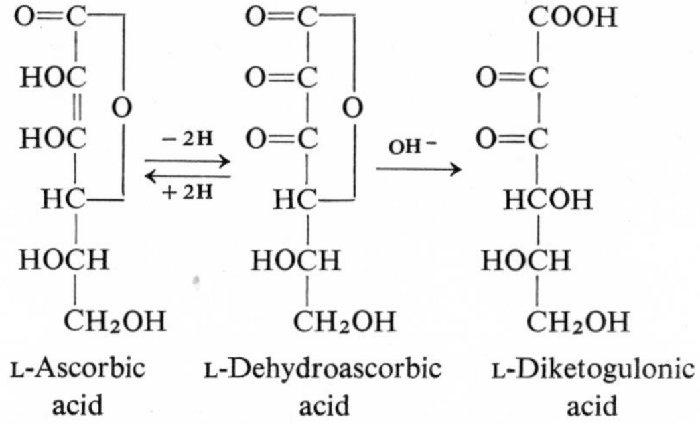

Figure 70 Ascorbic acid and the product of its oxidation

17*

L-ascorbic acid; the D-isomer is inactive in the body. The most important chemical property of vitamin C is its ability to act as a strong reducing agent. It can be oxidized readily to dehydro-ascorbic acid, a reaction which is reversible (see Figure 70). Further oxidation of dehydroascorbic acid produces an inactive compound, diketogulonic acid. The oxidative destruction of ascorbic acid is accelerated by high temperatures, alkalinity, and light.

Absorption and metabolism

Vitamin C is readily absorbed from the small intestine. Although it is not stored to any appreciable extent, the body nevertheless contains some mobilizable reserves. The concentration of vitamin C in tissues and organs approximates their metabolic activity. The plasma level is 0.4–1.0 mg per 100 ml and is influenced by recent dietary intake. The excess intake is excreted in the urine, or as end products of vitamin C metabolism such as oxalic acid and diketogulonic acid.

Functions

Vitamin C is required for the conversion of proline to hydroxyproline in collagen. In scurvy, hydroxyproline excretion increases which may represent either a reduced synthesis or an increase in degradation of collagen.

Vitamin C is also required for dentin formation. It is involved in the biosynthesis of progesterone by maintaining the required coenzyme (NAD^+) in an oxidized state. It is also involved in the synthesis of neurotransmitters, such as norepinephrine and serotonin. Vitamin C deficiency leads to enlargement of the adrenal gland which suggests that it is involved in the function of that organ. It is concerned with the oxidation of the amino acids phenylalanine and tyrosine, and it converts inactive folic acid to the active citrovorum factor. Since it undergoes reversible oxidation-reduction (ascorbic acid $\rightleftarrows$ dehydro-ascorbic acid), it may transport hydrogen from one compound to another in cellular oxidation-reduction reactions. It aids in the utilization of iron by reducing ferric ions to ferrous ions in which form it is absorbed. It also functions in incorporating iron in liver ferritin.

Deficiency of vitamin C

Vitamin C deficiency has so far been reported only in man and other animal species which cannot synthesize vitamin C from glucose.

The body stores of vitamin C are adequate to maintain health for about four months on a vitamin C free diet. Vitamin C deficiency disease is called scurvy (see page 42). In this disease there is a failure of various types of connective tissue cells to form collagen and dentin. Scurvy becomes obvious when the body pool of vitamin C falls from about 1500 mg to less than 300 mg and when the whole blood vitamin C is less than 0.3 mg per 100 ml.

The condition readily responds to treatment with dietary or synthetic sources.

The vitamin C intake of a population is best judged from vitamin C levels in the plasma.

Sources

Vitamin C is widely distributed in plant and animal tissues; raw liver, raw milk, citrus fruits, green leafy vegetables, green peppers, green peas and beans, tomatoes, potatoes, and strawberries are all good sources. Much of the vitamin C content of food is lost during cooking, processing, and storage procedures. Contact with heavy metals, particularly copper, is also deleterious to vitamin C.

Requirement

The requirements for vitamin C are discussed in Chapter 4.

Vitamin B$_1$

Chemistry

Vitamin B$_1$, or thiamine, consists of a pyrimidine and a thiazole ring and contains sulfur in its structure (see Figure 71). It is a white crystalline compound, usually prepared as a chloride which is more stable. It is resistant to heat and acids in the dry state but is very easily destroyed by moisture and heat in neutral and alkali solutions, which break the molecule up into its constituents, pyrimidine and thiazole.

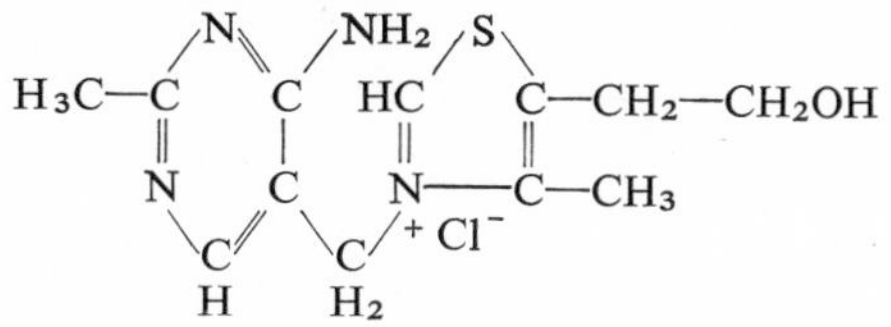

Thiamine chloride

Figure 71   Thiamine

Absorption and metabolism

Most of the thiamine in vegetables is in a free state and is readily absorbed from the small intestine. The molecule of the coenzyme of thiamine (thiamine pyrophosphate or cocarboxylase) is too large to be absorbed, so it is split prior to passage through the intestinal mucosa and subsequently phosphorylated wherever, and whenever needed.

The adult body contains 30–70 mg of thiamine. The concentration in plasma is 1 μg per 100 ml and 6–12 μg per 100 ml in blood, most is in the red blood cells as thiamine pyrophosphate combined with protein. Only limited amounts of thiamine can be stored. It is found mainly in the heart, liver, kidney, skeletal muscle, and brain. Any intake in excess of immediate needs is excreted in the urine. Because of this, a regular daily supply of thiamine is needed. Normally about 50 μg of thiamine is excreted in urine in a free form each day. This represents about 10 per cent of the total amount absorbed. Fecal thiamine is probably largely of bacterial origin.

Functions

Thiamine is a constituent of the coenzyeme thiamine pyrophosphate or, cocarboxylase. Cocarboxylase is required in three reactions in the intermediate metabolism of carbohydrates. First, in the decarboxylation of pyruvic acid to acetyl coenzyme A and secondly in the oxidative decarboxylation of alpha ketoglutaric acid in the Kreb's Cycle. It also activates the enzyme transketolase in the direct oxidation of glucose. The metabolic importance of this reaction is the synthesis of ribose, a sugar involved in the formation of nucleic acids and the production of the coenzyme of niacin (NADPH); this is required for synthesis of fatty acids. These three reactions are summarized as follows:

1. pyruvic acid $\xrightarrow{\text{cocarboxylase}}$ acetyl coenzyme A $\xrightarrow{\text{oxaloacetic acid}}$ Kreb's Cycle

2. alpha ketoglutaric acid $\xrightarrow{\text{cocarboxylase}}$ succinyl coenzyme A
(in Kreb's Cycle)

3. glucose $\xrightarrow{\text{transketolase}}$ ribose $\longrightarrow$ ribonucleic acid
$\quad\quad\vert\longrightarrow$ NADPH $\longrightarrow$ fatty acids

The signs and symptoms of thiamine deficiency may be a consequence of the accumulation of intermediate products of carbohydrate metabolism, such as pyruvic acid, in the blood and tissues.

Thiamine deficiency

Deficiency of thiamine causes the disease beri-beri which has been described in detail in Chapter 1.

Beri-beri can be treated by administering thiamine orally, intravenously or intramuscularly.

The urinary excretion of thiamine and erythrocyte transketolase activity reflect levels of thiamine intake and they are, therefore, good measurements of nutritional status. This subject is discussed in further detail in Chapter 5.

Sources

Thiamine is widely distributed in plant and animal tissues. The richest sources are pork meat, whole grain cereals, liver, egg yolk, green leafy vegetables, legumes, and yeast. Much of the thiamine in food is lost during processing and when the water in which the food is cooked is discarded. The thiamine content of foods is essentially unaffected by freezing. Some synthesis occurs by intestinal micro-organisms but the contribution to man is questionable.

Shellfish and certain fish contain a heat-labile enzyme, thiaminase, which splits thiamine. This enzyme is destroyed by cooking so that thiamine deficiency is unusual unless large quantities of raw fish or shell fish are ingested over a prolonged period of time.

Requirement

Thiamine is needed for carbohydrate metabolism so there is a direct relationship between thiamine requirements and the carbohydrate intake; the higher the intake the greater is the thiamine requirement. This also means more thiamine is required when excessive amounts of alcohol are consumed. As thiamine is required for the metabolism of carbohydrate but not fat, dietary sources of the latter have a sparing effect on thiamine.

The daily requirement of infants is 0.2–0.5 mg, for children 0.6–1.1 mg, for men 1.2–1.5, for women 1.0–1.2 mg per day. There is an additional requirement of 0.1 mg per day during pregnancy and 0.5 mg per day during lactation.

Riboflavin

Chemistry

Riboflavin is an orange-yellow compound which is resistant to heat, acid, and oxidation but sensitive to light and alkali solution. It consists of a flavin nucleus combined with the alcohol of ribose (ribitol) (see Figure 72).

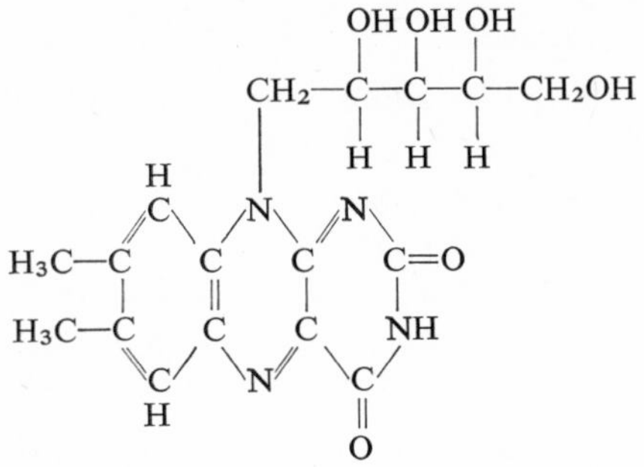

Riboflavin

Figure 72   Riboflavin

Absorption and metabolism

Riboflavin is chiefly absorbed from the small intestine by a process of passive diffusion. It is phosphorylated in the mucosa and then transported in the blood stream to all the cells of the body. In the tissues it is found in the form of the coenzymes, flavin mononucleotide (FMN) and flavin dinucleotide (FAD). Its concentration in plasma is 2.5–4 μg per 100 ml. It is not stored in the body to any degree but the highest concentrations occur in liver, kidney, and muscle. About 500–750 μg of riboflavin are excreted each day in the feces, most of this is of bacterial origin. However, the daily urinary excretion is 0.1–0.4 mg per day depending on the daily intake. A number of physiological stresses, such as negative nitrogen balance and acute starvation, increase the urinary excretion of riboflavin, whereas during rapid tissue growth or short periods of hard physiological work, it is decreased.

Functions

Riboflavin is an essential constituent of two coenzymes (FMN and FAD) which are involved in biological oxidation-reduction reactions. These coenzymes receive hydrogen atoms from the nicotinic acid coenzyme, NADH, and give them to iron-porphyrin cytochromes. Riboflavin enzymes are part of a complex enzyme system in the mitochondria of the cells. These bring about the transfer of hydrogen from the substrate to molecular oxygen; in this process, water is formed and energy released. Riboflavin is also an integral part of enzymes which are involved in the transfer of hydrogen atoms in protein and purine metabolism.

Deficiency

Riboflavin deficiency in man causes eye and skin changes which are described in Chapters 1 and 5.

Deficiency can be induced readily under experimental conditions in man by giving riboflavin antagonists and a riboflavin deficient diet.

Sources

Riboflavin is widely distributed in both animal and plant tissues. The richest sources are milk, yeast, germinating seeds, eggs, green vegetables, legumes, and offal.

Riboflavin is synthesized by micro-organisms in the intestinal tract. The amount produced in humans is greater when a vegetable diet is consumed than when the diet contains meat, but most of the synthesized vitamin is not available and is excreted in the feces.

Riboflavin is relatively stable under usual conditions of food preparation but it is destroyed in alkaline solutions and by light. Significant losses occur when cooking water is discarded since riboflavin is readily soluble in water.

Requirement

The daily requirement for infants is 0.4–0.6 mg, for children 0.6–1.2 mg, for men 1.3–1.7 mg, and for women 1.3–1.5 mg. The requirement increases to 1.8 per day during pregnancy and to 2 mg per day during lactation.

Niacin

Chemistry

Niacin (nicotinic acid) is a white crystalline compound which is one of the most stable vitamins, being resistant to heat, light, air, alkali, and acid. In tissues it occurs chiefly as nicotinamide. Its chemical structure is shown in Figure 73.

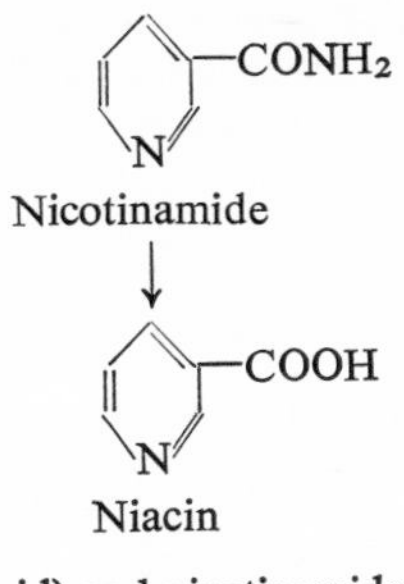

Nicotinamide

Niacin

Figure 73   Niacin (nicotinic acid) and nicotinamide

Biosynthesis

Niacin can be synthesized in the body from the amino acid *tryptophan*; however, this requires pyridoxal phosphate (the coenzyme of vitamin B_6) which means that the availability of tryptophan and the coenzyme affect the requirement for niacin. Sixty mg of dietary tryptophan is equivalent to one mg of niacin.

Absorption and metabolism

Both niacin and nicotinamide are readily absorbed from the intestine. Whole blood contains 0.2–0.9 mg of nicotinic acid per 100 ml, most of which is in red blood cells. There is little storage of this vitamin in the body. The major urinary metabolite is N'-methylnicotinamide of which 3–12.5 mg is excreted per day, but there is also some excretion of niacin (0.25–1.25 mg per day) and nicotinamide (0.5–4.0 mg per day).

Functions

Nicotinamide is a constituent of the coenzymes nicotinamide adenine dinucleotide (NAD) and nicotinamide adenine dinucleotide phosphate (NADP) (previously known as DPN and TPN, or coenzymes I and II). These coenzymes function in biological oxidation-reduction systems in which hydrogen is transferred from many substrates to oxygen, through a series of other coenzymes (FAD and cytochromes), to form water. They are therefore part of the intracellular respiratory mechanism of all cells.

Deficiency

Niacin deficiency in humans causes the disease pellagra (see page 36).

Measurement of the urinary excretion of N'-methylnicotinamide provides the most reliable diagnostic laboratory test for pellagra, urinary levels being subnormal in niacin deficiency.

In the treatment of niacin deficiency, nicotinamide is preferred to nicotinic acid because it is free from the unpleasant side effects of nicotinic acid such as flushing of the skin and tingling sensations.

Sources

Niacin is widely distributed in plant and animal tissues. The richest sources are yeast, whole grain cereals, liver, kidney, meat, fish, legumes, and some vegetables. Although certain foods such as milk and egg are poor sources of niacin, they have a high content of tryptophan which can be converted into niacin. A considerable amount of niacin is lost during milling.

Requirement

The daily requirement of niacin for infants is 5–8 mg, for children 8–15 mg, for men 14–20 mg, for women 12–16 mg, and for lactating mothers 20 mg of niacin or its equivalent are required per day.

Pyridoxine

Chemistry

Vitamin B_6 exists in nature as an alcohol (pyridoxol), and aldehyde (pyridoxal), and an amine (pyridoxamine) (see Figure 74). All three forms exhibit equal biological activity in animals. Pyridoxal and pyridoxamine occur in animal products while pyridoxol is the largest component of vegetable products. Only a small proportion of vitamin B_6 is found in the free state, where it is mainly in combination with protein.

Pyridoxine is a colorless crystalline solid, stable to heat, acid, and alkali but sensitive to light.

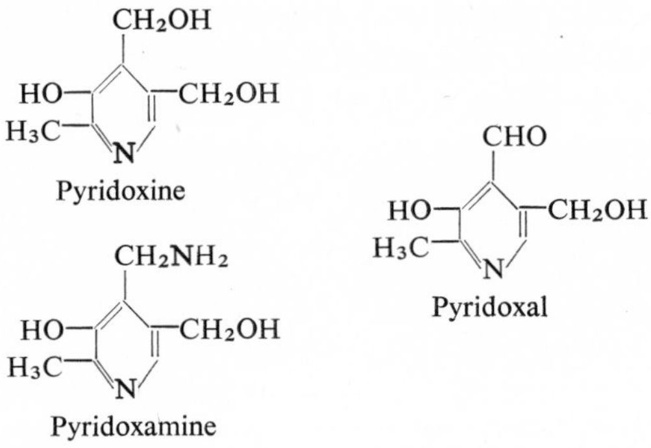

Figure 74   Pyridoxine

Absorption and metabolism

Pyridoxine is mostly absorbed from the upper gastrointestinal tract. Pyridoxol, pyrodoxal, and pyridoxamine, in the form of their phosphates, are interconvertible *in vivo*. The functional form of vitamin B_6 is pyridoxal phosphate which the body can make from any of the other three forms. However, pyridoxine cannot be stored in the body to any appreciable extent. The total body content of pyridoxine is 16–25 mg. The level in the blood is 5 µg per 100 ml, most of which is in red blood cells. The major urinary product is pyridoxic acid, but, in addition, a small quantity of pyridoxal and pyridoxamine are also lost in urine (0.5–0.7 mg per day) and some pyridoxine (0.7–0.9 mg per day) is lost in feces.

Functions

The functional form of vitamin B_6 is the coenzyme pyridoxal phosphate designated as co-decarboxylase. It is mainly concerned with amino acid metabolism.

It transfers an amino group from an amino acid to an alpha keto acid to form a different amino acid. This is the process of transamination. It is also concerned with deamination, or the removal of amino groups from amino acids. It removes carbon dioxide from amino acids, a process essential for formation of serotonin, norepinephrine, and histamine, and it removes sulfur from certain sulfur-containing amino acids such as cysteine. It is involved in the conversion of the amino acid tryptophan to niacin and it can convert D forms of amino acids into L forms. It is also concerned with the active transport of amino acids and certain metallic ions across the cell membrane. Vitamin B_6 is part of the enzyme phosphorylase, which facilitates the release of glycogen as glucose-1-phosphate from liver and muscle. It functions in the transfer of single carbon units because it is involved in the interconversion of serine and glycine, thus aiding in transfer of carbon units to tetrahydrofolic acid. It is also necessary for the production of antibodies and the synthesis of hemoglobin.

Deficiency of vitamin B_6

Vitamin B_6 deficiency, characterized by convulsions and anemia, has been noticed in children receiving a diet lacking in vitamin B_6. Adults given deoxypyridoxine, a vitamin B_6 antagonist, develop peripheral neuritis, hyperirritability, lymphocytopenia, naso-labial and other skin lesions, glossitis, stomatitis, weight loss, apathy, somnolence, and difficulty in walking. A defect in tryptophan metabolism also develops, therefore large quantities of xanthurenic acid appear in the urine after the ingestion of tryptophan. There is an increase in oxalate excretion and a reduction in pyridoxic acid excretion in the urine.

Although there is no satisfactory method of determining vitamin B_6 status, the determination of pyridoxic acid, oxalic acid, and pyridoxine in the urine may be useful.

Sources

Vitamin B_6 is widely distributed in foods. The richest sources are "royal jelly", yeast, whole grain cereals, egg yolk, muscle meat, fish, liver, and some vegetables. As much as 90 per cent of the vitamin B_6 content of rice and wheat is lost in milling and about 25 per cent of the vitamin B_6 activity of vegetables is lost in freezing.

It can be synthesized by intestinal bacteria but the extent to which it is available to man is not known.

Requirement

The daily requirement for vitamin B_6 in infants is 0.2–0.4 mg, in children 0.5–1.2 mg, in adults 1.4–2 mg, and pregnant and lactating women require 2.5 mg per day.

Factors which affect the bacterial synthesis of vitamin B_6 or have sparing effects on vitamin B_6 metabolism, influence the requirement for this vitamin. For instance, protein, linseed oil, and sucrose increase vitamin B_6 requirement, while choline, aureomycin, essential fatty acids, biotin, dextran, and pantothenic acid lower it.

Biotin

Chemistry

Biotin is a heterocyclic sulfur-containing compound with an empirical formula, $C_{10}H_{16}N_2O_3S$ (see Figure 75). The crystals are long, colorless, and needle-like. Biotin is stable to heat, acids, and bases but it is readily oxidized.

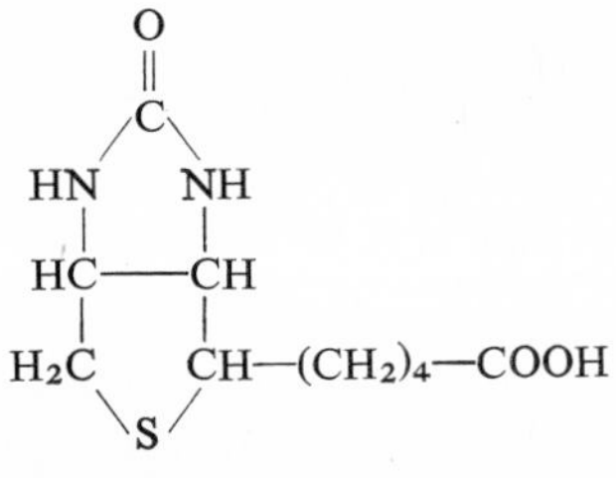

$$
\begin{array}{c}
O \\
\parallel \\
C \\
\diagup \quad \diagdown \\
HN \qquad NH \\
\mid \qquad \mid \\
HC\text{---}CH \\
\mid \qquad \mid \\
H_2C \qquad CH\text{---}(CH_2)_4\text{---}COOH \\
\diagdown S \diagup
\end{array}
$$

Biotin

Figure 75   Biotin

Metabolism

Biotin is stored to a limited extent in the liver and kidney. A considerable portion of biotin-active material in the tissues cannot be extracted with water, which indicates that it is probably existing in a bound form. The enzyme biotinidase, which is capable of liberating biotin from simple biotin esters and amides, is widely distributed in animal tissues. Normal adults excrete 10–180 μg of biotin per day in urine and 15–200 μg in the feces.

Functions

Biotin is involved in many reaction in which there is carbon dioxide fixation (carboxylation) and removal (decarboxylation). It is therefore concerned in carbohydrate metabolism with the addition of carbon dioxide to pyruvate to form malate, and the removal of carbon dioxide from oxalosuccinate to form alpha ketoglutarate. It also functions in the metabolism of fatty acids, the deamination of some amino acids, and the synthesis of nicotinic acid.

Deficiency of biotin

Biotin deficiency can be induced experimentally in man. The symptoms and signs are dermatitis, pallor of the skin and mucous membranes, depression, lassitude, somnolence, muscle pains, hyperesthesia, anorexia, nausea, anemia, and hypercholesterolemia. These symptoms disappear a few days after biotin is given by injection.

Sources

Biotin is widely distributed in nature in both plant and animal tissues. In the former, it is mainly found in a water-soluble form, but in animal tissues, animal products, and in yeast, it is chiefly in a bound, water-insoluble form. The richest sources are egg yolk, liver, kidney, milk, and yeast. "Royal jelly" is an exceptionally good source of biotin. Some biotin is also made available to the host through bacterial synthesis in the intestine.

Requirement

The requirement for biotin has not been established but as the body utilizes about 150 μg of biotin per day this amount appears to be adequate.

Pantothenic acid

Chemistry

Pantothenic acid is so designated because it is widely distributed in nature, in all forms of living matter.

It is a pale yellow, viscous oil. Its calcium salts are white and crystalline. Pantothenic acid is stable in neutral solution but it is destroyed by acids and alkalis; it is also quite stable at normal cooking temperatures. It is a peptide of beta alanine with dihydroxy-dimethylbutyric acid. The empirical formula is $C_9H_{17}NO_5$, the structural formula is shown in Figure 76.

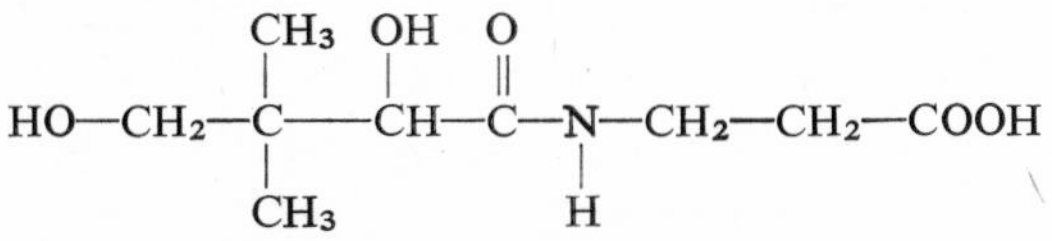

$$HO-CH_2-\underset{\underset{CH_3}{|}}{\overset{\overset{CH_3}{|}}{C}}-CH-\underset{\overset{||}{O}}{\overset{OH}{|}}\overset{O}{\underset{}{C}}-\underset{\underset{H}{|}}{N}-CH_2-CH_2-COOH$$

Pantothenic acid (pantoyl-ß-alanine)

Figure 76   Pantothenic acid

In tissues it is found as part of coenzyme A.

Functions

As part of coenzyme A, it functions in both the catabolism and anabolism of carbohydrates, fats, and proteins. Coenzyme A degrades these compounds by combining with their two carbon fragments to form acetyl coenzyme A, which enters the Kreb's Cycle for energy production. Coenzyme A is concerned therefore with maintaining the rate of phosphorylation which accompanies the cellular oxidation of foodstuffs.

Coenzyme A is also involved in the synthesis of cholesterol, adrenocortical hormones, porphyrin, and acetylcholine.

Deficiency

Pantothenic acid deficiency does not occur normally in man, but it can be induced experimentally. It is characterized by fatigue, headache, insomnia, nausea, abdominal cramps, muscle cramps, impaired coordination, burning sensation in the feet, numbness and tingling of hands and feet, and depression. All these symptoms disappear after administration of pantothenic acid.

Pantothenic acid deficiency can be produced in animals but the signs differ in various animals.

Metabolism

Pantothenic acid is found in all tissues in small quantities but its highest concentration is in the liver and kidney. Its concentration in whole blood is 14–45 µg per 100 ml with the cells having a higher concentration than the plasma. Normally 2.5–5 mg per day is excreted in urine. The products of its catabolism are not known.

Sources

"Royal jelly", yeast, liver and kidney, egg yolk, wheat and rice bran, milk, peas, and fresh vegetables are the richest sources of pantothenic acid. It is relatively stable under storage conditions and normal cooking procedures.

Requirement

The human requirement for pantothenic acid is not known but a daily intake of about 10 mg per 2500 calories has been recommended.

Folic acid

Chemistry

Folic acid (pteroylglutamic acid) derives its name from the fact that it was first found in the leaf of spinach.

Folic acids consists of a pteridine nucleus, para-amino-benzoic acid, and glutamic acid (see Figure 77). In nature it may exist as folic acid, pteroyl-monoglutamic acid, or as polyglutamic acid conjugates (having 3 or 7 glutamic acids). The enzymes, conjugases, liberate folic acid from its conjugates. The functionally active form of folic acid is the coenzyme tetra-hydrofolic acid or citrovorum factor.

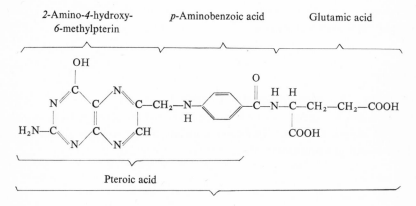

Pteroylglutamic acid   (folic acid, PGA)

Figure 77   Folic acid

Folic acid is light yellow in color and crystalline. It is sensitive to heat in an acid medium, and to light. It loses most of its activity during storage.

Absorption and metabolism

Folate is best absorbed in its monoglutamate and triglutamate forms; however, food folate consists largely of polyglutamic acid compounds. The intestinal secretions contain conjugases capable of reducing polyglutamate to simpler compounds; this enables absorption to take place in the upper and lower portions of the intestine. After absorption the body converts folic acid to the coenzyme form, tetrahydrofolic acid. This latter compound is abundant in the body but it is concentrated mostly in the liver. The normal serum folic acid level is 1.5 µg per ml. Normal adults excrete 2–6 µg per day in urine and 130–550 µg per day in feces.

Functions

Folic acid coenzymes function in reactions involving the transfer of single carbon units, such as methyl ($-CH_3$), hydroxymethyl ($-CH_2OH$), formyl ($-CHO$), and formimino ($-CH=NH$) groups, from one compound to another. Thus their role is analogous to that of pantothenic acid which functions in the transfer of two-carbon units.

The most important metabolic reactions carried out by folic acid coenzymes include the interconversion of glycine and serine, and the methylation of homocysteine to methionine and ethanolamine to cholesterol. It is involved in the synthesis of nucleic acids, the hydroxylation of phenylalanine to tyrosine, and the formation of the porphyrin ring which is a necessary part of hemoglobin synthesis.

Deficiency of folate

This subject has been discussed in Chapter 1.

Megaloblastic anemia in man is characterized by large red blood cells; there is also a reduction in blood platelets and polynuclear leucocytes, glossitis and gastrointestinal disturbances.

Therapeutic uses

Folic acid therapy is used in treating several clinical syndromes including the megaloblastic anemia caused by folic acid deficiency, and the anemia, glossitis, and gastrointestinal disturbances of tropical sprue. Folic acid relieves the anemia and glossitis of pernicious anemia but does not cure the neurologic degeneration associated with it.

Sources

Folic acid is widely distributed in nature, being present in many animal and plant tissues such as liver, kidney, yeast, and green leafy vegetables. Intestinal micro-organisms also produce folate which is available to the host.

Requirement

The daily requirement of folate for infants is 0.05–0.1 mg, for children 0.1–0.3 mg, for adults 0.4 mg, for pregnant women 0.8 mg, and for lactating mothers 0.5 mg per day.

Vitamin B_{12}

Chemistry

Vitamin B_{12} (cyanocobalamin) has a complex structure and an empirical formula of $C_{63}H_{88}N_{14}O_{14}PCo$. It is the only vitamin which has not been synthesized. It has a trivalent cobalt atom firmly bound in the center of a porphyrin-like structure, and is directly linked to a cyanide group. Vitamin B_{12} may exist in several different forms which have been given the generic name cobalamine. The cyanide group may be replaced by other anions, such as hydroxyl (hydroxycobalamin), nitrite (nitritocobalamin), chlorine (chlorocobalamin), or sulfate (sulfatocobalamin), all of which possess comparable activities. The coenzyme of vitamin B_{12}, the functional form in certain reactions, contains adenosine in place of the cyanide group. In animal tissues vitamin B_{12} is conjugated with protein. The needle-like crystals of vitamin B_{12} are deep red in color and they are sensitive to alkalis and are liable to be destroyed in cooking.

Absorption

Vitamin B_{12} (or extrinsic factor) requires the presence of a heat-labile mucoprotein, known as *intrinsic factor*, before it can be absorbed. The intrinsic factor is normally secreted in the gastric juice. In the ileum it removes vitamin B_{12} from complexes with animal proteins, attaches it to the intestinal mucosa, and releases it into the mucosal cells.

Metabolism

After absorption, vitamin B_{12} is bound by plasma proteins and circulates to where it is needed. Any unbound vitamin B_{12} in the circulation is rapidly excreted by the kidney and the excess over immediate body need is stored in the liver in combination with protein and is known as cobalamin coenzyme. Liver contains about 2000 μg of vitamin B_{12} and the total body content may vary from 7.5–12 mg. The normal blood level also varies between 0.1 and 1 mg per 100 ml.

Functions

Vitamin B_{12} is essential for maintenance of growth, neural function, and blood formation. In cells it is found in the mitochondria where it participates in the synthesis of labile methyl groups from glycine, serine, or formate. Unlike formic acid, it is not involved in the transfer of methyl groups but in their synthesis. The methyl groups are vital to the formation of many body compounds.

Vitamin B_{12} is involved in the biosynthesis of nucleic acids and the incorporation of amino acids into proteins. It also functions in the reduction of disulfides to sulfhydryl radicals. Since many important enzymes contain a sulfhydryl group, this action may explain its metabolic role in the metabolism of carbohydrates, fats, and proteins. Vitamin B_{12} reduces hydroxymethyl or methylene to methyl groups. It can therefore activate folic acid coenzymes and control reactions requiring folic acid.

Deficiency

Vitamin B_{12} deficiency causes pernicious anemia. This condition is not a primary dietary deficiency (except perhaps in *vegans*), but rather a secondary deficiency which may have several causes. These are associated with a failure to absorb the vitamin B_{12} present in adequate quantities in the gastrointestinal tract. The defects include the absence of the intrinsic factor in the gastric secretion and consequently a failure of intestinal absorption of vitamin B_{12}. The body may be infested with the fish tapeworm which competes with the host for dietary vitamin B_{12}.

Pernicious anemia is characterized by abnormalities in the alimentary tract, bone marrow, and the nervous system. Since hematopoiesis is inefficient, anemia results and may be accompanied by degenerative lesions of the spinal cord that cause peripheral sensory disturbances.

The disease can be treated with vitamin B_{12} administered intramuscularly or by a larger oral dose administered with a concentrate of intrinsic factor. Nutritional megaloblastic anemia responds to oral administration of vitamin B_{12}.

Sources

Vitamin B_{12} is found almost exclusively in foods of animal origin. Liver, kidney, meat, seafoods, and milk are the richest sources. Much of the vitamin B_{12} in food occurs in conjugation with protein and it must be released from the bound complex by proteolytic enzymes before it becomes active.

More than 70 per cent of vitamin B_{12} is retained after cooking. Large quantities are synthesized in the colon by bacteria but, as it is not absorbed from this segment of the alimentary tract, the contribution is negligible.

Requirement

The daily requirement of vitamin B_{12} for infants is 1–2 mg, for children 2–5 mg, for adults 5 mg, and for pregnant women 6 mg per day. The consumption of a small quantity of animal protein would supply this requirement.

Choline

Chemistry

Choline has three methyl groups attached to a nitrogenous base: $(CH_3)_3$—N—CH_2—CH_2OH. It is a colorless crystalline substance

|
OH

which readily decomposes, particularly when heated.

Biosynthesis

Choline can be synthesized in the body from glycine or by decarboxylating serine and because of this facility, it cannot be classified, in the strictest sense as a vitamin. It does not function moreover as a biological catalyst but as a structural component of phospholipids.

Functions

Choline has several important functions in the body.

It is a constituent of lecithin, a compound which aids in the transport of fats and contributes to cell structure, and of sphingomyelin found in nerve tissues.

It reacts with acetyl coenzyme to form acetylcholine which is responsible for transmission of nerve impulses.

It serves as source of labile methyl groups important in metabolic processes such as the formation of creatinine and the synthesis of epinephrine.

Deficiency of choline

In experimental choline deficiency, there is a deficiency of labile methyl groups, and development of a fatty liver. The deficiency state is less severe if folic acid and vitamin B_{12} are included in the diet and it can be largely alleviated by supplementing the diet with a source of labile methyl groups such as methionine or betaine.

In man, no specific disease has been associated with choline deficiency and further studies are required to establish the role of choline in the pathogenesis and the therapy of fatty liver.

Sources

Choline occurs in all plant and animal cells, either as free choline or as phospholipids; the richest sources are egg yolk, meat, fish, whole cereals, and legumes.

Requirement

Since choline can be synthesized in the body and because deficiency has not been observed in man, its requirement has not been established.

Myoinositol

Chemistry

Inositol is a cyclic compound whose empirical formula is similar to that of glucose ($C_6H_{12}O_6$). There are at least 9 isomers of inositol but only one of them has biological activity. It is designated myo-, meso-, or i-inositol. Because of its alcoholic nature (6 hydroxyl groups), it forms esters with phosphoric acid. The most important of these esters is phytic acid, the hexaphosphoric acid ester of inositol. Phytic acid forms a complex with

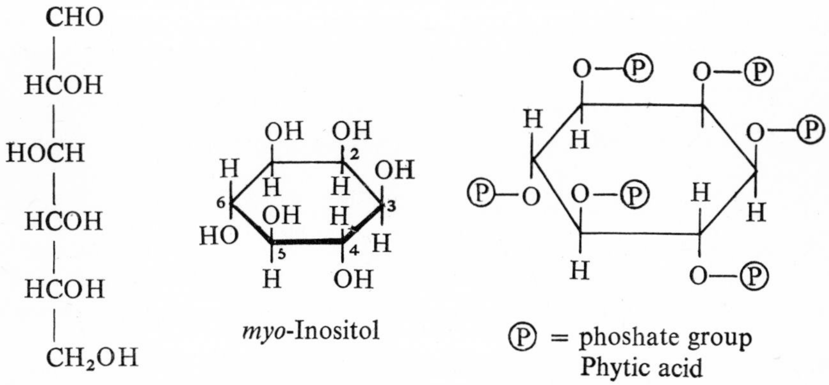

myo-Inositol

Ⓟ = phoshate group
Phytic acid

D-Glucose

Figure 78 The relationship of D-glucose, myoinsital and phytic acid calcium, magnesium, and other metals in the intestinal tract and renders them unavailable for absorption. The relationship of D-glucose, myoinositol and phytic acid can be seen in Figure 78.

Metabolism

Free inositol and phospholipids are readily absorbed from the intestine. Although the daily dietary intake is about 1 g per day, only a few mg appear in the urine. The blood level is 0.37–0.67 mg per 100 ml. In diabetes, the urinary excretion of inositol increases, perhaps as a result of competition with glucose for reabsorption by the kidney tubules. About 70 per cent of ingested inositol is converted to glucose in the body.

Functions

Inositol is a growth factor for certain strains of yeasts and molds and it is a constituent of certain cephalins. As it can be synthesized in the body and is present in large concentrations in tissues, it may have some function in man, but its metabolic role is not known yet.

Deficiency

Deficiency of inositol in man is unknown.

Sources

Inositol occurs in plants and animals in quantities greater than substances classified as vitamins. Fruits, vegetables, whole grains, and organ meats are particularly good sources. In cereals it occurs as phytates. In some animals, including man, bacterial synthesis in the intestine provides an adequate supply of inositol to the host.

Requirement

No specific disease has been associated with lack of inositol and its requirement is not known, but has been estimated to be 1 g per day per 2500 Calories.

The functions of vitamins and the characteristics of vitamin deficiency are summarized in Table 27.

The role of minerals in the diet

The nutrients discussed so far (carbohydrates, fats, proteins, and vitamins) are organic compounds composed of the elements carbon, oxygen, hydrogen, and nitrogen. Minerals are inorganic elements that comprise less than 5 per cent of body weight. After complete oxidization of organic

Table 27 Summary of functions of vitamins and manifestations of vitamin Deficiencies

Vitamin	Function	Characteristics of the Deficiency State
Fat Soluble		
A	vision, membrane structure, health of epithelia, bone formation, reproduction, growth, synthesis of mucopolysaccharides, glycogen and RNA	night blindness xerophthalmia keratomalacia bone malformation growth retardation
D	calcium absorption, mobilization of calcium from bone, phosphorus retention, citric acid oxidation	rickets
E	antioxidant, cellular respiration, heme synthesis	anemia
K	blood coagulation, oxidative phosphorylation	hemorrhage
Water Soluble		
ascorbic acid	formation of collagen and dentin, oxidation of phenylalanine and tyrosine, utilization of folic acid and iron, synthesis of progesterone, neutrotransmitters and catecholamines, cellular respiration	scurvy
thiamine	carbohydrate metabolism	beri-beri
riboflavin	biological oxidation-reduction reactions	cheilosis, glossitis, angular stomatitis, eye changes
niacin	biological oxidation-reduction reactions	pellagra
pyridoxine	amino acid metabolism	anemia, convulsions, dermatitis
biotin	fixation and removal of carbon dioxide	dermatitis, muscle pain, anemia, somnolence
pantothenic acid	transfer of acyl groups and maintaining rate of phosphorylation	cramps, depression, insomnia, burning sensation in feet
folic acid	transfer of single-carbon compounds	megaloblastic anemia
B_{12}	synthesis of single-carbon compounds	pernicious anemia
choline	constituent of lecithins, sphingomyelin and acetylcholine, methyl donor	fatty liver in animals
inositol	constituent of certain cephalins	weight and hair loss and fatty liver in animals

compounds, minerals may be left as a residue and they are referred to as ash. In food and in the body, most minerals are found as components of organic compounds; for example, iron is included in the hemoglobin molecule, cobalt in vitamin B_{12}, and phosphorus in phospholipids.

According to their levels in the body, minerals are divided into two groups:

Macroelements

These are present in relatively large quantities in the body and they include calcium, phosphorus, magnesium, sodium, potassium, chlorine, and sulphur.

Microelements or trace elements

These are present in very small quantities in the body and they include iron, copper, manganese, cobalt, zinc, iodine, fluorine, molybdenum, selenium, and chromium.

There are other elements which participate in biological reactions but they have not been proved essential to life as yet; these include vanadium, barium, bromine, strontium, cadmium, and nickel. According to their function, minerals can be classified in one of the following groups:

Structural   Skeletal rigidity depends on the insoluble compounds of calcium and phosphorus which are deposited in the matrix of bone and teeth as hydroxyapatite crystals. Some magnesium and fluorine also occur in the skeleton where they are found mainly in the outer layers.

Homeostatic   The chief electrolytes in the body fluids and tissues are sodium and potassium salts of chloride, sulphate, phosphate, and carbonate. While potassium and phosphorus are found mainly within the cells, sodium and chlorine are found mainly in the extra-cellular fluid. These electrolytes regulate the acid-base balance of the body and help to maintain a proper osmotic pressure.

Catalytic   All trace elements and some of the macromolecules are either parts of hormones (for example, sulfur and zinc are part of the insulin molecule, iodine is found in thyroxine), vitamins (sulfur in thiamine and biotin, cobalt in vitamin B_{12}), metalloenzymes, or metal-enzyme complexes (see Table 28).

Metalloenzymes   These contain a fixed amount of a metal which is firmly bound to, and is not easily removed from, the protein moiety. If the metal should be removed from the protein, the enzyme loses its biological activity and it is not restored when the metal is replaced. These metals have either a catalytic or a structural role, or fulfill both functions.

Table 28 The catalytic function of metals in enzyme systems

Enzyme	Reaction	Metal
pancreatic lipase	triglycerides $+ H_2O \rightarrow$ glycerol $+$ fatty acids	calcium
phosphatase	$ATP + H_2O \rightarrow ADP + H_3PO_4$	magnesium
amylase	starch $+ H_2O \rightarrow$ maltose	chlorine
catalase	$2H_2O_2 \rightarrow 2H_2O + O_2$	iron
tyrosinase	tyrosine $\rightarrow$ melanin	copper
ascorbic acid oxidase	ascorbic acid $\rightarrow$ dehydroascorbic acid	copper
arginase	arginine $+ H_2O \rightarrow$ urea $+$ ornithine	manganese
mevalonic kinase	mevalonic acid $\rightarrow$ cholesterol	manganese, vanadium
carbonic anhydrase	$H_2CO_3 \rightarrow CO_2 + H_2O$	zinc
xanthine oxidase	xanthine $+ O_2 \rightarrow$ uric acid $+ H_2O_2$	molybdenum

Metal-enzyme complexes In these, the metal is loosely bound to protein and can be removed easily from it. The enzyme is also reactivated if the same, or even a different metal, is added to the protein. Carbonic anhydrase which binds zinc firmly and specifically is an example of a metalloenzyme, while dipeptidases and arginase which bind zinc loosely and unspecifically are examples of metal-enzyme complexes.

Calcium

Body distribution

Calcium is the largest cation in the body and it comprises 1.5–2 per cent of total body weight. In the adult body there is 1.0–1.2 kg of calcium; 99 per cent of the mineral is concentrated in the hard structure of bones and teeth as hydroxyapatite crystals, $Ca_{10}(PO_4)_6(CH)_2$. The remaining one per cent is in the soft tissues and the extracellular fluid. Blood serum contains 9–12 mg of calcium per 100 ml of blood; 60 per cent of the calcium is ionic, diffusible, and present principally as salts of phosphate and carbonate. The other 40 per cent is nondiffusible and is bound to serum proteins. Equilibrium exists between the ionic and protein-bound forms, and redistribution between the two forms is a continuous process.

Absorption

The major site of calcium absorption is the proximal part of the small intestine. Although the ileum has the lowest rate of absorption, the movement of the ingested food through this segment is so slow that the ileum is, in effect, the most important segment of the gut in calcium absorption. The mineral crosses into the intestinal mucosa by an active transport mechanism; normally about 20–30 per cent of dietary calcium is taken into the body but there is a great variation in the efficiency of absorption which seems to depend on body needs, the type of food, and the amount of calcium ingested.

Absorption of calcium is favored by an acid medium because it keeps calcium in solution; for this reason, vitamin C and lactose facilitate absorption. Vitamin D or its metabolite, 25-hydroxycholecalciferol, increases calcium absorption by inducing synthesis of a calcium-binding protein that facilitates transport of calcium across the mucosal membrane. Other factors which aid absorption of calcium are protein, some amino acids (L-lysine and L-arginine), parathyroid hormone, estrogen, growth hormone, antibiotics, and bile. Fats, whose constituent fatty acids are mostly long and saturated (such as mutton fat), decrease the absorption of calcium by forming insoluble calcium soaps. Phosphates and oxalates found in certain vegetables such as rhubarb and spinach, and phytates found in the bran of cereal grains, decrease absorption by binding the calcium in an insoluble complex.

Metabolism

After absorption through the intestinal wall, calcium is transported in the blood stream and released to the extra-cellular fluid, which bathes the cells. Some calcium is taken up by the soft tissues but mostly it is deposited in the bone where it is stored and called upon in times of need; the most labile supply being the bone *trabeculae*. The deposition of calcium in bone depends on vitamin D.

The calcium concentration in the extra-cellular fluid is maintained relatively constant under the influence of parathyroid hormone, calcitonin, and vitamin D. Parathyroid hormone and vitamin D facilitate calcium absorption from the intestine and reabsorption from the kidney tubules; they also stimulate release of calcium from bone. Calcitonin, secreted by the thyroid gland, lowers the serum calcium level. The kidneys seem to play a major role in maintaining calcium homeostasis.

Excretion

Calcium is excreted mainly via feces which contain both unabsorbed and endogenous calcium. About 150 mg of endogenous fecal calcium is secreted in the bile and pancreatic juice. About 20 mg is lost as a result of desquamation and perspiration; only a very small quantity is excreted via the kidneys. Approximately 23 g of calcium is passed from the mother to fetus during gestation. During lactation the mother loses calcium in her milk.

Functions

In addition to its function in the formation of bones and teeth, calcium serves several other vital functions.

It helps to maintain the normal rhythm of the heart beat and it stimulates contraction of muscle fibers, thereby balancing the action of potassium which relaxes muscles. It controls neuromuscular irritability by the formation of acetylcholine for transmission of nerve impulses.

Calcium is bound to the lecithin of cell membrane. This allows the regulation of the transport of ions across the cell membrane by controlling the permeability of the membrane to nutrients.

Calcium activates several enzymes including pancreatic lipase, succinic dehydrogenase of the Kreb's Cycle, and some of the proteolytic enzymes.

It serves an important role in the blood clotting mechanism by stimulating the release of thromboplastin which catalyzes the conversion of prothrombin to thrombin. Thrombin then polymerizes fibrinogen to fibrin, the basis of blood clot.

$$\text{prothrombin} \xrightarrow[\text{thromboplastin}]{\text{calcium}} \text{thrombin} \quad \begin{array}{c} \text{fibrinogen} \\ \downarrow \\ \text{fibrin} \end{array}$$

Calcium deficiency

This may be caused primarily by an inadequate intake or it may be secondary to other conditions; for example, in the malabsorption syndrome, unabsorbed fat and calcium form insoluble soaps. Calcium deficiency may also be associated with vitamin D inadequacy since this vitamin facilitates the absorption of calcium. Calcium deficiency can also be caused by excessive demands in the presence of a low intake, for example, in pregnancy and lactation or when the secretion of parathyroid hormone is diminished. The clinical manifestations of calcium deficiency are rickets, osteomalacia, and osteoporosis described in Chapter 1. Infantile or neonatal tetany has also been recognized as a danger in formula fed babies (see pages 72 and 116).

Sources

The best sources of calcium are milk, hard cheeses, green leafy vegetables, and eleusine millet.

Requirements

These are discussed in Chapter 4.

Phosphorus

The adult body contains approximately 650 grams of phosphorus; this represents about one per cent of the total body weight. Eight per cent of the phosphorus is in hydroxyapatite crystals in the skeleton; the remainder is in the soft tissues and body fluids. Whole blood contains 35–45 mg of phosphorus per 100 ml; of this, approximately one-half is contained in the red cells; serum contains 3–4 mg per 100 ml. Four to nine mg of the whole blood phosphorus is inorganic phosphorus; this is most readily affected by dietary intake and is in constant exchange with the organic phosphate of the blood. An inverse relationship exists between calcium and phosphorus; an increase in the concentration of one is accompanied by a compensatory decrease in the other, and vice versa.

Absorption

Phosphate compounds are hydrolyzed to free phosphate ions prior to absorption; approximately 70 per cent of the phosphate in the diet is absorbed. Although the duodenum absorbs phosphate more rapidly than the rest of the alimentary tract, the ingested food passes through the duodenum very rapidly so the ileum is of more importance in phosphate absorption, a process achieved by an active transport mechanism. An excessive intake of calcium, magnesium, aluminum, or iron, hinders the absorption by forming insoluble phosphates which are then excreted. The absorption of phosphate unlike calcium, is independent of dietary fat.

Functions

Phosphorus, in association with calcium, is necessary for the formation of teeth and bones. It is part of the high-energy compounds such as ATP which are involved in the catabolism and anabolism of carbohydrates, fats, and protein. It is also a part of creatine phosphate which is necessary for muscle metabolism. Phosphorus is essential therefore for the energy metabolism of all cellular activities. Phosphorus is an important constituent of nucleoproteins and nucleic acids (DNA and RNA), which are responsible for cell division, reproduction, transmission of hereditary characteristics, and protein synthesis. It is a component of several enzyme or coenzyme systems such as thiamine pyrophosphate. Phosphorus facilitates the absorption and transport of nutrients through the cell membrane and their uptake by cells by combining with substances such as glucose to form glucose-6-phosphate and fatty acids to form phospholipids. Inorganic phosphates in the blood act as buffers for the regulation of the acid-base balance thereby helping to maintain neutrality in the tissue fluids.

Deficiency of phosphorus

Because of its metabolic significance in both animal and plant tissues, phosphorus is widely distributed in foodstuffs and a dietary deficiency of phosphorus does not occur in humans.

Requirement

Children and adults require 0.8 grams per day but adolescents and pregnant or lactating women require 1.3 grams per day. These requirements can easily be met from a normal diet.

Sources

Egg, meat, fish, poultry, cheese, milk, nuts, legumes, and whole grains are all rich phosphorus sources.

Magnesium

Body distribution

The adult body contains 25 grams of magnesium, 70 per cent of this is incorporated in bone where it is mostly found on bone surfaces in the form of phosphates and carbonates. In the soft tissues it is concentrated intra-cellularly and little is found outside the cells. Blood contains 1–3 mg per 100 ml. About 35 per cent of serum magnesium is bound to proteins while the rest is in the form of ions.

Absorption

Magnesium absorption can occur throughout the small intestine. Like calcium and phosphorus, magnesium is absorbed across the intestinal membrane by an active transport mechanism. A number of factors such as high intakes of calcium, phosphate, phytate, and poorly digestible fats interfere with magnesium absorption, while protein, lactose, vitamin D, growth hormone, and antibiotics facilitate its absorption.

The proportion of magnesium which is absorbed, and magnesium levels in the serum show a progressive decline when the calcium or phosphate intake is increased. Both minerals have this effect alone or in combination; singly, a high phosphate intake has a greater inhibitory effect on magnesium absorption. Increasing the calcium to phosphorus ratio increases the proportion of magnesium absorbed. Both magnesium and calcium form an insoluble salt with phosphate which is then unavailable to the body. A high calcium intake may depress magnesium absorption by competing with it for the site of absorption, or perhaps by competing for the carrier of the active transport system which takes it across the intestinal wall. The increase in magnesium absorption occuring when the calcium to phosphorus ratio is raised may be due to the fact that excess calcium will combine with phosphate, thus liberating magnesium which would have otherwise formed an insoluble compound with phosphate.

The absorption and fecal excretion of magnesium are correlated with those of fats suggesting a quantitative relationship between the two. When absorption of one is impaired, the absorption of the other is impaired at the same time. When a diet contains long chain saturated fatty acids which are poorly absorbed, magnesium absorption may be impaired and the serum and bone levels of magnesium may be lowered in consequence.

Functions

Magnesium activates many enzymes including those splitting and transfering phosphate groups (phosphatases) and others which are concerned with oxidative phosphorylation and the production of ATP. Magnesium relaxes nerve impulses and muscle contraction. In this respect it is antagonistic to calcium which is stimulatory.

Deficiency of magnesium

Magnesium deficiency has been observed in alcoholics, in severe renal disease, and in kwashiorkor. It is characterized by neuromuscular hyperirritability, hypo-magnesemic tetany, vasodilation, calcification of soft tissues, and atheromata.

Requirement

The magnesium requirement of infants is 40–70 mg per day, for children 100–250 mg, for adults 300–400 mg, and for pregnant and lactating women it is 450 mg per day. The requirement is met from a normal diet.

Sources

Nuts, whole grains, legumes, and dark green vegetables are rich sources of magnesium.

Sodium

Body distribution

About 0.2 per cent of the body consists of sodium of which half is in the extra-cellular fluid, 40 per cent in the skeleton, and only about 10 per cent is within the cells. Sodium diffuses into cells by passive diffusion but the body works continuously pumping intra-cellular sodium out across the cell membrane into the extra-cellular fluid. This pumping is achieved by an active transport mechanism. In the blood most of the sodium is in the plasma which contains 320 mg per 100 ml.

Metabolism

About 95 per cent of ingested sodium is absorbed; this is achieved by an active transport mechanism. Sodium is mostly excreted in urine as chloride and phosphate. In hot weather, losses through the skin are important as a means of sodium excretion because each litre of sweat contains 0.5–3.0 g of sodium. Where sweating is excessive, the ingestion of sodium is essential if heat exhaustion is to be avoided.

Aldosterone, a hormone of the adrenal cortex controls the reabsorption of sodium by the renal tubule. It also increases the conservation of sodium in the body by decreasing its excretion in sweat and by increasing its absorption from the intestine. A deficiency of this hormone, known as *Addison's disease*, leads to excessive losses of sodium in the urine.

Functions

About 90 per cent of the basic ions in plasma are sodium ions and hence it is the predominant basic element concerned in neutralizing excess acid and so regulating the pH of the body. It maintains osmotic pressure outside the cell membrane as well as the normal water balance within the cell. Together with potassium, sodium is involved in the transmission of nerve impulses and it is concerned with active transport of glucose and amino acids across cell membranes.

Deficiency of sodium

Sodium deficiency due to inadequate dietary intake is not seen but it may arise from excess losses caused by diarrhea, vomiting, intense sweating in hot weather, or adrenal cortical insufficiency. Loss of sodium leads to a reduction in the osmotic pressure of the extra-cellular fluid compartment. As a result, water moves into the cells causing a reduction in the extra-cellular fluid volume. In order to equalize the osmotic pressure on either side of the cell membrane, potassium diffuses out of the cell into the extra-cellular fluid. The symptoms of sodium deficiency are nausea, anorexia, apathy, muscular weakness, and cramps. In later stages of the disease there is respiratory failure and peripheral circulatory collapse.

Excess

The ingestion of too much sodium or an excess of aldosterone therapy leads to sodium retention. A high sodium concentration in the extra-cellular fluid will increase osmotic pressure and as a result water will move out of the cell, leading to an elevation in the volume of the body fluids. Estrogen promotes sodium retention, which is the reason why there is water retention by some women prior to menstruation and during pregnancy.

A prolonged high salt intake in humans is correlated with hypertension. In ra's, excessive sodium produces hypertension as well as degenerative vascular disease affecting the arterioles and glomeruli of the kidney. An increase in potassium appears to have a protective effect. In hypertensive patients, sodium levels in the tissues increase; this may be countered by restricting the sodium intake which also tends to lower the blood pressure. In cardiac failure and nephritis, sodium is retained in the body and thus water is held in the tissues.

Requirement

The sodium requirement is probably half a gram per day; the normal diet contains more than four times this amount.

Sources

Rich sources of sodium include table salt, sea foods, meat, egg, and milk.

Potassium

Body distribution

The total body potassium content is somewhat less than that of sodium but unlike that mineral it is concentrated inside the cells. The plasma level is only 16 mg per 100 ml.

Metabolism

About 90 per cent of ingested potassium is absorbed from the alimentary tract and it is almost completely excreted in urine; the renal mechanism for conservation of potassium is less efficient than it is for sodium.

Functions

Potassium maintains the proper osmotic pressure and acid-base relationship inside the cell.

It activates a number of intra-cellular enzymes involved in carbohydrate metabolism and oxidative phosphorylation.

Potassium regulates nervous and muscular irritability by diffusing out of muscle cells and nerve fibers into the extra-cellular fluid during muscle contraction and nerve stimulation; it re-enters the cells during rest.

Potassium relaxes heart muscle, and it therefore has a function opposite to that of calcium which is stimulatory.

Potassium is associated with glycogen formation, tissue protein synthesis, and cellular hydration.

Deficiency of potassium

Because it is widespread in foods, potassium deficiency does not occur under normal circumstances but it is found in starvation, kwashiorkor, vomiting, diarrhea, and diabetic acidosis. It may follow extensive tissue damage as in severe burns; it may be a feature of renal tubular disease or hyperaldosteroneism. The symptoms of potassium deficiency are extreme muscular weakness, loss of gastrointestinal tone leading to abdominal distention, anorexia, myocardial degeneration, and pulmonary edema.

Excess of potassium

An excess of potassium in the body occurs in renal failure or severe acidosis. Treatment lies in potassium restriction, removal of potassium by gastrointestinal sodium-exchange resins, correction of the acidosis, and administration of glucose with insulin.

Requirement

The potassium requirement may be about one mg per day but the normal diet provides 15 times this amount.

Sources

Meat, fish, poultry, cereals, fruits, and vegetables are rich sources of potassium.

19   Robson I (0314)

Chlorine

Body distribution

Chlorine constitutes about 0.15 per cent of total body weight. It readily crosses cell membranes and it is found both within cells as potassium chloride and in the extra-cellular fluid as sodium chloride. About 88 per cent of body chlorine is extra-cellular and it is the chief anion of extra-cellular fluid. The highest concentration is found in cerebrospinal fluid; lower concentrations exist in the lymph and gastric secretions. The chloride level of plasma is 340–370 mg per 100 ml; the level in the blood cells is about half this amount. Chlorine is rapidly absorbed from the gastro-intestinal tract and it is excreted in association with sodium.

Functions

It activates salivary and intestinal amylase which breakdown starches into maltose and it is also a constituent of the hydrochloric acid of the stomach.

Approximately two-thirds of the acidic ions in blood are chloride and they play an important role in maintaining the acid-base balance of body fluids. Finally, potassium participates in the regulation of osmotic pressure.

Deficiency of chlorine

Chlorine deficiency does not occur in humans except as a consequence of prolonged vomiting.

Requirement

Chlorine requirement is probably about 0.5 g per day but the normal diet supplies more than 6 times this amount.

Sources

Table salt, meat, milk, egg, and seafoods are all rich sources of chlorine.

Sulfur

Body distribution

About 0.15–0.25 per cent of body weight is made up of sulfur. It is found in every cell but there are high concentrations in hair, skin, and nails where it is found in the molecules of the amino acids, methionine and cystine.

Inorganic sulfur is poorly absorbed and the body relies on methionine and cystine as a source of this element. Excess sulfur is eliminated in the urine as sulfates.

Functions

Sulfur forms part of the molecule of the amino acids, cystine, cysteine, methionine, and taurine. Methionine is an essential amino acid and plays a role in the transfer of methyl ($-CH_3$) groups. It is also part of the vitamins, thiamine, biotin, pantothenic acid, and lipoic acid. Sulfur is a constituent of the hormone insulin, the pigment melanin, bile, and glutathione which functions in the biological systems of oxidation. It is involved in the synthesis of sulfomucopolysaccharides such as chondroitin sulfate. The deficiency of this compound impedes the collagen-producing activity of fibroblasts. It is also involved in mucoitin sulfate synthesis which functions as a gut lubricant and heparin which inhibits blood coagulation. Sulfur compounds combine with toxic substances; after detoxification they are excreted.

Sources

Sulfur is found in about 1 per cent of proteins, the content depending on the sulfur-containing amino acids. Sulfur rich sources are therefore those foods which are rich in proteins such as meat, fish, egg, cheese, legumes, and nuts.

Iron

Body distribution

The adult body contains about 4 g of iron, two-thirds of this amount is in hemoglobin. The iron content of muscle hemoglobin (myohemoglobin) and oxidative enzymes amounts to only 150 mg. The remainder is stored in the liver, spleen, and bone marrow as ferritin and hemosiderin.

Absorption

Iron is absorbed almost entirely from the duodenum and jejunum. There is little absorption from the ileum and almost none from the stomach and colon. Absorption takes place in the ferrous state. The presence of reducing substances such as vitamin C converts the iron from the ferric (Fe^{+++}) to the ferrous (Fe^{++}) state and keeps more iron in solution at the alkaline pH of the duodenum. On the other hand, carbonates, phosphates, phytate, and oxalate form insoluble compounds which are not readily absorbed. Normally about 10 per cent of ingested iron is taken into the body, the actual amount depending on the level of the tissue iron stores and the rate of hemoglobin synthesis. The greater the rate of hemoglobin formation and the lower the level of tissue iron stores, the more iron is absorbed; anemic patients, for example, absorb more than 20 per cent of the ingested iron.

Hemoglobin-iron in the form of heme is absorbed from food more efficiently than inorganic iron and is independent of vitamin C or iron-binding chelating agents. Unlike inorganic iron, heme is more soluble in alkaline media, so that the duodenal pH is more advantageous for heme iron absorption than it is for inorganic iron.

Feces contain relatively large amounts of iron whereas the urine contains very little. It has been established that the passage of iron in the body is a one way affair and there is no satisfactory method of excreting iron either in the gut, or in the urine. Iron balance is therefore, maintained by controlling absorption.

Excess iron accumulates in the cells in the intestinal mucosa; as they grow older they become filled with iron but they eventually slough off into the gut. This mechanism not only eliminates iron but the presence of iron-loaded cells serves as a block to further iron absorption. This homeostatic mechanism is unique to iron.

Iron is transported through the mucosal cell, perhaps as an iron-amino acid complex, but the exact mechanism is not known.

Metabolism

(See Figure 79.)

In the blood, 2 atoms of ferric iron are bound to each molecule of a beta globulin protein called *transferrin*; the combination forms transferritin. Iron is transported in this form to the bone marrow where it may be incorporated into newly synthesized hemoglobin molecules. Alternatively it may go to the storage depots in the liver, spleen, and bone marrow, where it combines with a protein and is deposited as ferritin. When excessive amounts of ferritin accumulate in the tissues they form a colloid material which is granular and much larger than the ferritin molecule; in this form it is known as *hemosiderin*. Hemosiderin can not be excreted and its accumulation in the tissues eventually interferes with body functions and causes the disease known as *hemosiderosis*.

Free iron which has dissociated into ions is very toxic, so the iron molecule always travels within the body in combination with protein. When the levels of these ions exceeds the binding capacity of the transferrin iron toxemia occurs. Normally the amount of iron in plasma is sufficient to bind only one-third of the transferrin. The remaining two-thirds represents the unbound reserve.

The normal red cell has a life of about 120 days; at the end of its life the hemoglobin is broken down in the liver or spleen. From these organs it is transported to the bone marrow where it is synthesized once more into hemoglobin which will enter newly formed red blood cells. Twenty to twenty-five mg of iron are used for hemoglobin synthesis each day.

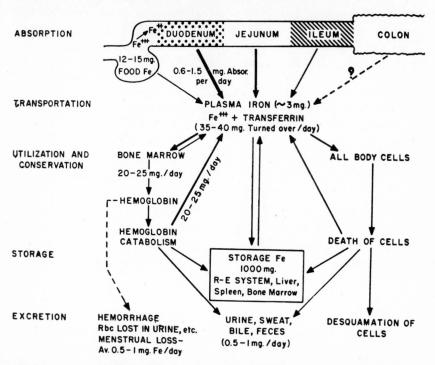

Figure 79 A diagrammatic summary of iron metabolism. (Originally published by the University of California Press; reprinted by permission of the Regents of the University of California)

Excretion

Approximately 0.3–0.5 mg of iron are lost daily in the feces. These losses consist of blood losses into the gastro-intestinal tract, unabsorbed iron, biliary iron, and desquamated intestinal mucosal cells. There is also a small amount lost in the urine (0.1 mg per day) and there are losses from the skin that are hard to estimate; they could, however, be substantial in hot climates. The total excretion is about one mg per day.

Females also experience a loss of approximately 0.5 mg of iron per day during menstruation. The cost of iron during pregnancy is 0.5 mg per day on an average and another 0.5 mg is lost in the milk during lactation.

Functions

Iron is a component of hemoglobin, myoglobin, cytochromes, catalase, and peroxidase. The iron is incorporated with porphyrin in the molecule of protoporphyrin or heme. When heme combines with amino acids and proteins it produces hemoglobin, myoglobin, and heme enzymes. Iron functions as part of these heme complexes by transporting oxygen in hemoglobin and in cellular respiration. Iron is also incorporated in myoglobin which acts as a store for oxygen in the cells.

Requirement

Iron requirements are discussed in detail in Chapter 4. Children, men, and postmenopausal women require one mg per day. Pregnant and lactating women 2 mg per day. Since only 10 per cent of ingested iron is absorbed, it is recommended that the diet should provide the former group with 10 mg and the latter with 20 mg of iron per day.

Sources

The best source of iron is liver but meat, egg yoke, dark green vegetables such as spinach; molasses, and legumes, also contain useful amounts of iron.

Iron deficiency

The effects of iron deficiency are discussed in Chapter 1 (see page 48).

Iron overload

Iron cannot be excreted readily from the body, so once excess iron is absorbed or introduced by any other means, the body is faced with a disposal problem. Iron overload may occur as a result of metabolic defects or high intakes of iron. Idiopathic hemochromatosis is an inherited disease which permits the absorption of large amounts of iron. The excess is then deposited in the organs which are eventually damaged. A variety of clinical symptoms and signs may occur, including hyperpigmentation of the skin, cirrhosis of the liver, diabetes, and myocardial failure.

Excess intake may be the result of naturally high intakes, or artificaly high or prolonged, intakes of iron.

Excessive intakes of iron from natural sources occur in the *Bantu* of South Africa who cook their food in iron pots and ferment beer in iron utensils. These processes add considerable amounts of iron to the diet and the intake may be as high as 100 mg per day. Hemosiderosis and *cirrhosis* of the liver tend to develop in these individuals. The ingestion of iron tonics over prolonged periods of time and repeated blood transfusions can also lead to excessive iron storage.

Copper

Body distribution

The total copper content of the body in adults is 100–150 mg; in the newborn it is considerably higher. It is mainly stored in the liver where copper levels reflect the dietary intake; however, it is also widely distributed in other tissues and organs. The blood plasma level is 50–190 μg per 100 ml.

Metabolism

After absorption in the intestine the copper reaches the blood stream where about 93 per cent of it becomes firmly bound to ceruloplasmin, a compound consisting of a globulin bound to 8 atoms of copper and whose function is obscure. Of the remainder, some is bound to albumin with which it is transported to the various tissues. The balance is bound to amino acids believed to be involved in the movement of copper through membranes.

Excretion

About 80 per cent of absorbed copper is excreted through the bile. About 16 per cent is emptied directly back into the intestine through the gut wall and the remainder is excreted in the urine. A high dietary intake of zinc, or an excessive ingestion of molybdenum in the presence of sulfates, increases copper excretion.

Functions

Copper facilitates iron absorption and the release of iron in storage in the liver, thereby aiding hemoglobin formation. Copper is concerned with energy metabolism because it is a constituent of cytochrome oxidase in the electron transport chain, from which ATP is derived. It is also a constituent part of the enzyme tyrosinase which is essential for conversion of tyrosine to melanin, a compound responsible for the pigmentation of the skin.

Since copper is involved in the formation of phosphatidic acid and phospholipids, it plays a role in the formation of myelin surrounding the nerve fibers. Copper is associated with an enzyme essential for the synthesis of elastin in the aorta. It is also a constituent of the enzyme ascorbic acid oxidase and is therefore involved in the metabolism of vitamin C.

Deficiency

Up to now copper deficiency in man has not been shown to be due to dietary deficiency alone. In animals it produces low ceruloplasmin levels, low plasma iron, high iron storage in liver and spleen, a hypochromic microcytic anemia, hair depigmentation or bleaching, demyelination of spinal cord, bone disorders, and reduced reproductive capacity. Some of these abnormalities are due to reduced activity of copper-containing enzyme systems.

Wilson's disease or hepatolenticular degeneration

This is a genetically determined inborn error of metabolism characterized by hepatic cirrhosis, brain damage, and demyelination, kidney defects, and the deposition of copper in the cornea as brown or green rings. The primary defect may be a deficiency of an enzyme system in the liver which removes the albumin-bound copper from the plasma and incorporates it in ceruloplasmin. The condition can be reversed by controlling dietary copper, and by the administration of chelating agents such as penicillamine which binds the free copper and excretes it in the urine.

Requirement

The copper requirement of adults is about 2 mg per day; infants require about 0.05 mg of copper per kg of body weight.

Sources

Shell fish, liver, meat, fish, nuts, legumes, cocoa, dried fruits, and whole grain cereals are all rich sources of copper.

Manganese

Body distribution

The human body contains about 12–20 mg manganese. It is found in all the tissues but it is concentrated in bones, liver, kidney, pancreas, and pituitary gland. Within the cells it is concentrated in the mitochondria.

The bones, and to a lesser extent the liver, serve as storage sites and are influenced by the dietary intake. Blood contains 12–18 µg per 100 ml, about two-thirds of which is in the cells.

Absorption and excretion

Manganese is poorly absorbed and retained. It is transported in the plasma by binding to a β_1-globulin, known as transmanganin. It is mainly excreted in the feces via bile and is reabsorbed as bile-bound manganese. High intakes of calcium and phosphorus increase manganese excretion, presumably by adsorption to the surface of insoluble calcium phosphate in the gut.

Functions

Manganese functions as a catalyst in a number of enzyme systems. It activates some of the enzymes (polymerase and galactotransferase) involved in the synthesis of chondroitin sulfates in connective tissues; it also activates bone alkaline phosphatase. It activates liver arginase and is therefore involved in urea formation.

Along with vitamin B_6, it forms a chelate with amino acids which facilitate the transport of amino acids.

$$\text{amino acid} \xrightarrow[\text{vitamin } B_6]{\text{manganese}} \text{amino acid-manganese-vitamin } B_6 \text{ complex}$$

Manganese and choline are both lipotropic agents; this means that they are effective in reducing liver fat.

Manganese increases the activity of mevalonic kinase, which is involved in cholesterol biosynthesis.

$$\text{acetyl coenzyme A} \longrightarrow \text{mevalonic acid} \xrightarrow{\text{mevalonic kinase}} \text{squalene} \longrightarrow \text{cholesterol}$$

Manganese is involved in oxidative phosphorylation in the mitochondria by activating the enzymes in the Kreb's Cycle.

Deficiency

Manganese deficiency in man has not been yet demonstrated but in animals there are nervous system manifestations, bone abnormalities, and reduced fertility.

Requirement

About 3–5 mg per day has been recommended.

Sources

Meat, fish, poultry, whole grain cereals, legumes, green leafy vegetables, and tea are rich sources of manganese.

Zinc

Body distribution

The total amount of zinc in the human body is 2.2 g. It is widely distributed in all organs and tissues but relatively high levels are found in skin, hair, nails, eye, and the prostate gland. The concentration of zinc in whole blood is about 900 μg per 100 ml, of which about 120 μg per 100 ml are in the serum. Approximately 3 per cent of all the blood zinc is found in leukocytes where it is associated with alkaline phosphatase. In erythrocytes, it is mostly associated with carbonic anhydrase. Serum zinc may be firmly bound to globulins in which state it has an unknown function. Alternatively it may be loosely bound to other proteins; in this form it is concerned with zinc transport.

Absorption and excretion

Zinc is poorly absorbed and it is primarily excreted through the intestinal mucosa, pancreatic secretions, and urine. High dietary calcium levels in the presence of phosphate or phytate favors chelation; this inhibits zinc absorption and promotes its excretion in the feces.

Functions

Zinc is a constituent of carbonic anhydrase; this enzyme catalyzes the following reaction.

$$H_2CO_3 \rightleftharpoons CO_2 + H_2O$$

Carbonic anhydrase is essential for the acid-base equilibrium of the body and the release of carbon dioxide in the lung. It is also vital for cell respiration and carbon dioxide transport. A number of dehydrogenases such as alcohol, glutamic, lactic, and malic dehydrogenase depend on zinc for their activities and structural integrity. Zinc is necessary for carboxypeptidase; this enzyme hydrolyzes peptide bonds and liberates amino acids from the carboxy terminal of proteins.

Zinc is associated with insulin in the pancreas and hence it is involved in carbohydrate metabolism. The enzyme alkaline phosphatase cannot function without zinc.

Zinc is firmly bound to RNA, stabilizing its secondary and tertiary structures. It is concerned therefore with the metabolism of nucleic acids and proteins. DNA synthesis has been observed to be impaired in zinc deficient rats.

Zinc salts accelerate wound healing after surgery.

Iodine

Body distribution

The total iodine content of the human body is about 25 mg; 10 mg of this is found in the thyroid gland. Normal blood levels lie in the range of 4–10 μg of iodine per 100 ml of blood; all of the iodine is in plasma.

Absorption

Iodine is absorbed as iodide. Most of the iodine which is present in food is in this form. Free iodine and iodate are converted to iodide to facilitate absorption. Organic iodine such as that in the hormone thyroxine is partly absorbed in that form, the remainder is broken down into iodide. Absorption takes place in the small intestine; about 30 per cent of the total amount absorbed is removed from the blood stream by the thyroid gland.

Excretion

Iodine is mainly excreted via the kidneys but there is some loss through the intestine, lungs, saliva, bile, and milk.

Biosynthesis of thyroid hormone

In the thyroid gland, iodide is oxidized to iodine by peroxidase; this is then combined with the amino acid tyrosine to form mono-iodotyrosine (MIT) and di-iodotyrosine (DIT). Two molecules of DIT conjugate and form thyroxine. Tri-iodothyronine may be formed from either the conjugation of DIT with MIT or from the de-iodination of thyroxine. Thyroxine and tri-iodothyronine are incorporated in a protein known as thyroglobulin which is then stored as iodothyroglubulins in the colloid matter of thyroid follicles.

Metabolism

Thyroxine and tri-iodothyronine are released into the circulation on demand. This is achieved by the action of proteolytic enzymes. In the plasma, thyroxine and tri-iodothyronine bind loosely to globulin, any excess binds

20*

to albumin. Iodine in the plasma is known as protein bound iodine (PBI) and measurements of iodine in the circulation are achieved by determining PBI levels in the plasma. In hyperthyroidism the PBI level is higher than 11 μg per 100 ml and in hypothyroidism its level is less than 3 μg per 100 ml. Thyroglobulin can not penetrate the tissues so the component thyroxine and tri-iodothyronine separate from the protein and enter the cells. Part of the thyroxine is converted into tri-iodothyronine which is about four times as potent as thyroxine. When the hormones are used up, the iodine is released to the blood; approximately half of the iodine is re-utilized and the remainder is excreted in the urine (40 per cent) and the feces (10 per cent). Iodine metabolism is summarized in Figure 80.

Functions

Iodine functions as a constituent of thyroxine, a hormone that regulates the rate of energy exchange, growth and development, and the metabolism of various other nutrients.

Deficiency of iodine

Iodine deficiency results in several clinical conditions which are discussed in Chapter 1.

Simple, or endemic goiter This is caused by iodine deficiency. It is usually the result of a lack of the element in water and soil. Certain cases of goiter may be due to the ingestion of drugs which interfere with the synthesis of thyroxine. For example, thiocyanate and perchlorate inhibit the uptake, concentration, and accumulation of iodine by the thyroid gland, while thiourea, thiouracil, and sulfonamides interfere with the oxidation of iodide to iodine. Certain seeds and vegetables, including those of the cabbage family, contain progoitrin and the enzyme which converts it to goitrin; this last substance prevents the synthesis of thyroxine. Fortunately progoitrin is heat labile and is inactivated by cooking. With the exception of vegetarians and foods faddists, the normal intake of goitrin is not high.

The thyroid gland responds to the lack of iodine by enlargement, a clinical condition known as a goiter. The enlargement subsides if the cause is removed. Clinical improvement is more rapid if thyroxine is also given, as plasma thyroxine levels are low in goitrous states. Endemic goiter is best controlled by iodating table salt.

Cretinism This occurs in infants whose mothers have been depleted during pregnancy.

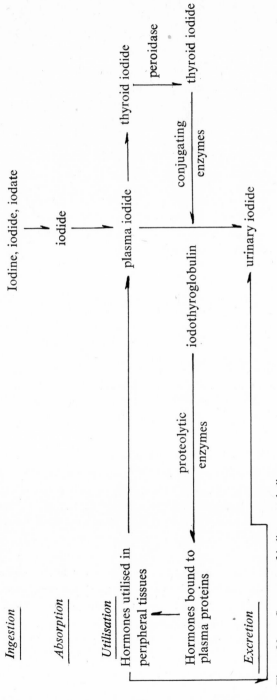

Figure 80   Summary of iodine metabolism

Myxoedema   This is a metabolic disorder caused by inadequate thyroid function (*hypothyroidism*), and occurs in adults. Patients with hypothyroidism have a lowered basal metabolic rate and exhibit skin and hair changes.

Hyperthyroidism   This is the result of overactivity of the thyroid gland. It is also known as *exopthalmic goiter* or *Graves Disease*. It is characterized by an increase in the basal metabolic rate; there may be a fine tremor of the hands, nervousness, protuberance of the eyeballs, heat intolerance, and loss of weight.

Requirement

The iodine requirement for children is 0.05–0.10 mg per day, and for adults 0.1–0.15 mg per day. During pregnancy it is 0.125 mg per day and during lactation 0.15 mg per day.

Sources

Iodized salt, seafoods, and seaweeds are all rich sources of iodine.

Fluorine

Body distribution

The fluorine content of the adult body is less than 1.4 mg and is found mainly in bones and teeth.

Absorption and excretion

Ninety per cent of ingested fluorine is absorbed from the intestine and probably also from the stomach. About 75 per cent of the ingested fluorine is excreted in the urine and some also appears in the sweat and feces.

Functions

There is an inverse relationship between the incidence of dental caries as indicated by teeth decayed, missing or filled (*DMF*) and the fluorine content of water. When children less than 5 years old consume drinking water containing 1 ppm fluorine, the teeth are protected against dental caries not only during childhood and adolescence but alo throughout adult life. This has led to fluoridation of water supplies in many countries which has had good effects on dental public health. There is as yet no scientific evidence to indicate that the intentional fluoridation of water has been harmful to anybody at any age, but the effects of fluoride intakes from several sources are the cause of concern (see page 26).

Fluorine is probably adsorbed to the enamel surfaces of hydroxy-apatite crystals producing fluoroapatite which is more resistant to the action of mouth acids. Fluorine may also inactivate oral bacterial enzymes which create acids from carbohydrates. The fact that fluorine stimulates new bone formation is utilized therapeutically in osteoporosis, but adequate calcification can only take place if vitamin D and calcium are administered at the same time.

Although fluoridation of water supplies is the most effective method of controlling dental caries; it is possible to add fluorine to a number of other food materials such as milk, cereals, and salt. It may be taken also in tablet form as sodium fluoride, or it may be applied topically to the gums.

Mottled enamel or dental fluorosis

When the fluoride content of drinking water of a community exceeds 2.5 ppm, the dental enamel is likely to become mottled, a sign of dental fluorosis. It is confined to the permanent teeth and develops only during their period of formation. The fully formed teeth are not affected and decidous teeth are only affected at very high intakes. The degree of mottling of the enamel may be mild, moderate, or severe, depending upon the level of fluorine intake and individual susceptibility. In areas where the fluoride content of water is high, mottling can be prevented by treating the water supply with phosphate.

Sources

In addition to drinking water, seafoods and tea are excellent sources of fluorine.

Cobalt

Metabolism

Cobalt is readily absorbed from the intestine. It is not stored in the body to any appreciable degree but it is concentrated in the liver and kidney. Approximately two-thirds of ingested cobalt is excreted in the urine while the rest appears in the feces. The cobalt content of whole blood is 80–300 $\mu\mu$g per 100 ml, of which 60–80 $\mu\mu$g is in plasma.

Function

Cobalt comprises 4.5 per cent of vitamin B_{12} (cyanocobalamin) which prevents pernicious anemia. Vitamin B_{12} cannot be synthesized in human tissues, and the micro-organisms in the colon cannot make sufficient vitamin B_{12} to meet human requirements, so a dietary source of vitamin B_{12} is required.

Cobalt cycle

Plants remove cobalt from the soil and ruminants ingest the plants. Subsequently, bacteria in the rumen incorporate plant cobalt into vitamin B_{12}. This vitamin is absorbed and taken up by the tissues from the blood stream. Man obtains cobalt by eating the flesh of ruminants. Upon the death of animals and man, vitamin B_{12} returns to the soil; after degradation the cobalt is released and the cycle repeats itself. This cycle is schematically shown in Figure 81.

Deficiency

Cobalt deficiency has not been found in humans.

Sources

Cobalt must be supplied as vitamin B_{12}. Humans obtain their requirement from animal tissues, especially liver, kidney, and seafoods. But the content of these foods depends on the quantity of cobalt in the soil and in the plants on which the animals feed.

Chromium

Metabolism

Only a small part of ingested chromium is absorbed and it is mainly excreted in the urine. It is found in the blood in two forms; trivalent chromium which is bound to transferrin, and hexavalent chromium which has a selective affinity for red blood cells.

Deficiency

Recent studies in Jordan and Nigeria have revealed impaired glucose tolerance in children who drink water with a low chromium content.[9] The ability of the body to deal with high glucose levels correlates with the

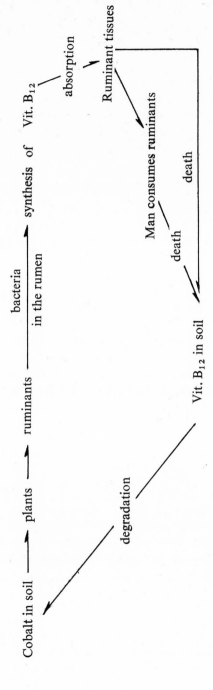

Figure 81   The Cobalt Cycle

chromium content of drinking water. Further evidence of the role of chromium in glucose metabolism is provided by reports that oral supplementation of the diet with chromium leads to improvements in glucose tolerance.

Function

Chromium is not a hypoglycemic agent but it increases the effectiveness of insulin by forming a bridge between the sulfydryl groups (SH) of insulin and the insulin receptor groups of cell membranes:

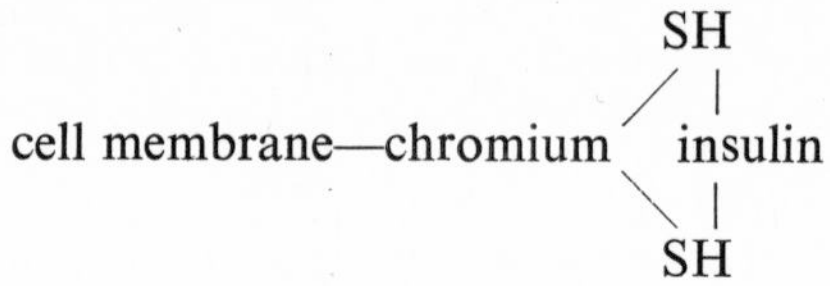

$$
\text{cell membrane—chromium}
\begin{array}{c}
\text{SH} \\
\diagup \quad | \\
\text{insulin} \\
\diagdown \quad | \\
\text{SH}
\end{array}
$$

Molybdenum

Metabolism

Molybdenum is readily absorbed from the intestine and rapidly excreted in the urine. A small quantity is also excreted in feces and bile. There is little retention of this element except in bones, liver, kidney, and skin. The metabolism of molybdenum is apparently related to that of copper and sulphur. An increase in dietary sulfate and copper is accompanied by an increase in the excretion of molybdenum in the urine and its depletion in blood and tissues.

Function

Molybdenum activates the enzyme xanthine oxidase which is necessary for the conversion of xanthine to uric acid. It also activates the enzyme aldehyde oxidase.

Deficiency

The requirement for molybdenum is very low and molybdenum deficiency has not been found yet in humans. However, deficient animals such as rats have poor growth and produce weak and malformed young.

Sources

Legumes, cereals, offal, and dark green leafy vegetables are good sources of this metal.

Selenium

Metabolism

Absorption of selenium depends on two factors; the solubility of the compounds ingested and the dietary ratio of selenium to sulfur. Ingested selenium is deposited in all tissues of the body except fat. It is found in the highest concentration in liver, kidney, heart, and spleen. It is mainly excreted in the urine but small quantities are also lost in the feces, sweat, and lungs. Ingested selenium is quickly taken up by serum albumin in which form it is transported; it is then gradually transferred to serum globulin. A large percentage of ingested selenium is incorporated into the tissues as selenocystine and selenomethionine.

Selenium competes with sulfur where it has a vital metabolic role such as in the amino acids, cystine and methionine, or enzymes containing sulfhydryl groups or other sulfur-linkages.

Function

Selenium can replace vitamin E completely or partially in treating some vitamin E deficiency diseases. It may therefore function by maintaining the stability of biological membranes of structures such as the mitochondria, microsomes, and lysosomes within the cells. It is believed that selenium may be a biological carrier for vitamin E, enhancing its activity by increasing its retention and transport across membrane.

Deficiency

Selenium deficiency is not known in man, but some children with kwashiorkor with low serum selenium levels failed to gain weight until they were given selenium.

Sources

The selenium content of foodstuffs depends on the selenium content of the soil in which the plants are grown. Cereals are better sources than vegetables.

Vanadium

Vanadium inhibits the biosynthesis of cholesterol by lowering the activity of the enzyme mevalonic kinase. Vanadium is therefore antagonistic to manganese which increases the activity of this enzyme. In animals, inhi-

bition of cholesterol biosynthesis is accompanied by low plasma phospholipids and cholesterol concentration, and retardation of the development
of atheromata. In one study the average serum cholesterol levels of workmen
exposed to industrial sources of vanadium were lower than those in controls.
The toxicity of absorbed vanadium is high and much more needs to be
learned of its action and function before it can be used for therapeutic
purposes.

Toxicity of trace elements

Although small quantities of trace elements are essential for normal body
function, they become toxic when they are ingested in large quantities.
For example, an excessive intake of fluorine causes mottled enamel and
bone changes, iron absorbed in large quantities leads to hemosiderosis,
high levels of intake of copper and manganese cause hemolytic anemia
and encephalitis, respectively.

Zinc, in excess causes a loss of iron and copper from the liver, and a high
intake of molybdenum results in bone abnormalities. It should be remembered that although these nutrients are useful to the body, they are safe
only within a limited range of intake.

Interrelationship of minerals

One of the factors which complicates studies of the function and needs
of minerals, is their interrelationship with each other during absorption,
utilization, and excretion. Only a few examples of interaction of minerals
can be mentioned here. The relative amounts of calcium and phosphorus in
the diet (calcium to phosphorus ratio) influence absorption of both minerals
from the intestines. High intakes of calcium and phosphorus interfere with absorption of a number of elements such as magnesium, manganese, and iron.
Selenium is antagonistic to sulfur metabolism replacing that element in
many important enzymes. High intakes of zinc cause anemia by depleting
the liver of iron and copper. Excess manganese interferes with hemoglobin
synthesis. The metabolism of molybdenum, copper, and sulfur are all
related. Because of these interrelationships, supplementing the diet with
minerals must be viewed with caution.

The functions of minerals and manifestations of deficiency are summarized
in Table 29.

Table 29 Summary of functions of minerals and manifestations of mineral deficiencies

Mineral	Function	Characteristics of the deficiency state
calcium	formation of bones and teeth regulation of muscle contraction, nerve irritability and the rhythm of the heartbeat activation of some enzymes blood clotting	rickets osteomalacia osteoporosis tetany
phosphorus	formation of bones and teeth constituent of high-energy compounds, nucleoproteins, phospholipids, enzyme systems and buffer salts	emaciation fragile bones rickets
magnesium	activation of phosphatases and oxidative phosphorylation enzymes relaxation of nerve impulses and muscle contraction a constituent of chlorophyll	vasodilation soft tissue calcification atherosclerosis tetany
sodium	regulation of pH, osmotic pressure and water balance transmission of nerve impulses active transport of glucose and amino acids	nausea anorexia muscular weakness and cramps
potassium	regulation of osmotic pressure and acid-base balance activation of a number of intracellular enzymes regulation of nerve and muscle irritability	weakness, anorexia, abdominal distention tachycardia pulmonary edema adrenal hypertrophy
chlorine	activation of amylase a constituent of hydrochloric acid regulation of osmotic pressure and acid-base balance	poor growth in rats
sulfur	part of some amino acids, some vitamins, some hormones, bile, melanin synthesis of sulfomucopolysaccharides detoxifying agents	not found
iron	part of hemoglobin, myoglobin and heme enzymes	anemia
copper	hemopoiesis, metabolism of vitamin C and energy, formation of melanin, phospholipids and elastin	anemia depigmentation of hair (in animals) demyelination of nerve bone disorders

Table continues

Table 29 (*cont.*)

Mineral	Function	Characteristics of the deficiency state
manganese	synthesis of chondroitin sulfates, bone formation, urea formation, amino acid transport, lipotropic agent, cholesterol synthesis, oxidative phosphorylation	ataxia infertility (in animals)
zinc	activation of carbonic anhydrase and several dehydrogenases alkaline phosphatase, carboxypeptidase wound healing, metabolism of nucleic acids associated with insulin	hepatosplenomegaly dwarfism hypogonadism
iodine	constituent of thyroxine which regulates metabolism	goiter cretinism
fluorine	imparts greater resistance to tooth decay stimulates new bone formation	dental caries
cobalt	constituent of vitamin B_{12}	anemia wasting disease (in ruminants)
chromium	increases effectiveness of insulin	impaired glucose tolerance curve
molyb-denum	activation of xanthine oxidase	poor growth malformed young (in rats)
selenium	maintaining stability of membranes increasing retention of vitamin E	growth retardation

References

1. Keys, A. "The Diet and the Development of Coronary Heart Disease." *J. Chron. Dis.* **4:** 364, 1956.
2. Jolliffe, N., Archer, M. "Statistical Associations Between International Coronary Heart Disease Death Rates and Certain Environmental Factors." *J. Chron. Dis.* **9:** 636, 1959.
3. Fredrickson, D. S., Levy, R. I., Lees, R. S. "Fat Transport in Lipoproteins." *New Eng. J. Med.* **276:** 148, 1967.
4. Langman, M. J. S., Elwood, P. C., Foote, J., Ryrie, D. R. "ABO and Lewis Blood-Groups and Serum-Cholesterol." *The Lancet* **2:** 607, Sept. 1969.
5. "Prostaglandins." *Proceedings Nobel Symposium No.* 2. Stockholm 1966. London: Interscience Publishers, 1966.

6. Crawford, M. D., Gardner, M. J., Morriss, J. N. "Mortality and Hardness of Local Water-Supplies." *The Lancet* **1**: 827, April 1968.

7. Platt, B. S., Heard, C. R. C., Stewart, R. J. C. Experimental Protein-Calorie Deficiency. In *Mammalian Protein Metabolism*, **2**: 446, London: Academic Press, 1964.

8. Waterlow, J. C. "Observations on the Mechanism of Adaption to Low Protein Intakes." *The Lancet* **2**: 1091, November 1968.

9. "Chromium and Carbohydrate Metabolism in Infantile Malnutrition." *Nutr. Rev.* **26**: 235, 1968.

10. "Vanadium Inhibition of Cholesterol Synthesis." *Nutr. Rev.* **17**: 231, 1959.